New Security Challenges

Series Editor
George Christou, University of Warwick, Coventry, UK

The last decade has demonstrated that threats to security vary greatly in their causes and manifestations and that they invite interest and demand responses from the social sciences, civil society, and a very broad policy community. In the past, the avoidance of war was the primary objective, but with the end of the Cold War the retention of military defence as the centrepiece of international security agenda became untenable. There has been, therefore, a significant shift in emphasis away from traditional approaches to security to a new agenda that talks of the softer side of security, in terms of human security, economic security, and environmental security. The topical New Security Challenges series reflects this pressing political and research agenda.

For an informal discussion for a book in the series, please contact the series editor George Christou (G.Christou@warwick.ac.uk), or Palgrave editor Alina Yurova (alina.yurova@palgrave-usa.com).

This book series is indexed by Scopus.

More information about this series at
https://link.springer.com/bookseries/14732

Caroline Varin
Editor

Global Security in Times of Covid-19

Brave New World?

palgrave
macmillan

Editor
Caroline Varin
Professors Without Borders
Regent's University London
London, UK

ISSN 2731-0329 ISSN 2731-0337 (electronic)
New Security Challenges
ISBN 978-3-030-82229-3 ISBN 978-3-030-82230-9 (eBook)
https://doi.org/10.1007/978-3-030-82230-9

This Palgrave Macmillan imprint is published by the registered company Springer Nature Switzerland AG
The registered company address is: Gewerbestrasse 11, 6330 Cham, Switzerland

To those who were lost in this pandemic.
And to Alexia and Adi, for a safer world.

—Caroline Varin

Foreword: COVID-19 and Security

How Has COVID-19 Undermined Security?

Has the pandemic of COVID-19 undermined global security, the security of countries and the security of individuals? Whilst these are diverse definitions of security, they share a common concern—on the one hand for a peaceful world and on the other for individuals to live freely in a tolerant society. The pandemic has posed challenges to security in each of these forms. From the global perspective, it has first raised tensions between the superpowers of China and the US and second demonstrated that the will of rich countries to help much poorer countries is strictly limited when their own public's health is at risk. At the level of individual countries, it has in some cases increased their tendency to fragment and in others led to an authoritarian regime which may well outlast the pandemic. In the case of individuals, it has led to unprecedented forms of monitoring, which accentuate the growth of the 'surveillance state'. In each of these three areas, it has also accentuated the growth of various forms of corruption and in many countries set back the agenda to address climate change. This book provides an analysis of these issues from the perspective of society in a range of countries and is therefore a crucial contribution to understanding the pandemic's immediate and longer-term impact.

International Cooperation

The fight against the pandemic started badly as China, the physical origin of the virus, identified it on 30 December 2019 and reported it to the WHO on 2 January 2020, which published the information. However, China seems to have been reluctant to take on board the scale of the problem until 23 January when the city of Wuhan was completely locked down, but by this time Chinese sources were quoting case numbers at about 2300 a multiple of four in four days.[1] Nonetheless the response amongst several countries of the region, such as Taiwan, Thailand and Singapore was strong and quickly extended to viral testing.

However, once notified by the WHO of a 'Public Health Emergency of International Concern' on 30 January,[2] most OECD countries delayed a response proportionate to the risk, and countries such as Italy, France and the UK initiated responses which—in terms of mortalities—proved to be tragically too late.

The response of the US, which in theory had a well-developed strategic response to a potential pandemic, was a disaster. This reflected the bombastic claims of the Trump Presidency in which the actual pandemic was wished away as a diversion, a position which led to at least 600,000 deaths. The surge in the pandemic in mid-2020 coincided with a decision by the US to withdraw from the WHO, at a time when this UN body was crucial to inspiring an international co-ordinated response. Further, the tensions created by President Trump's consistent references to the 'Chinese' virus further raised the stakes in relations between China and the US, at a time when both countries were sliding into a tariff war, which would certainly affect the stability and security of the world trading system. It would also exacerbate tensions in the South China Sea.

Whilst the two superpowers railed at each other's failures, the richer countries of the OECD were very slow to support COVID-related strategies in the low-income countries, which are the target of their development aid programmes. In mid-2020 the form of support that was most urgent included Personal Protective (PPE) equipment and ventilators, for both of which the demand was critical within the donor countries themselves and for which international supplies were very limited. China was the country which had the greatest capacity to deliver these products to poorer countries but not surprisingly did so in limited amounts with the maximum publicity.

Until late 2020 it remained uncertain as to whether there would be sufficient vaccines available to have a global impact, but an international procurement and distribution body, COVAX,[3] was established in anticipation of their availability. By early 2021, it was clear that there were at least six effective vaccines available from different companies with bases in the US, the UK, Germany, Russia and China. However, whilst the EU and the UK made substantial grants to COVAX, the availability of vaccines, as a result of manufacturing hitches, proved far more limited than anticipated. The US and the UK, with relatively robust supplies, adopted a policy of vaccinating all those who were willing to be vaccinated before engaging in international distribution. The EU's procurement strategy proved very inadequate and the international distribution which it allowed, though substantial by mid-2021, was limited in relation to the need in low-income countries. In fact, the world's largest corporate manufacturer of vaccines, the Serum Institute, is in Pune, India, but as global demand for vaccines increased, the government of India, faced with an escalating pandemic, banned vaccine exports in March 2021. This cut off supplies to a range of countries both on a bilateral basis and through COVAX. These shortfalls, which could have been avoided by more effective and balanced international action, accentuated a sense of global injustice and of insecurity.

The Domestic Front

For some low- and middle-income countries, the pandemic significantly weakened the grip of the government as public services became overwhelmed by the acceleration of the virus, and created a vacuum into which mafia and quasi-mafia groups inserted themselves. This was particularly true in some countries, where the informal sector is large, and may account for more than 40% of GDP. Thus, the phenomenon was strong in contexts such as Colombia, Peru and Brazil. In these cases, existing groups with a capacity for violence used the pandemic both to enforce lockdowns and to win support from the population by supplying food and medical equipment, and in these cases the writ of the government was seriously weakened.

In some very large countries such as the US and India, the federal nature of government made it difficult to that lockdown ensure that lockdown rules were applied across the country and that PPE equipment was available on an equal basis across constituent states. In fact, in the US

State Governors adopted very different approaches to lockdown, group gatherings and mask wearing. This meant that they had a 'bigger impact on the direction of pandemic policies than the federal government', and states with more preventive measures had lower rates of infections and deaths.[4] This played directly into the tensions in interparty relationships, which were on display in the riot at the Capitol on 6 January 2021.

Although the Biden Presidency was ultimately able to orchestrate and accelerate an equitable vaccine rollout, the huge mortality figures confirmed the cost of earlier delays at the state level. The historian and lawyer Roger Babbit has argued that this has further undermined the viability of the current US constitution.[5]

In India, the credibility of the central government was seriously undermined when a 'third wave' of the virus broke out in early 2021 and a new lockdown was imposed, necessitated by the clear rejection in some states of rules on social distancing. Furthermore, when the central government finally recognised the priority of mass vaccination, final orders were only placed in March 2021 although the Serum Institute is located in Pune.

Key Examples

Contributors to this book describe in detail the impact on security of these and related outcomes of the pandemic. I refer here to some outstanding and dramatic examples. The influence of mafia groups is illustrated in the case of Mexico by the fact that the daughter of 'El Chapo' (Shorty) Guzman, the sometime boss of *La Linea* (one of the two largest drug dealing cartels in the early 2000s), was active in handing out boxes with food and medical supplies with El Chapo's picture on it.[6] This can only have strengthened the hand of the cartel in the course of the pandemic. In Sicily, it was the *Cosa Nostra* who were active in distributing food parcels and in Calabria it was the powerful mafia group, the *N'drangheta*, who enforced the lockdown.[7]

In some cases, governments used the excuse of lockdown to control the opposition and implemented draconian measures. In Thailand, where political opposition exploded in late 2020, the military government could present crowd control measures as a response to the pandemic, effectively limiting the growth of the burgeoning Future Forward party [8]—a position which would certainly threaten security in the longer run. In China, where citizen surveillance is already well-developed, the central government ensured that in Wuhan and all over Hubei Province the administration took exceptional measures to ensure a tough lockdown, to the extent of only allowing one person with an ID card to leave a residence each day to buy food. This was monitored by drones equipped with loudspeakers for the police to speak from the sky. The film *Coronation* by Ai Wei Wei, released in August 2020, has shown how much resentment this created.

Corruption in procurement is always resented by the public, even if welcomed by a small number of fixers and beneficiaries. The COVID pandemic has seen many billions of dollars spent on equipment purchase and the IMF has provided very large loans to low-income countries to facilitate such purchases. Thus, Cameroun received an 'Emergency Loan' of $256M from the IMF to respond to COVID-19 in May 2020, with a commitment by the IMF to lend a further $570M over the following three years. Both loans were subject to conventional requirements for open reporting on the identity of selected bidders for the relevant contracts, a commitment on which Cameroun subsequently sought and obtained a reversal by the end of the year. Similar loans from the IMF, totalling $7.97 Bn, were obtained by Egypt in 2020 but by mid-2021, only $286M of procurement had been accounted for publicly.[9]

Yet such lapses were not unique to low- and middle-income countries. The UK government allowed a huge procurement programme to be managed without regard for long-standing procedures, although it is an active member of the international 'Open Government Procurement' initiative. In the course of 2020, the government disbursed £18Bn in COVID-related expenditure, of which £3.7 Bn was directed to the purchase of equipment with contracts issued to 73 suppliers. Detailed analysis by Transparency International UK (TI) has shown that 24 of these were issued to companies with known connections to the Conservative Party, and of these 13 had been formed less than ten days before the contract award[10]. The award system was dependent on a dual list system of potential suppliers divided into a 'fast track' and a standard track, with the former acquiring a much higher proportion of the contracts. Elements of these apparently corrupt processes occurred in a range of countries, accentuating the lack of confidence in the public sector.

Further, equipment acquired through dubious bidding procedures could be counterfeit. This danger was already highlighted by Interpol in March 2020, specifying the 'dark web' as a key source of counterfeit products. Later in the year, Interpol organised 'Operation Rangers' a co-operative exercise between 90 countries which identified many thousand shipments of such products. The US Department of Home Security is particularly active in relation to potential counterfeit vaccines, and by May 2021 had already recovered $48M in all types of counterfeit vaccines, and closed down 80 sites on the 'dark web' purporting to sell these products. Such websites were focused on customers in countries such as Mexico and Brazil with a record in dealing with counterfeit drugs.

On a global basis, there was a fall of seven per cent in GDP in 2020, with a more acute fall in some low-income countries with a dependence on commodity exports. As a consequence, the pressure for migration to both the EU, from Africa and the Middle East, and to the US from Central America was acute, and organised crime gangs were quick to respond to this, in some cases promoting ever more dangerous routes. One survey of Arab youth found that nearly a third were more likely to seek to migrate after COVID-19.[11]

In the case of countries in the Sahel where large scale violence orchestrated by jihadist and ethnic minority groups has been active for more than a decade, the additional spread of COVID-19 raised the pressure to 'escape', with sea routes attracting larger flows than those across the Sahara had done in the recent past. In the spring of 2021, attempted arrivals in Italy from Libya and Tunisia by sea could reach as many as a thousand per day. In the US, an attempt by President Biden to restrict new entries to 15,000 per day were almost immediately rescinded as domestic political pressure forced him to double this, whilst illegal crossings greatly exceeded either figure. Intense pressure for immigration, facilitated by organised crime, is bound to heighten the public's sense of insecurity.

Questions of Corruption, Climate Change and Inequality

Each of the factors discussed feed into the questions of corruption on a global basis and the fight to accommodate climate change, both of which accelerate the perception of a decrease in public security. TI's annual 'Corruption Perception Index' regularly places the UK fairly high in the group of 'least corrupt countries'.[12] Given that the index is particularly geared to capturing the interface between government and business, the scandal of equipment procurement undermines the credibility of this ranking. However, other OECD countries have experienced comparable cases: in Germany in mid-2020, two elected MPs were exposed as having been directly associated with equipment purchase worth several million Euros.[13] Elsewhere, huge upward price movements in PPE equipment in mid-2020 offered opportunities for organised crime—and well-placed individuals—to take a cut on the transactions involved. Counterfeiting was not limited to masks and PPE equipment but eventually extended to vaccines.

Climate change was recognised by 2020 as the key issue of our time, with the COP26 Conference due in 2021. But in the course of the year, the pandemic had become profound enough to raise questions about whether this could indeed be a face to face event, suggesting a less resilient and so more insecure outcome.

This was a minor question in relation to the huge expenditure, which OECD governments expended or planned to expend to fight the pandemic. The EU put together a fund of Euros 750 Bn, to assist member states, which was for the first time subject to a joint guarantee. This was partly in the form of a loan to governments and so a slow recovery from the pandemic will endanger financial stability in Europe.

All G7 member states expanded their public debt to an aggregate 130% of GDP, previously regarded as quite unacceptable. It was widely agreed that this was only sustainable if interest rates remained at a level close to one per cent, and that they would in any case put huge pressure on government budgets. Thus, the projected annual support to low-income developing countries of $100 Bn per year in support of climate change action might well be in jeopardy, with grave implications for security. A further and little recognised consequence of the quantitative easing employed by most G7 central banks was the explosion of billionaire wealth triggered by an increase in the global stock market valuation of thirty percent in 2020.[14] In the course of that year, the share of GDP held by billionaires increased dramatically across a range of countries. From an average of 10% in 2010, it grew to 20% in the US, 30% in Sweden and an amazing 15% even in China in 2020. This was concurrent with a widespread debate about ‘inequality’ within countries, which had already been encapsulated by the Presidential primary campaign of Bernie Sanders who identified the ‘billionaire class’ as a target for the next US administration. The fact that financial measures to counter COVID-19 exacerbated this only added to profound public doubts about the fairness and security of the financial system.

Conclusion

There is plenty in this book to guide us to some insights into the questions I mentioned at the beginning of this Foreword, though real answers will not be available for many years, given the unique nature of the experience of the pandemic. In relation to international security, it is clear that the institutional system has been weakened by a failure to collaborate effectively at every stage of the crisis, a position confirmed by WHO's own report of May 2021.[15] COVAX failed in its prime task of being the global agency for the purchase and distribution of vaccines, leaving much of this to ad hoc decisions by governments and companies. In spite of a specific initiative by President Biden to make vaccine manufacturing patents a public good, this was rejected by the EU and other relevant governments in mid-2021. Whilst the crisis has highlighted the need for a global approach to public health, it has also shown how far the world has to go to achieve it.

There are few countries that emerge with a heightened sense of security from the crisis. This is especially true of those already designated as 'fragile states' (notably those of the Sahel), where COVID-19 has intersected with ongoing civil conflicts and increased the pressure for migration. But it is also true in larger middle-income countries such as Mexico, Brazil and Colombia, where the weak administration of public health, the active role of coercive violent groups and populist politics have converged to further inflate the consequences of the pandemic. In high-income countries such as France, Germany and the UK the incidence of corruption in procurement scandals has weakened the credibility of governments (though the UK's successful vaccine roll-out was recognised in regional elections in mid-2021).

The question of individuals' willingness to be subject to 'surveillance for the public good' has been sorely tested. Where it has been used to subdue the opposition, as in Thailand, it has been very unpopular. In China, it appears to have been widely accepted, in spite of some determined protests. In Europe, whilst political leaders have been surprised by the willingness of the public to be 'locked down' in some countries (such as France), there has been a deep resentment at the policing of these arrangements. In the US, the popular objection to such measures has rendered them rather ineffective, but also prevented the extensive use of surveillance systems. Overall, the international experience appears to suggest that individuals will accept a higher degree of surveillance for a sense of public security than was expected.

Overall this book confirms that the pandemic has weakened both actual and perceived security. It also shows the scale of the action needed to reverse this consequence at every level. A repeat of this pandemic or the failure to constrain another one would be a further blow from the security which arises from international solidarity.

Laurence Cockcroft

Notes

1. Michael Lewis, *The Premonition: A Pandemic Story* (London: Allen Lane, 2021), p 170.
2. The defining moments of the COVID 19 pandemic, in How an Outbreak became a Pandemic, Independent Panel for Preparedness and Response, *March 2021, Geneva*, "WHO Coronavirus Disease (COVID-19) Dashboard," *World Health* Organization, May 4, 2021, https://covid19.who.int/table?tableChartType=heat.
3. Covid-19 Vaccines Global Access.
4. Julie VanDusky-Allen and Olga Shvetsova, "How America's Partisan Divide over Pandemic Responses Played Out in the States," *The Conversation*, May 13, 2021, https://theconversation.com/how-americas-partisan-divide-over-pandemic-responses-played-out-in-the-states-157565.
5. Philip Babbit, "We Are All Failed States Now," in *Covid-19 and The Future of Conflict*, ed. Hal Brands and Francis J. Gavin (Maryland: John Hopkins Press, 2020).
6. Chapter 2, Dr. Oscar Palma, University of Rosario, Colombia.
7. Chapter 12, Organised Crime during and after the pandemic, Virginia Comelli, Global Initiative against Transnational Organised Crime.
8. *Securitisation of the corona virus in Asian countries*, Dr. Sipim Sornbanlang.
9. 'IMF Covid-19 Emergency Loans, A view from Four Countries', *Transparency International*, March 30, 2021, https://www.transparency.org/en/news/imf-covid-19-emergency-loans-cameroon-ecuador-egypt-nigeria.
10. "Track and Trace," *Transparency International UK*, March April, 2021, https://www.transparency.org.uk/track-and-trace-uk-PPE-procurement-corruption-risk-VIP-lane-research.
11. Chapter 3, *Europe a Geographical Expression*? Arthur de Lied Kirke, Mathew Robinson.

12. CPI report shows the UK came 9th; Andy King, "Consumer Price Inflation, UK: December 2020," *Office for National Statistics*, January 20, 2021, https://www.ons.gov.uk/economy/inflationandpriceindices/bulletins/consumerpriceinflation/december2020.
13. Georg Nuesslein acted as an intermediary for a China based PPE manufacturing company and Nikolas Loebel earned Euros 250,000 in a parallel deal; Guy Chazan, "Germany's CDU Rocked by a Pandemic Procurement Scandal," *Financial Times*, March 7, 2021, https://www.ft.com/content/85c06c2d-2c80-4e94-a792-1539ad306a5b.
14. Richir Shama, "The Billionaire Boom," *Financial Times*, May 14, 2021, https://www.ft.com/content/747a76dd-f018-4d0d-a9f3-4069bf2f5a93.
15. How an Outbreak became a Pandemic, Independent Panel for Preparedness and Response, *March 2021, Geneva.*

Bibliography

Babbit, Philip. "We Are All Failed States Now." In *Covid-19 and the Future of Conflict*, edited by Hal Brands and Francis J., Gavin, Maryland: John Hopkins Press, 2020.

Brands, Hal, and Francis J. Gavin, ed. *Covid-19 and the World Order*. Maryland: John Hopkins University Press, 2020.

Chazan, Guy. "Germany's CDU Rocked by a Pandemic Procurement Scandal." *Financial Times*, March 7, 2021. https://www.ft.com/content/85c06c2d-2c80-4e94-a792-1539ad306a5b.

How an Outbreak became a Pandemic, Independent Panel for Preparedness and Response, *March 2021, Geneva.*

"IMF Covid-19 Emergency Loans, A view from Four Countries." *Transparency International*, March 30, 2021. https://www.transparency.org/en/news/imf-covid-19-emergency-loans-cameroon-ecuador-egypt-nigeria#.

Lewis, Michael. *The Premonition: A Pandemic Story.* London: Allen Lane, 2021.

Shama, Richir. "The Billionaire Boom." *Financial Times*, May 14, 2021. https://www.ft.com/content/747a76dd-f018-4d0d-a9f3-4069bf2f5a93.

"Track and Trace." *Transparency International UK*, March April, 2021. https://www.transparency.org.uk/track-and-trace-uk-PPE-procurement-corruption-risk-VIP-lane-research.

VanDusky-Allen, Julie, and Olga Shvetsova. "How America's Partisan Divide over Pandemic Responses Played Out in the States." *The Conversation*, May 13, 2021. https://theconversation.com/how-americas-partisan-divide-over-pandemic-responses-played-out-in-the-states-157565.

Laurence Cockcroft is a development economist who has worked across Africa for governments, companies, international organisations and charitable foundations. He is a co-founder of Transparency International and a former Chairman of Transparency International (UK). He has written widely on corruption-related issues and is the author of '*Global Corruption: Money Power and Ethics in the Modern World*' and '*Unmasked: Corruption in the West*' (co-authored with Anne-Christine Wegener) (Published by IB Tauris in 2012 and 2017 respectively).

Acknowledgements

This book would not have been possible without all the contributors who were willing to take the time to share their experiences and analysis on the COVID crisis in this highly unusual year. We hope that with these lessons learnt, we can be better prepared to safeguard our future and put in place the policies needed to protect those most vulnerable, wherever they may be.

I am particularly grateful to:

Mitchell, for all the brainstorming sessions since March 2020.

Njomeza Blakcori, Jeanette Batchelor and Keaton McGruder for reviewing these chapters with me.

My team at Professors Without Borders, George, Colin, Rachel, Kasia, Richard, Hannah, Tessy, Rebekah, Sam … for keeping me optimistic about the future, no matter how grim it sometimes looks.

And to Alexia, Daniel and Adi, for making it all matter.

Praise for *Global Security in Times of Covid-19*

"Will the twenty-first be the century of global pandemics as the twentieth was the century of world wars and revolutions? Is this the sobering reality of the 'brave new world' which lies ahead of us? This timely and provocative collection of essays provides an acute and sustained analysis by an outstanding group of scholars of how Covid-19 has begun to reshape our thinking about security. One of the very few books whose own scale matches that of the challenge it describes."

—Christopher Coker, *Director, LSE IDEAS, London, UK*

"The team which Caroline Varin has assembled demonstrates both the deep implications of covid for national and international institutions and its likely impact on all our futures. It is particularly strong in assessing the impact of covid at the grass roots across a range of countries. Whether we consider personal security, the security of the state or the ability of the world to secure a path through climate change, the epidemic has opened a new and dangerous prospect. This is a thought provoking read shot through with original insights."

—Laurence Cockcroft, *Co-founder Transparency International*

Contents

List of Contributors

Mitchell Belfer Euro-Gulf Information Centre, Rome, Italy

Virginia Comolli The Global Initiative against Transnational Organized Crime, London, UK

Lewis Herrington Regent's University, London, UK

Arthur de Liedekerke Rasmussen Global, Brussels, Belgium

Casmir Chukwuka Mbaegbu Department of Political Science, University of Nigeria, Nsukka, Nigeria

Oliver Geffen Obregon Freelance Epidemiologist, London, UK

Freedom Chukwudi Onuoha Department of Political Science, University of Nigeria, Nsukka, Nigeria

Oscar Palma Faculty of International, Political and Urban Studies, Universidad del Rosario, Bogotá, Colombia

George E. Richards Edinboro University, Edinboro, PA, USA; PROWIBO Online, London, UK

Matthew Robinson Euro-Gulf Information Centre, Rome, Italy

Sipim Sornbanlang Department of Political Science, Faculty of Social Sciences, Srinakharinwirot University, Bangkok, Thailand

Michael Stephens Foreign Policy Research Institute, Philadelphia, PA, USA

Caroline Varin Professors Without Borders, Regent's University London, London, UK

Alexandre Vautravers Department of Security, Employment and Health (DSES), Geneva, Switzerland

Acronyms

5G	Fifth Generation of Technology
ACLED	Armed Conflict Location and Event Data
AFCFTA	African Continental Free Trade Area
AFCOR	Africa Task Force for Novel Coronavirus
AFRICOM	United States Africa Command
AMISOM	African Union Mission in Somalia
AU	African Union
BEC	Business Email Compromise
BLM	Black Lives Matter
BWC	Biological Weapons Convention
CCDC	Chinese Center for Disease Control and Prevention
CCSA	Center of COVID-19 Situational Administration
CDC	Centers for Disease Control and Prevention
CDU	Christian Democratic Union of Germany
CECC	Central Epidemic Command Center
CJNG	Cartel de Jalisco Nueva Generacion
COVID	Coronavirus
CSDP	Common Security and Defence Policy
CSIS	Center for Strategic and International Studies
DHSC	Department of Health and Social Care
DRC	Democratic Republic of Congo
E3	European 3: France, Germany and the United Kingdom
ECFR	European Council on Foreign Relations
ECRIS	European Criminal Records Information System
ELN	National Liberation Army (Colombia)
EU	European Union

EVD	Ebola Virus Disease
FAFF	Financial Action Task Force
FAO	Food and Agriculture Organization
FARC	Revolutionary Armed Forces of Colombia
FBI	Federal Bureau of Investigation
FCAS	Future Combat Aircraft System
FTA	Free-Trade Agreement
GCC	Gulf Cooperation Council
GDP	Gross Domestic Product
GIs	Geographical Indications
GOP	Grand Old Party
HDR	Human Development Report
HTS	Hayat Tahrir Al-Sham
ICCPR	International Covenant on Civil and Political Rights
ICESCR	International Covenants on Economic, Social, and Cultural Rights
ICSVE	International Centre for the Study of Violent Extremism
ICUs	Intensive Care Units
IFAD	International Fund for Agricultural Development
IMF	International Monetary Fund
IRA	Irish Republican Army
IRGC	Islamic Revolutionary Guard Corps
ISIS	Islamic State of Iraq and Syria
ISWAP	Islamic State West Africa Province
IUU	Illegal, Unreported and Unregulated
JCPOA	Joint Comprehensive Plan of Action
LRFs	Local Resilience Forums
MENA	Middle East and North Africa
MERS	Middle East Respiratory Syndrome
MFF	Multiannual Financial Framework
MINUSMA	Multidimensional Integrated Stabilization Mission in Mali
MP	Member of Parliament
MRCA	Multi-Role Combat Aircraft
NATO	North Atlantic Treaty Organization
NCSC	National Cyber Security Centre
NHS	National Health Service
OCCRP	The Organized Crime and Corruption Reporting Project
OCHA	United Nations Office for the Coordination of Humanitarian Affairs
OECD	Organisation for Economic Co-operation and Development
ONS	Office of National Statistics
OSCT	Office for Security and Counter Terrorism
PCC	Primeiro Comando da Capital
PESCO	Permanent Structured Cooperation

PHE	Public Health England
PM	Prime Minister
PNR	Passenger Name Records
PPE	Personal Protective Equipment
RARCSS	Revitalized Agreement Resolution of the Conflict in the Republic of South Sudan
RWCPS	Reasonable Worst-Case Planning Scenario
SAGE	Scientific Advisory Group for Emergencies
SARS	Severe acute respiratory syndrome
SCG	Strategic Coordination Group
SGBV	Sexual and Gender-based Violence
SGSS	Second-Generation Surveillance System
SIPRI	Stockholm Institute Peace Research Institute
SIS	Schengen Information System
SIS II	Schengen Information System II
SNA	Somali National Army
SPD	Social Democratic Party of Germany
TCA	Trade and Cooperation Agreement
TI	Transparency International
TPP	Trans Pacific Partnership
UAE	Violent Non-State Actors
UDHR	Universal Declaration of Human Rights
UK	United Arab Emirates
UN	United Kingdom
UNAMID	United Nations African–Union Mission in Darfur
UNCTED	United Nations Counter Terrorism Executive Directorate
UNDPKO	United Nation's Department of Peacekeeping Operations
UNECA	United Nations Economic Commission for Africa
UNESCO	United Nations Educational, Scientific and Cultural Organization
UNICEF	The United Nations International Children's Emergency Fund
UNSC	United Nations Security Council
US	United States
US AID	US Agency for International Development
VNSAs	Violent Non-State Actors
WFP	United Nations World Food Programme
WHO	World Health Organization
WMD	Weapons of Mass Destruction
WWII	World War II
XUAR	Xinjiang Uyghur Autonomous Region

List of Figures

List of Tables

CHAPTER 1

Introduction

Caroline Varin

Introduction

Human beings have lived with diseases since the dawn of time. The Black Plague, Cholera, Typhoid, Malaria, Leprosy, Tuberculosis, Smallpox, Rabies, Influenza and HIV/AIDS each managed to kill more people than wars have. The competition between microparasites[1] and humans appeared to be over, however, with the scientific advances of the late twentieth century. The first antibiotic drug became available in 1944. This was followed by a half century of successful vaccination campaigns,[2] genetic engineering, medical discoveries and improved hygienic practices that reduced our perceived and actual risk of illness and early death. As Coronavirus SARS-CoV-2 (COVID-19) emerged in late 2019, modern society, armed with a false sense of invincibility, reacted first with complacency, non-chalance, disdain and "an almost pathological sense of mass denial."[3]

COVID-19 was not an existential threat to human beings. With a mortality rate of 0.23% in low-income countries, 1.15% in high-income

C. Varin (✉)
Professors Without Borders, Regent's University London, London, UK
e-mail: varinc@regents.ac.uk

C. Varin (ed.), *Global Security in Times of Covid-19*, New Security Challenges, https://doi.org/10.1007/978-3-030-82230-9_1

countries and climbing to 5% among individuals over 80 years old,[4] this pales in comparison to the 2003 SARS outbreak, with a 9.6% mortality rate and 34.3% rate for the 2012 MERS epidemic.[5] COVID's virulence took many by surprise. Indeed, at least four million people died from the disease within 18 months of the first case recorded in Wuhan, China in December 2019. Yet when compared to the 20 to 50 million people killed in the Spanish flu outbreak in 1917–1918, this virus looks relatively manageable. And it is. Taiwan recorded 224 deaths in the first 18 months of the epidemic. China officially 4,636. Australia 910 deaths. Most African countries excluding South Africa reported very low cases and few deaths. On the other hand, the United States lost over half a million people in the same timeframe; Europe including the UK roughly 679,000 people.[6] Comparable numbers were found in Brazil and India by mid-2021.

A pandemic was long expected, well-documented in public policy and scientific research papers.[7] We have had plenty of warnings and time to prepare. In vain. Arguably, it was pure luck that COVID had such a relatively low mortality rate, considering the less than stellar responses of many policy-makers and of the international organisations responsible for promoting cooperation and ensuring the security of nations and their people. Rather than viewing COVID as a once-in-a-century epidemic, it is very likely that we have entered a century of infectious diseases, exacerbated by the increasing rate of man-made environmental degradation and climate change.[8] One fortuitously optimistic note in all this is the emergence of successful mRNA vaccines which may hold the key to fighting all future diseases. Conversely, COVID "might be one of the easiest targets we've seen in modern times,"[9] pointing to a bleak century ahead. We believe it is critical now to look back at the state of the world in December 2019 and assess how COVID affected it, both in order to address the security threats that have emerged in the wake of this disease and to anticipate the next crisis.

In addition to creating new problems, COVID-19 appears to have aggravated existing weaknesses in the system of states that was created by the Allies after-World War II. An increasingly globalised world promoted interdependence and trade, travel and cooperation. There was a sense, if not a reality, of communal responsibility for ensuring global security, guaranteed by the United States and its traditional partners. International organisations such as the United Nations and later the European Union were promoted as successful models for cooperation, peace and democracy. There was a general reliance on the under-funded and politicised

World Health Organisation to anticipate any disease outbreak with an early warning-system as it did with both SARS and MERS.

At the same time, the world experienced the rise of other countries, namely China and a re-emerging Russia, with alternative views of how the international system should be managed, thereby challenging the balance of powers and Western hegemony. This was accompanied by new models of governance, including populism, nationalism and authoritarianism. Today, more than half the world's population "live under some form of authoritarian rule."[10] Some of these countries have managed the disease far more successfully than the Great Democracies.[11] Other nations[12] have become more authoritarian through their management of the crisis, rolling back on fundamental and hard-won freedoms in the name of public health. Conversely, the hardest-hit countries are democratic nations that have been reluctant to implement WHO-recommended measures to slow down disease transmission. This reluctance stemmed both out of concern for said freedoms and to safeguard their own economies with little consideration to the cost to others.

As the disease spread around the world, we watched the international system of states erode. In March 2020 Italy, a member of the European Union, was left struggling for medical supplies as France and Germany announced bans on exports of protective gear.[13] In April 2021, India ran out of oxygen leading to thousands of excess deaths as it exported critical vaccine supplies abroad and maintained a 12% tax on the import of critical drugs and oxygen.[14] Nations have erected measures to safeguard their own populations, freezing diplomatic accords with their neighbours. Nationalism and national sovereignty replaced solidarity as successful vaccines became available only to those who could access them, principally higher-income countries. The old lines of the Cold War were redrawn as Sputnik and Sinovac were spurned by Europeans, despite their own lack of vaccines and the threat of another wave cresting over the continent. To make matters worse, the World Health Organisation (WHO) responded over-cautiously throughout the entire outbreak; sanitising information, misreading the disease and failing to alert its members to the impact it could have until, too late, the WHO declared a pandemic on 11 March 2020, having lost credibility in the eyes of the world.

With the temporary breakdown of international relations, nations were largely left to their own devises. The COVID-19 outbreak was not an existential threat, but its securitisation[15] (and lack of) transformed the security environment in all corners of the planet, regardless of the prevalence of the disease. COVID evolved from being a biological threat to health to a politically induced socio-economic crisis and threat to human security with a knock-on effect on the most vulnerable nations.

This book invites security and health experts from around the world to share their analysis of the COVID-19 outbreak and its impact on regional and global security. In publishing this edited volume, we hope to highlight the lessons learnt from around the world, in particular the need for regional and international cooperation and solidarity when it comes to combating a transnational security threat that does not respect political boundaries.

COVID and Global Security

Although each chapter addresses a particular aspect of the COVID-19 crisis, the themes explored inevitably overlap. This edited volume is organised into two parts. In the first, authors discuss the regional experience of the outbreak, focusing on Latin America (Chapter 2), the United States (Chapter 3), Europe (Chapter 4), Africa (Chapter 5), the Middle East (Chapter 6) and Asia (Chapter 7). The second half of this book develops the security threats mentioned in the regional chapters, highlighting the impact of COVID on the new world order (Chapter 8), civil unrest (Chapter 9), terrorism (Chapter 10), organised crime (Chapter 11) and global health systems (Chapter 12). The final chapter assesses the role of international institutions in managing this crisis.

The Social Contract and State Failure

The COVID-19 epidemic eventually forced states to take action to avoid their health systems becoming overwhelmed, unable to cope with the influx of patients. In the first year of the outbreak, at least 94 countries covering over half the world's population had experienced some kind of lockdown mandated by the government. These lockdowns immediately and, sometimes indefinitely, restricted the rights of citizens: freedom of movement, freedom of assembly, in some cases freedom to work, which inevitably disrupted earnings and food security. The right to a family life, to marry and to an education were brushed aside to protect the right to life, while handing over more power to each nations' political establishment.

As time passed and the epidemic persevered, many lost faith in their governments' ability to manage the health crisis and looming economic disaster; new frustrations, compounded with old societal rifts, prompted the public to protest on the streets of Colombia, Chile, Brazil, Peru, Guinea, Senegal, India, Iran and Israel, Russia and Belarus, the United States and across Europe. Police responded forcefully, leading to more protests against what was widely perceived as systemic police violence carried out on behalf of an increasingly authoritarian and unaccountable state. The use of state security services to enforce frontier closures, lockdowns and curfews also led to human rights abuses including extrajudicial killings as evidenced in Colombia (Chapter 2), Nigeria, South Africa and Mozambique,[16] where more people were killed by the police than by the disease (Chapter 5), further weakening the delicate balance between the state, the army and society.

Civil unrest and the breakdown of the social contract reappear in each chapter of Part I and is further explored by Dr. George Richards of Edinboro University in Chapter 9. Richards shows how the COVID epidemic affected the social contract by exacerbating existing fissures in the state system, especially in the United States. Despite a general increase in public sector spending to shield individuals from the gravest economic consequences of the lockdown[17]—itself the result of government policies—growing social, economic and demographic[18] inequalities have revealed who is not fully covered by the social contract promised by the state. Moreover, manifesting discontent through mass protests is in direct contradiction with state-mandated social distancing measures to avoid contagion from COVID-19. Richards concludes that this pandemic has effectively suppressed political dissent, thereby strengthening the power of the state but weakening the contract with its people.

However, not all countries moved to shut their borders and set controls over their citizens' freedoms. Brazil and Mexico openly denied the threat of COVID-19 and failed to implement any policies to safeguard their populations (Chapter 2). As the number of cases—and deaths—rose in Latin America, Asia, Africa and Europe, drug cartels and organised crime stepped in to fill the void left by the state, declaring local lockdowns, imposing curfews, distributing victuals and other essential items including soap and disinfectant. Dr Oscar Palma from Rosario University, Colombia (Chapter 2) and Virginia Comolli from the Global Initiative against Transnational Organized Crime (Chapter 10) found that countries which refused to properly securitise the epidemic also weakened their social contract, leading to a loss of state legitimacy and an opportunity for violent non-state actors to capture the state. The subsequent growth and resilience of these groups will prove to be a long-term challenge to stability and security in the region.

The Rise of Violent Non-state Actors

COVID-19 has severely disrupted the ability of states to address existing and growing threats from violent non-state actors (VNSAs). Border closures have limited regional and international cooperation and peace-building efforts, halted multi-national military operations, and have slowed down the supply chain of military equipment. Outbreaks, quarantine and social distancing measures have affected the deployment of security forces and intelligence-gathering. This has enabled a rise in maritime piracy, cybersecurity attacks, terrorist recruitment, criminal operations and illegal transnational activities from VNSAs eager to exploit any opportunity to expand their reach and undermine the state.

Terrorism expert Dr Lewis Herrington argues that frustration against nationwide lockdowns and resentment towards economic policies and resulting hardships have led to an increase in extremist ideology and radicalisation (Chapter 10). Terrorist groups have maintained and even increased their tempo of attacks. In the first year of the pandemic, attacks were up 16.5% from the previous year. These groups are looking to expand their arsenal to include biological weapons, inspired by the near-apocalyptic impact COVID appears to have had on modern society. Furthermore, as governments look inwards and focus on their cities, designated terrorist groups like Hebzollah in Lebanon, Hayat Tahrir Al-Sham (HTS) in Syria and Islamic State West Africa Province (ISWAP) in Nigeria (see Chapters 5 and 6) have also grasped the opportunity to increase their relevance and political legitimacy in rural areas.

In Chapter 11, Virginia Comolli describes how criminal networks have similarly prospered by exploiting quarantine measures to multiply their operations in cybercrime, fraud, trafficking and counterfeiting. Cybercrime has increased exponentially with a 30% uptick in scams in the first six months of the pandemic costing an estimated US$30 billion according to the U.S. Secret Service.[19] Cyber-terrorism in the form of disinformation campaigns have further undermined the state, promoting vaccine hesitancy and an increase in civilian attacks on critical infrastructure. This was evident when a conspiracy theory linking 5G technology to COVID inspired over 150 arson attacks on telecommunication masts across Europe in 2020.[20] In May 2021, a cyber-criminal gang succeeded in taking a major U.S. pipeline offline, affecting fuel supply and prices, highlighting the threat VNSAs pose in a digital world.

Herrington argues that the COVID epidemic overshadowed the threat of terrorism and organised crime worldwide and led to a redistribution of funding away from security and counterterrorism budgets, which is likely to endure in the foreseeable future. Indeed, the 2021–2027 European Multiannual Financial Framework (MFF) has already seen a 40% drop in security defence allocation as the EU focuses on its economic recovery.[21]

A Return to Realpolitik

The pandemic has been a test of legitimacy for each nation-state and for the international system designed 75 years before this pandemic's outbreak. It has also accentuated the divide between the global North and the global South. In 2020, nations retrenched into their borders, abandoning any pretence of collaboration or solidarity in their response to the outbreak. A lack of leadership, epitomised by Trump and then Biden's America-First approach as well as Europe's nationalisation of healthcare both created an uncontested space on the global platform for China and Russia to assert themselves regionally and globally. Indeed, the policies adopted by the global North epitomise a return of *Realpolitik*, where each nation embraces a position towards COVID based on their own calculations of power and the national interest.[22]

In Chapter 8, security advisor Dr Alexandre Vautravers examines how the breakdown of European unity and solidarity since the outbreak, in addition to the rift in EU–US relations during Trump's Presidency, have created a strategic vacuum in the international system. EU-experts Arthur de Liedekerke and Matthew Robinson argue in Chapter 4 that great power competition and shared enemies, Russia and Iran, could push the EU and UK to a closer alliance post-Brexit than would otherwise have occurred. This is compounded by America's retreat from world affairs throughout the Trump presidency and as a result of its health and socio-economic crisis, which has forced the United States to focus on domestic priorities (see Chapters 2 and 9).

EU and U.S. peacekeeping and peace-enforcing missions, military training operations, humanitarian operations, crisis management and counterterrorism efforts have all been deescalated in the last 18 months of the outbreak. Although a leading donor to the COVAX scheme, both the EU and U.S. have demonstrated their indifference towards the fate of other nations, especially former colonies in Africa, Asia and the Middle East. Thus, they were left to struggle with the pandemic, a dearth of vaccines and an economic disaster largely caused by the breakdown in trade and tourism originating from the global North.

On the other hand, China has successfully mastered the art of health diplomacy. With a near monopoly of the supply of facemasks and medical kits and early experience managing the outbreak, Beijing sent medical aid, experts and financial assistance to over 150 countries, positioning itself as the world's doctor and the single dominant political player, despite being the suspected source of the virus.[23] In Chapter 3, Senior Fellow at Foreign Policy Research Institute Michael Stephens disagrees with the apparent Chinese supremacy on the world stage: Despite Chinese diplomatic successes during the outbreak, there is rampant distrust towards the Asian giant due to its human rights record and secretive behaviour early in the pandemic. Stephens argues American leadership is still possible, providing it wants such a role and is able to balance it against Russia and China's recent ascent.

Human Security

Until this pandemic, security studies focused largely on national security in terms of peace and conflict. A growing interest in human security, which includes political freedoms and economic security, was not sufficient to spark an interest in political (and business) leaders to prepare for a seriously disruptive viral outbreak, despite receiving adequate warnings from the scientific community that such an event was imminent and inevitable.[24]

Early securitisation of the disease and the ensuing measures implemented in many Asian countries, in Australia and in New Zealand were successful at safeguarding their citizens from the health and economic crises that have plagued the rest of the world. In Chapter 6, Dr Sipim Sornbanlang from Srinakharinwirot University in Thailand maintains strategies adopted in Asia not only served to protect national security, however, they also deliberately infringed on human security, affecting the freedoms and livelihoods of individuals.

Digital platforms have been developed around the world to oversee and control the movements of visitors and citizens whose rights to assemble, protest and speak have been strictly curtailed Examples of countries that have truncated the rights of citizens are China, Thailand, Iran and Turkey. Facial recognition in particular has lifted the surveillance debate to a new level, tracking the movements of people in an indelible manner. With "Big Brother" constantly watching under the guise of protecting humanity, this Orwellian use of technology and the invasion of privacy by unaccountable governments and potential hackers has raised a number of serious security dilemmas including the protection of civil liberties.

Government measures restricting movement and therefore economic activity inevitably had a profound effect on economic security and food security, not only inside their own countries but across the globe. In 2020, over 100 million people, principally in Asia, lost their jobs as the tourist industry ground to a halt.[25] The countries that could afford to, provided some financial support measures safeguarding businesses, industries and people affected by the economic impact of shutting down human activity. Others, the majority maybe, were unable to protect their own citizens from the impact of policies adopted half a world away. Some two billion people working in the informal sectors lost their daily incomes and received limited, if any, government support, despite their plight being the direct result of lockdown measures at home and abroad. For many people, lockdowns represented a bigger challenge than the virus itself. Similarly, migrant workers everywhere found themselves in a no-man's land, unable to make a living or to travel back to their homes.

In Chapter 5, Freedom Onuoha and Casmir Mbaegbu of the University of Nigeria describe the economic impact of the outbreak on the African continent, despite successful mitigation methods implemented as early as January 2020. COVID-19 and its associated measures pushed 124 million people into poverty and a further 62 million into extreme poverty,[26] 80% of which are in Sub-Saharan Africa and South Asia. Furthermore, reduced incomes and disrupted supply chains pushed increased global food prices by 38% between January 2020 and May 2021. Responses to the locust outbreak in 23 countries across East Africa and the Middle East in 2020 were also disrupted by the COVID outbreak, exacerbating an already dire food supply situation. Despite the apparent resilience of the global food system,[27] a combination of lockdown measures and diseases that have affected workers, the loss of jobs and ensuing income and the volatility of food prices have together exacerbated hunger and food insecurity around the world.[28] This in turn is likely to push migration to new heights, further empowering the smuggling of people and human trafficking and straining political tensions in Western countries with a knock-on effect on the risk of populism and nationalist support.

Conclusion

Throughout history, epidemics have disrupted human civilisations, changing the structure of societies, deciding the outcome of wars and prompting incredible technological innovation.[29] Studying the impact of a pandemic, in the midst of its outbreak, is a risky endeavour that opens up our contributors to criticism and error. Nonetheless, a rare consensus appears among our authors: COVID-19 has not changed our world—yet—but it certainly has exposed existing faults in the international system.

Unsurprisingly, most governments have responded to this emergency by prioritising the lives of their own citizens. By doing this, we have rolled back years of progress in institution-building and collective responsibility, and instead returned to a primitive form of *Realpolitik* dominant before the twentieth century. With a transnational threat of this nature, wouldn't a concerted response led by a proactive U.S. have been in everyone's best interest? That is what institutions such as the United Nations and World Health Organisation were designed to facilitate. In the case of COVID-19, their failure has had catastrophic results.

The age of information, epitomised by social media and the 24/7 news coverage, could have contributed to the solution, Instead, it led to increased societal anxiety. Governments shamelessly capitalised on this by grabbing extraordinary powers and denying basic human rights in both democratic and authoritarian countries. In Chapter 12, WHO consultant Oliver Geffen Obregon acknowledges the epidemiological reasoning for political measures such as curfews, postponing of elections and restrictions on the right to protest, but queries their eventual impact on the spread of the virus, given approaches to implementation. Obregon blames a lack of transparency and accountability for exacerbating an already deadly situation. Politicising the virus, both domestically and internationally, has been a force-multiplier for COVID-19 and its variants. These conditions all point to an ominous century ahead.

Notes

1. Microparasites include viruses, bacteria and multi-celled creatures.
2. In 1980 the World Health Assembly declared Smallpox eradicated thanks to a successful global vaccination programme.
3. Laurie Garrett, *The Coming Plague* (New York: Farrar, Straus and Giroux, 1995).
4. Sabine Elsland, "COVID-19 Deaths: Infection Fatality Ratio Is About 1% Says New Report," *Imperial College London*, October 29, 2020, https://www.imperial.ac.uk/news/207273/covid-19-deaths-infection-fatality-ratio-about/.
5. Yella Hewings-Martin, "How do SARS and MERS compare with COVID-19?," *Medical News Today*, April 10, 2020, https://www.medicalnewstoday.com/articles/how-do-sars-and-mers-compare-with-covid-19#MERS.
6. "COVID-19 Data Repository," *Center for Systems Science and Engineering (CSSE),* https://github.com/CSSEGISandData/COVID-19.
7. Samuel Brannen and Kathleen Hicks, "We Predicted a Coronavirus Pandemic: Here's What Policymakers Could Have Seen Coming," *Politico Magazine*, March 7, 2020, https://www.politico.com/news/magazine/2020/03/07/coronavirus-epidemic-prediction-policy-advice-121172; Bronwyn Fryer and Jonathan Quick, *The End of Epidemics: How to Stop Viruses and Save Humanity Now,* 1st ed. (London: Scribe, 2020); Laurie Garrett, *The Coming Plague* (New York: Farrar, Straus and Giroux, 1995); William McNeil, *Plagues and People*, (New York: Anchor Books, 1998).
8. Bronwyn Fryer and Jonathan Quick, *The End of Epidemics: How to Stop Viruses and Save Humanity Now,* 1st ed. (London: Scribe, 2020); William McNeil, *Plagues and People* (New York: Anchor Books, 1998).
9. Derek Thompson, "How mRNA Technology Could Change the World," *The Atlantic*, March 29, 2020, https://www.theatlantic.com/ideas/archive/2021/03/how-mrna-technology-could-change-world/618431/.
10. Hal Brands and Francis J. Gavin, ed., *COVID-19 and World Order* (Baltimore: Johns Hopkins University Press, 2020).
11. USA, Brazil, India, European nations all share a democratic system and the highest infection rates of COVID-19.

12. Such as Hungary and Thailand
13. Francesco Guarascio and Philip Blenkinsop, "EU Fails To Persuade France, Germany To Lift Coronavirus Health Gear Control," *U.S.*, March 26, 2020, https://www.reuters.com/article/us-health-coronavirus-eu-idUSKBN20T166.
14. "Government Slashes IGST On Oxygen Concentrators For Personal Use To 12%," *The Economic Times*, May 1, 2021, https://economictimes.indiatimes.com/news/india/government-slashes-igst-on-oxygen-concentrators-for-personal-use-to-12/articleshow/82346790.cms.
15. Securitisation is the process by which states legislate on issues and thereby address the urgency of finding a solution including, but not exclusively, releasing funds or mobilising security forces to deal with the matter at hand.
16. Amnesty International, "Mozambique 2020," *Amnesty International,* https://www.amnesty.org/en/countries/africa/mozambique/report-mozambique.
17. Anu Madgavkar, et al., "COVID-19 Has Revived the Social Contract in Advanced Economies—For Now. What Will Stick Once the Crisis Abates?" *McKinsey Global Institute*, December 10, 2020, https://www.mckinsey.com/industries/public-and-social-sector/our-insights/covid-19-has-revived-the-social-contract-in-advanced-economies-for-now-what-will-stick-once-the-crisis-abates#.
18. According to both ethnic and age group.
19. Allison Peters, et al., "The COVID-19 Pandemic and Trends in Technology," *Chatham House*, February 16, 2021, https://www.chathamhouse.org/2021/02/covid-19-pandemic-and-trends-technology/03-covid-19-changing-cybercrime-landscape.
20. Anthony Cuthbertson, "5G Conspiracy Theory Threatens Economies and Risks Leaving People with Slow Connections, EU Countries Warn," *The Independent*, October 19, 2020, https://www.independent.co.uk/life-style/gadgets-and-tech/5g-conspiracy-theory-masts-tower-coronavirus-b1154406.html.
21. Niklas Novaky, "The Budget Deal and EU Defence Cooperation: What Are the Implications?," *Euractiv*, July 23, 2020, https://www.euractiv.com/section/defence-and-security/opinion/the-budget-deal-and-eu-defence-cooperation-what-are-the-implications/.
22. Henry Kissinger, *Diplomacy* (New York: Touchstone, 1994).

23. Moritz Rudolf, "China's Health Diplomacy during Covid-19," *SWP Comments*, no. 9 (2021): 1–7. https://www.swp-berlin.org/fileadmin/contents/products/comments/2021C09_ChinaHealthDiplomacy.pdf.
24. Samuel Brannen and Kathleen Hicks, "We Predicted a Coronavirus Pandemic: Here's What Policymakers Could Have Seen Coming," *Politico Magazine*, March 7, 2020, https://www.politico.com/news/magazine/2020/03/07/coronavirus-epidemic-prediction-policy-advice-121172; Bronwyn Fryer and Jonathan Quick, *The End of Epidemics: How to Stop Viruses and Save Humanity Now*, 1st ed. (London: Scribe, 2020); Laurie Garrett, *The Coming Plague* (New York: Farrar, Straus and Giroux, 1995); William McNeil, *Plagues and People* (New York: Anchor Books, 1998).
25. "Employment Loss in the Travel and Tourism Industry Due to the Coronavirus (COVID-19) Pandemic Worldwide in 2020, by Region," *Statista,* https://www.statista.com/statistics/1104835/coronavirus-travel-tourism-employment-loss/.
26. Christoph Lakner, "Updated Estimates of the Impact of COVID-19 on Global Poverty: Looking Back at 2020 and the Outlook for 2021," *World Bank Blogs*, January 11, 2021, https://blogs.worldbank.org/opendata/updated-estimates-impact-covid-19-global-poverty-looking-back-2020-and-outlook-2021.
27. Economist Editorial Board, "Keeping Things Cornucopious: The World's Food System Has So Far Weathered the Challenge of Covid-19." *The Economist*, May 9, 2020, https://www.economist.com/briefing/2020/05/09/the-worlds-food-system-has-so-far-weathered-the-challenge-of-covid-19.
28. Jennifer Clapp, and William G. Moseley, "This Food Crisis Is Different: COVID-19 and the Fragility of the Neoliberal Food Security Order," *The Journal of Peasant Studies* 47, no. 7 (2020): 1393–1417, https://www.tandfonline.com/doi/full/10.1080/03066150.2020.1823838#.
29. William McNeil, *Plagues and People* (New York: Anchor Books, 1998).

Bibliography

"Employment Loss in the Travel and Tourism Industry Due to the Coronavirus (COVID-19) Pandemic Worldwide in 2020, by Region," *Statista*. https://www.statista.com/statistics/1104835/coronavirus-travel-tourism-employment-loss/.

"Government Slashes IGST on Oxygen Concentrators For Personal Use To 12%." *The Economic Times,* May 1, 2021. https://economictimes.indiatimes.com/news/india/government-slashes-igst-on-oxygen-concentrators-for-personal-use-to-12/articleshow/82346790.cms.

"Mozambique 2020," *Amnesty International*, https://www.amnesty.org/en/countries/africa/mozambique/report-mozambique.

Brands, Hal, and Francis J. Gavin. *COVID-19 and World Order.* Baltimore: Johns Hopkins University Press, 2020.

Brannen, Samuel, and Kathleen Hicks. "We Predicted a Coronavirus Pandemic: Here's What Policymakers Could Have Seen Coming." Politico *Magazine*, March 7, 2020. https://www.politico.com/news/magazine/2020/03/07/coronavirus-epidemic-prediction-policy-advice-121172

Clapp, Jennifer, and William G. Moseley. "This Food Crisis Is Different: COVID-19 and the Fragility of the Neoliberal Food Security Order." *The Journal of Peasant Studies* 47, no. 7 (2020): 1393–1417. https://www.tandfonline.com/doi/full/https://doi.org/10.1080/03066150.2020.1823838#.

Cuthbertson, Anthony. "5G Conspiracy Theory Threatens Economies and Risks Leaving People with Slow Connections, EU Countries Warn." *The Independent*, October 19, 2020. https://www.independent.co.uk/life-style/gadgets-and-tech/5g-conspiracy-theory-masts-tower-coronavirus-b1154406.html

Economist Editorial Board. "Keeping Things Cornucopious: The World's Food System Has So Far Weathered the Challenge of Covid-19." *The Economist*, May 9, 2020. https://www.economist.com/briefing/2020/05/09/the-worlds-food-system-has-so-far-weathered-the-challenge-of-covid-19

Elsland, Sabine. "COVID-19 Deaths: Infection Fatality Ratio Is About 1% Says New Report." *Imperial College London*, March 29, 2020. https://www.imperial.ac.uk/news/207273/covid-19-deaths-infection-fatality-ratio-about/

Garrett, Laurie. *The Coming Plague*. New York: Farrar, Straus and Giroux, 1995.

Guarascio, Francesco, and Philip Blenkinsop. "EU Fails To Persuade France, Germany To Lift Coronavirus Health Gear Controls." *U.S.*, March 26, 2020. https://www.reuters.com/article/us-health-coronavirus-eu-idUSKBN20T166.

Hewings-Martin, Yella. "How do SARS and MERS Compare with COVID-19?." *Medical News Today*, April 10, 2020. https://www.medicalnewstoday.com/articles/how-do-sars-and-mers-compare-with-covid-19#MERS

Kissinger, Henry. *Diplomacy*. New York: Touchstone, 1994.

Lakner, Christoph. “Updated Estimates of the Impact of COVID-19 on Global Poverty: Looking Back at 2020 and the Outlook for 2021.” *World Bank Blogs*, January 11, 2021. https://blogs.worldbank.org/opendata/updated-estimates-impact-covid-19-global-poverty-looking-back-2020-and-outlook-2021.

Madgavkar, Anu, Tilman Tacke, Sven Smit, and James Manyika, et al. "COVID-19 Has Revived the Social Contract in Advanced Economies—For Now. What Will Stick Once the Crisis Abates?” *McKinsey Global Institute*, December 10, 2020. https://www.mckinsey.com/industries/public-and-social-sector/our-insights/covid-19-has-revived-the-social-contract-in-advanced-economies-for-now-what-will-stick-once-the-crisis-abates.

McNeil, William. *Plagues and People*. New York: Anchor Books, 1998

Novaky, Niklas. “The Budget Deal and EU Defence Cooperation: What Are the Implications?” *Euractiv*, July 23, 2020. https://www.euractiv.com/section/defence-and-security/opinion/the-budget-deal-and-eu-defence-cooperation-what-are-the-implications/.

Peters, Allison, et al., Sophia Ignatidou, Joyce Hakemh, and Emily Taylor. “The COVID-19 Pandemic and Trends in Technology.” *Chatham House*, February 16, 2021. https://www.chathamhouse.org/2021/02/covid-19-pandemic-and-trends-technology/03-covid-19-changing-cybercrime-landscape.

Quick, Jonathan D., and Bronwyn Fryer. *The End of Epidemics*. London: Scribe, 2020.

Rudolf, Moritz. “China’s Health Diplomacy during Covid-19.” *SWP Comments,* no. 9 (2021): 1–7. https://www.swp-berlin.org/fileadmin/contents/products/comments/2021C09_ChinaHealthDiplomacy.pdf.

Thompson, Derek. "How mRNA Technology Could Change the World." *The Atlantic*, March 29, 2020. https://www.theatlantic.com/ideas/archive/2021/03/how-mrna-technology-could-change-world/618431/.

CHAPTER 2

Latin America: The Covid-19 Pandemic and Security in Latin America

Oscar Palma

Introduction

The security agenda in Latin America has historically focused on confronting internal challenges rather than on conventional clashes between states. The absence, with only minor exceptions, of interstate conflicts, has led to a belief that Latin America is peaceful. In reality, internal conditions in each Latin American state have triggered different factors disrupting security at many levels: the illicit flows of narcotics, persons, gold, minerals, wildlife species and weapons, among other things, sustain a myriad of armed groups. Their actions affect the lives of people, communities and, in some cases, the stability of the state.[1]

Homicide, kidnapping, extortion, and internal displacement are indicators of pervasive actors that continue to operate under the radar of states that have not been able to solve these problems effectively. Institutional

O. Palma (✉)
Faculty of International, Political and Urban Studies, Universidad del Rosario, Bogotá, Colombia
e-mail: oscar.palma@urosario.edu.co

C. Varin (ed.), *Global Security in Times of Covid-19*, New Security Challenges, https://doi.org/10.1007/978-3-030-82230-9_2

weakness and the lack of state presence in specific areas have contributed to the emergence and consolidation of non-state actors which, through the consolidation of illicit economies, are able to control territories and even gain a relative support of the population.[2]

The pandemic is unlikely to change this historical situation dramatically, but it is demonstrating that non-state agents are more adaptable, innovative, and flexible, than more rigid and slow state institutions, which have been entangled in their responses to the crisis. The duty of states to strengthen their institutions, throughout their territories, is still ongoing in Latin America, and with the pandemic more obstacles appear. Adding to the flexible character of armed groups, states must face both their possible increase of support in some regions, a more rabid violence in others, the worsening social and economic conditions caused by COVID-19, and their own history with corruption.

COVID-19 and Latin America

The COVID-19 crisis has not been easy for Latin America. A year after the first cases were announced, a lack of clarity as to how to control contagion remains. It is true that a solution to the pandemic is globally elusive, but countries in other regions have fared considerably better. Trying to avoid the scenarios of Spain and Italy, several Latin American countries decided to implement lockdowns very early, with the detection of the first cases. Most health systems in the region could not cope with the demand that European countries have had to face.

Lockdowns and social distancing were implemented in March 2020 with mixed results. Countries like Peru and Chile quickly jumped to the global top 10 list by cases. By mid-August, Peru was 6th (451,493 cases) and Chile 9th (388,855) globally. Colombia initially fared well, with 43,000 cases in June, but after lockdowns were relaxed, it quickly climbed to 8th position worldwide by August (476,660). Others did relatively better in the initial months: Argentina (299,126), Bolivia (101,223), and Ecuador (102,941).[3] A year after the pandemic, Latin American countries were still among the most affected, but no longer on the top 10. Argentina climbed up to the 11th position (3′005,259 cases), Colombia on the 12th (2′893,355), Peru 16th (1′810,998), and Chile 22nd (1′215,815).[4]

The cases of Brazil and Mexico deserve special attention as their presidents—Jair Bolsonaro and Manuel Lopez Obrador respectively—reacted curiously; denying the existence of the pandemic and downplaying its impact. By mid-August, Brazil was ranked the second country with most cases worldwide (3,359,570) with Mexico jumping to 7th (525,763). The Americas quickly became the continent with the highest number of COVID-19 cases[5] in the world. By May 2021, Brazil had become one of the most concerning cases globally, because a more contagious strain of the virus, which emerged in the Brazilian Amazon, drove a considerable increase in the number of cases, up to 14′754,910.[6] After the outstanding surge in India, Brazil became third in the world. Mexico became the 15th country with the most cases, with 2′348,873.[7]

Lockdowns in Latin America have proven to be an enormous challenge. The amount of people who live on the informal economy, whose income depends on the movement of people on the streets every day, is simply too high. For example, the informal economy in Colombia—in 23 metropolitan areas—is estimated at 47.9%,[8] in Peru its 65.7%,[9] Brazil 41.1%,[10] and in Bolivia 62.3%. For many people, then, lockdown represented a bigger challenge than the virus itself.

Although governments, national and local, and even concerned citizens, launched different campaigns to attend to the needs of this wide sector of society, people still needed to leave their homes. In Peru, for example, only 21.9% of homes have a refrigerator, meaning that people needed to go to the markets often, and markets were usually crowded. Subsidies provided by the government, which were among the highest on the continent, had to be claimed in crowded banks, given low banking membership standards, without mentioning the fact that many people lived in overcrowded homes, in Peru and other countries in the region.[11]

Security Before the Pandemic

Security conditions were already difficult before the pandemic, but with the crisis they were at risk of becoming more pressing for the people, for communities and the states. Armed groups had the chance to increase their control in specific areas, whereas the economic impact of the restriction of movement destroyed employment and a source of income for many. Urban insecurity and a continuing flow of migrants from Venezuela made the security picture more concerning.

In 2019, all but 8 from the top 50 most violent cities in the world were in Latin America and the Caribbean. Most of them are in Mexico, Brazil, Venezuela, and the northern triangle (Guatemala, Honduras, El

Salvador).[12] Tijuana, Mexico counted 134.24 homicides per 100,000 annually, compared to rates below 1 per 100,000 in Western European countries and Japan.[13] A considerable amount of this violence is explained by armed groups and criminal gangs, which are a pervasive threat to security in most Latin American countries: a threat to individuals, a threat to local order, and even a threat to national security.

Mexico has seen years of evolution of cartels and criminal groups: Sinaloa, Los Zetas, Cartel de Jalisco Nueva Generación (CJNG), La Familia Michoacana, Cartel de los Carrillo Fuente, Cartel del Golfo, Cartel de los Beltrán Leyva, and Caballeros Templarios, are the result of processes of adaptation and evolution, following clashes among different criminal groups and state forces, for years.

Further south, the Central American *maras* disrupt security on different levels. Mara Salvatrucha (MS-18) and Barrio 18 (La 18) emerged from the Hispanic gang culture in Los Angeles, mainly Salvadorean, spreading later throughout the Northern Triangle. The high insecurity levels and murder rates in Honduras, El Salvador, and Guatemala are explained by these *maras* and a network of smaller associated criminal groups.

In Colombia, the demobilization of the main insurgent group, the Revolutionary Armed Forces of Colombia (FARC) in 2016, did not bring an end to armed groups. If anything, there is now a more complex web of major and minor groups, struggling to capture territory and the rents of illicit economies. Major organizations like the National Liberation Army (ELN), FARC's dissidents and Clan del Golfo, are considered threats to national security, with others disturbing regional order: Pelusos, Caparros, Rastrojos, Puntilleros, etc. A myriad of local gangs, violent outsourcing groups and minor organized groups threaten the lives and rights of Colombians in diverse regions and cities.

The vacuum left by FARC in specific areas was an opportunity for others. The ELN and *Clan del Golfo* quickly moved in, while Mexican and Brazilian organizations started controlling wider sections of transnational routes. Mexican groups seem to have extended their presence in Colombia, while Brazilian groups became some of the biggest on the continent.

In Brazil, these include Primeiro Comando da Capital (PCC), Familia do Norte, and Comando Vermelho. PCC might even be the biggest in South America, with about 30,000 members.[14] Although it is based in Sao Paulo, its activity extends to almost every state in Brazil, and to Peru,

Venezuela, Paraguay, Ecuador, and Bolivia. Comando Vermelho has its base in Rio de Janeiro, while Familia do Norte operates in the Amazon, closer to the border with Colombia.

The final piece in this puzzle is Venezuela. The crisis in the country has triggered an amount of security challenges in different dimensions. Social and economic conditions have motivated a massive exodus, never seen before in Latin America. Neighboring countries, especially Colombia, have found it hard to cope with hordes of Venezuelans crossing the border. But tensions between Venezuela and other governments, especially Colombia, United States, Brazil, and Ecuador, also pose a more conventional state-to-state threat. Venezuela has become a hub for criminal networks. Several officials in the regime, most notoriously Diosdado Cabello, Tareck-el-Aissami, and Vladimir Padrino,[15] have been accused of being members of a drug-trafficking ring, commonly known as *Cartel de los Soles*. Even if this is not the case, Venezuelan territory is a hotbed for criminal activity. Colombian, Venezuelan and even groups from other continents, Hezbollah for example, operate with relative ease.

There are, of course, more groups in other countries. Throughout the Caribbean, Dominican Republic, Puerto Rico, Jamaica, there are also smaller criminal groups and networks connected to transnational illicit flows, making this a truly transnational system.

Most of these groups participate in drug trafficking networks. Cocaine produced in Colombia, and to a smaller extent Peru and Bolivia, is transported through different routes involving several actors to main consuming markets in North America, Europe, and the Far East. In Mexico, several opiates, meth, and marihuana are produced and shipped to the United States. But like most criminal groups worldwide, their portfolio is wider than narcotics. Some of them also traffic persons, illicit mining goods, and wildlife species. Local activities like loan sharking, extortion, and kidnapping are also common.

Given state weaknesses throughout the region, both in rural and urban spaces, many of these groups manage to control swaths of territory, imposing their own order. They regulate the economy, provide public goods, control the movement of people, charge taxes, provide "protection," and fight the state for this control. In some cases, they gain relative support from the population, strengthening their legitimacy. This is mainly because through illicit economies, they provide a source of income, while the state's plans to destroy these economies puts people's income and survival at risk. Of course, in many cases, order is imposed by force, clashing violently with the population, raising homicide levels and causing displacement.

Criminal and armed groups are thus a threat to security in different ways. They have an impact on human security: on people's lives, liberties, and political, social, cultural, and economic rights. As seen in Colombia and Mexico, those who challenge their authority, those who think differently, end up murdered. They also challenge local or public order, affecting the lives of communities. Concepts like "criminal governance" or "rebelocracy" give us an idea about the functions that non-state groups have in the administration of a territory, competing with state institutions, or sometimes exploiting them to their advantage. "They develop those activities that typically characterize a collective decision-maker's intervention on the economy: levying of taxes, coercive provision of public goods, and regulation of private agents through non-fiscal tools."[16]

They can also be understood as a threat to national security when they have the capacity to rival security forces. The ELN and FARC's dissidents in Colombia are not only criminal organizations, they also have a political agenda, pursuing state transformation. They fight the Military and the Police Forces, so they challenge institutions and the polity itself.

State Capture

Probably the clearest way that armed groups have been exploiting the COVID-19 pandemic, paralleling and at times rivalling the state, is related to response-time. Indeed, often such groups mobilize faster and are able to provide assistance in areas where the established institutions are historically weak. Through the provision of services, the regulation of flows of people, and the control of commerce and businesses, they are building more social capital and gaining legitimacy.

Colectivos in Caracas and groups in Rio de Janeiro outpaced the state in declaring lockdowns in their areas of control.[17] Bolsonaro's passive approach to the problem facilitated local actors to react to the pandemic unhindered. *Comando Vermelho* imposed a lockdown in the favela *Cidade de Deus*, knocking on doors, making public messages through speakers, and threatening punishment for those not complying.[18] A sign in a favela wall proclaimed that "If the government won't do the right thing, organized crime will."[19] Other favelas were placed in similar lockdowns by other groups and militias.[20] This was not restricted to Brazil and Venezuela with similar messages reported in Mexico. In Guerrero, for instance, a series of billboards placed by the cartels read "People of Iguala, we ask you to please stay inside your home, we do not want chaos outside. You have to respect the lockdown, we will seriously hurt those who we catch outside."[21]

Colectivos in the famous *23 de Enero* and *Petare* neighborhoods in Caracas enforced quarantine and hygienic protocols. Since they are aligned to the regime's forces, President Maduro called on them to control these zones along with security forces and other militias.[22] In Southwest Colombia, dissidents of FARC's 25th front were distributing pamphlets threatening those who defied the lockdown and setting illegal checkpoints to enforce this control.[23] Maras in San Salvador, both MS-13 and Barrio 18, threatened to kill those who did not comply with the lockdown.[24]

Also, some groups became service providers and handed out basic, highly valued, products, especially food and hygienic goods. In Mexico, a wide range of groups distributed food packages and essential items, even with a stamp or brand of the organization.[25] Such is the case of the *Cartel de Jalisco Nueva Generación (CJNG),* the *Cartel del Golfo,* and *Los Viagras.*[26] The former distributed boxes with a message: "From your CJNG friends, supporting [*sic* you] in the COVID-19 crisis."[27] Similar cases were observed in Tamaulipas with *Cartel del Golfo,* in Veracruz with *Los Zetas,* in Mexico and Guerrero with *Familia Michoacana,* and in Tierra Caliente with *Los Viagras.*[28] It was curious to see El Chapo Guzman's daughter handing out boxes with food and supplies with the Chapo's photo in it.[29] In Rio de Janeiro, criminal groups in favelas were distributing soap and disinfectant, threatening those who would try to increase prices because of the high demand and forbidding entrance to tourists.[30]

In the interest of alleviating some pressure on the population, some groups decided to postpone the charging of extortion rackets to local businesses, hoping to build sympathy. It is the case of Barrio 18 in Guatemala, although others, like *Unión de Tepito* in Mexico City continued charging extortion.[31] This is significant for criminal groups, since extortion permits a regular cash flow. Compared to March 2019, extortion fell 9% in Guatemala, 17% in El Salvador, and 80% in Honduras.[32] In a similar vein, some of these cartels loaned money to small businesses in difficulty.[33]

This "kindness" may come with a heavy price as aid will hardly be free. Criminals might charge people afterwards or they could demand their cooperation, providing information, money laundering, or loyalty against security institutions.[34] Honduran gangs have warned that once the quarantine ends, protection money will have to be paid retrospectively.[35]

This is one of the challenges states will face after the pandemic. The acts of some armed groups and criminals might make them more popular, but in other circumstances they pose a deeper threat to people's lives and rights.

And the State?

Latin American states tend to be weak. Institutional fragility in the region is expressed in many forms: constitutional checks and balances which do not constrain presidents, nominally independent judiciaries and central banks with no teeth, failed electoral reforms, weak party systems, enshrined social rights which are seldom respected, presidential term limits circumvented, and civil service laws, tax laws, and labor and environmental regulation enforced unevenly.[36]

Some elements of this institutional weakness are factors driving insecurity and violence, mainly because they allow state capture by armed groups:

- The inability of the state to control the territory, or large parts of the territory, and guarantee the security of citizens because it has lost the monopoly of the use of force.
- Its incapacity to uphold its internal legal order.
- Its inability to deliver public services to its population or to create the conditions for such delivery.[37]

This is especially evident in vast territories, particularly those with difficult topographies, but it's also a condition in deprived urban areas, with difficult social and economic standards. The pandemic has made this more visible. In Brazil, (former) Minister of Health, Luis Henrique Mandetta, suggested the local authorities get in touch with cartels to define how to control the pandemic.[38] In Mexico, the shortage of health supplies motivated hospitals to seek the help of cartels to get the necessary equipment.[39] This raised the profile of criminal groups further legitimizing their actions in the eyes of the public, demonstrating also the weakness of the state.

Besides state capture, the pandemic may also be proving that armed actors are more resilient, innovative, and adaptable than the state in critical regions. Restrictions of movement affected the plantation of the coca leaf, but it did not reduce trade. In regions of Peru and Colombia, communities decided to stop growing the leaf and set up roadblocks to stop the spread of the virus. In Colombia, authorities have increased the eradication of coca bushes since the beginning of lockdowns. However, major groups like *Clan del Golfo* seem to have been unaffected, resorting both to stockpiles and smaller coca farms requiring a smaller workforce. In Bolivia, the pandemic has actually limited the capacity of authorities to control the cultivation since they are now preoccupied with other more urgent issues.[40] Similarly, the amount of seizures registered in Peru, particularly in Ucayali, prove that cocaine continues to be moved through the country's borders with Brazil and Bolivia. Tonnes are transported via air and land routes despite the enhanced border controls.[41]

Similarly, because lockdowns have made common means of transport difficult, speed and fishing boats have given way to caravans of more than 20 people, in mules, moving through older routes. This is the case in the Colombian–Panamanian border.[42] Mexican cartels increased the use of tunnels and drone deliveries to the United States.[43] In Brazil, cocaine from Peru and Colombia—which is ultimately shipped to Africa and Europe—was brought through on boats traveling down the Amazon instead of the usual land routes.[44]

Adaptability and innovation are not limited to the drug market. Armed groups have also turned to other illicit flows, especially those stimulated by the pandemic. Black markets trading in medicine and medical equipment, including face masks, have opened in countries like Mexico, Guatemala, Colombia, Brazil, Peru, Cuba, Mexico, and Venezuela.[45] Local prohibitions motivated the smuggling of alcohol, from Costa Rica to Panama, and cigarettes from Paraguay to Argentina[46] and if criminals still see their income reduced, they are likely to resort to kidnapping, extortion, and protection rackets.[47]

Further concern relates to the trafficking of wildlife species. Latin America is home to some of the most biodiverse countries in the world. Brazil and Colombia are among the global top two, with Peru, Ecuador, Mexico, and Venezuela in the top ten.[48] Unfortunately, this has motivated the trafficking of species and timber, especially from the Amazon. These flows are also an opportunity for criminal organizations. Concern that such flows will profit major armed organizations has motivated a more careful observation of the phenomenon. In Colombia, for the first time, biodiversity and water resources were included as national security issues in the most recent National Security Policy.[49]

Cyberspace has also seen an increase in criminal activity, an area in which criminals are constantly outpacing security institutions, and private companies, in their response. Latin America is ranked as the third region in the world in the number of malware attacks, with 14% of global cases.[50] The lives of Latin Americans have become more dependent on the internet during the pandemic, inviting more opportunities for cybercrime. Most activities and transactions have moved to cyberspace, from banking to buying groceries and medicines. Email phishing schemes and apps exploiting the pandemic have appeared throughout the region. Some of these schemes, for example, promised free COVID-19 testing, or money from government aid programmes, while others demanded contributions for research, medicine kits, and vaccines.[51]

In Costa Rica, a data theft app called COVIDLock spread through the country in March 2020. As with many apps in other countries, it offered interactive virus-spread maps, supposedly helpful to slow contagion. Instead, the app hijacked mobiles and computers, to demand a ransom payment from victims through bitcoin.[52] Colombian authorities registered 160 complaints of cyberfraud, just on the weekend before lockdown—a 60% spike compared to the same period in 2019.[53]

A more meaningful problem of Latin American states, that has always existed, with a profound impact on security, is corruption, which has been a systemic feature of societies in the region. Most Latin American countries are ranked low on the transparency perception index. With a few exceptions, all countries are below 93rd place, with eight among the worst 50 cases: Venezuela (in the top 5), Honduras, Nicaragua, Guatemala, Paraguay, Mexico, and Dominican Republic.[54]

In a wider understanding of security, corruption is a threat. In developing countries still requiring considerable investment to achieve regional development, especially in more distant regions, corruption has been a major obstacle. Colombia, for example, has struggled to bring all the necessary infrastructure to remote conflict regions, where the illicit coca economy has defined the social and economic order for decades. But corruption has been an obstacle: funds are stolen or diverted, contracts are tailored to overcharge the state, politicians work for self-interest and projects go unfinished. Isolated regions continue to be isolated allowing non-state actors to thrive and to impose their own security conditions. Distrust of national authorities is widespread, rendering progress difficult.

The pandemic has proven that even when these countries face awful social and humanitarian conditions, state officials still exploit the situation for personal gain. In Honduras, the Attorney General's Office launched an investigation into irregularities in the purchasing of products and award of contracts by a Commission specifically created to address the COVID-19 pandemic. The National Anti-Corruption Council warned about Government corruption in the purchases of overpriced medical supplies.[55] In Ecuador, a mafia ring trading COVID medicines donated to hospitals was uncovered in July, while in Colombia, 56 contracts adding up to US$35 million were under investigation for alleged corrupt practices of local authorities in their response to the crisis.[56] The extent of corruption in Latin America was so alarming that the UN created an Observatory to keep an eye on the price of medicines in the region, motivated by scandals in Brazil, Bolivia, Paraguay, Colombia, Ecuador, Guatemala, Mexico, Peru, and Dominican Republic.[57]

Serious corruption problems have always been an obstacle in the fight against crime, they thwart states' responses to organized crime.[58] Evidently, cartels, mobsters, and kingpins have always had a strong corruptive power. They can pay members of police forces much more than the state can. There is a myriad of examples throughout Latin America, especially in Brazil, Mexico, Colombia, and the Northern Triangle, of how members of security institutions have helped cartels with their activities.

Concern with corruption during the pandemic is justified. Governments are likely to channel funds to local authorities, even at the municipal level, to sustain recovery schemes for communities facing difficult conditions. In regions where armed groups have some influence, they might be able to capture the rents coming from lucrative contracts.[59] For decades, groups like the ELN and FARC in Colombia have extracted capital from municipal budgets where they had been strong.

This corruptive power is not limited to security agencies. In recent years, an intensive campaign by several Latin American military and police forces have fought maritime drug trafficking both in the Caribbean and the Pacific successfully. Common modes of trafficking like go-fast, fishing and submarine boats have thus given way to the shipment of drugs in containers together with licit cargo, departing and arriving in different ports worldwide. Corruption, then, also reaches exporters in the private sector, and maybe even port authorities. During the pandemic, there might have been an added risk since some enforcement agencies occupied in the fight against COVID have eased controls at sea and ports, favoring the circulation of narcotics.[60]

Public Security and the State

In the analysis of public security, the pandemic has raised the question about the clash between illicit actors and the state. COVID-19 weakened national economies in Latin America profoundly, more than in other regions. One year after the pandemic, the GDP in the region had contracted 7.7%, with more than three million businesses closing. Latin America accounted for 27.8% of total deaths globally, with only 8.7% of the population.[61] In the context of state weakness this represents a significant peril for security.

If there was a high motivation to join gangs, armed groups, and criminal organizations before the pandemic, then the current circumstances could only push people further, especially in areas where the state is weakest. There is, therefore, concern of a possible increase in the recruitment of vulnerable people by criminal groups.[62] In Colombia, the recruitment of minors increased 113% between January and May 2020 and in the case of the ELN alone, 31 cases of youth recruitment were reported.[63] Concern is not limited to minors, but to the entire population, and opportunities are offered by armed groups in marginal areas, and cities where major and minor groups operate.[64]

Unemployment has also been driven by the closure of many businesses, especially small and medium enterprises unable to survive amid long lockdowns and decreased demand in certain goods and services. Concern here is that criminal groups could take over these businesses to launder illicit gains.[65]

In conflict regions, where armed actors are stronger than state institutions, the lives of people are affected by their operations. As discussed above, they might support the criminals, in others they might clash with them, meaning homicide, torture, extortion, and violently imposed curfews. Less violent areas have seen mixed results during the pandemic; some have experienced a reduction in crime and others an increase. In general terms, common criminality in Latin America—theft, robbery, and armed assault—decreased during the first months of the lockdowns because fewer people were in the streets. Buenos Aires, for example, reported a drop of 90% in street crime by mid-April, from 225 down to 30 cases daily.[66] The end of lockdowns, however, came with a spike in crime and violence, reaching "regular" levels as recorded before the pandemic.[67]

Femicide and domestic violence have also been on the rise since the pandemic began. Latin America has had a deep "machismo" culture for centuries.[68] Fourteen out of 25 of the countries with the highest reports of gender violence are in Latin America, with Mexico (for instance) counting an average of 10 women murdered daily.[69] Evidently, confining families in houses with tough environments, in many cases overcrowded, triggered a spiral of domestic violence. In Colombia alone, by May 2020 and since the beginning of the lockdown, authorities had reported 4,300 emergency calls related to gender violence, an increase of 175%.[70] Similar trends were spotted in Chile.[71] In Bolivia, there were more cases of violence against women than thefts and robbery and safe refuge houses had more demand in Peru and Mexico.[72]

Homicide, however, seems to have a different story. The struggle between armed groups to capture routes, markets, and drug production areas, in the context of weak state institutions, has caused an increase of violence in some regions. This seems to be the case in Mexico, which witnessed the highest monthly crime-related homicides in 13 years in March 2020.[73] On the other hand, in the same month, El Salvador, with the highest amount of murder rates in the world, experienced four days free of homicides, which is very rare for the Central American state.[74]

Colombia, however, has experienced several months, during the pandemic, with a worrying amount of homicide cases, many of them related to armed groups competing to control territories. In 2020, 310 "social leaders" were killed, adding up to a long list of leaders murdered in the last five years.[75] Numbers are disputed, the government speaks of 37 cases with another 49 being investigated, while social organizations reference 349 cases.[76] Social leaders are local community leaders fighting for many causes, from the environment to fair land distribution, who generally clash with the criminals' interests. The UN Human Rights Office in Colombia confirmed that by August 2020, it had registered 37 massacres, with 7 more to assess.[77] In only the second week of August, three different massacres committed against minors and young adults, in different regions, killing 16, shook the country, and increased the pressure against the government. All these cases speak about a weak state, which still does not have the capacity to control its territory. The pandemic has not changed this, and these problems are likely to persist even after the pandemic.

Conclusion

The competing dynamics between armed groups and the state are not new. Most of these dynamics are independent from the pandemic, they have always existed and will continue to exist for years. Lockdowns, however, have demonstrated that non-state agents are more adaptable, innovative, and flexible than the rigid and slow state institutions, which have seen yet more urgent problems to resolve, reducing its capacity to maneuver. Since some of the criminals' actions during the lockdowns might have built a stronger bond with communities, states will have to cope with this scenario, while they also fight groups in areas where they continue to threaten people's lives and rights. The struggle is never limited to military means and the use of force alone, it requires a comprehensive set of actions ranging from the diffusion of norms and values, to human and economic development.

A major concern is related to economics and employment. Human security standards are likely to degrade with the pandemic, and states will face hard conditions in the next months, maybe years, to improve access to jobs, housing, health, quality food, and security. Particular concern is raised by Latin Americans in sensitive areas and marginal regions, who might feel tempted to join armed groups to make a living. Of course, the history of widespread corruption in the state and through societies will continue to be a major obstacle to the construction of solutions.

In the years to come, the most pressing security threats in the region are likely to arise from the internal circumstances in each of the states, and not from the rivalry among states, like it has been for decades. Drug trafficking, homicide, wildlife smuggling, illicit mining, trafficking in persons, gangs, femicide, and the like, will crowd the security agenda. The Venezuela issue will still be a cause for concern, but more than the conventional threat it poses to others, like Colombia, it will continue to be worrying as a hub for illicit networks and armed groups, and a catalyst of immigration, with Venezuelans escaping to find better lives elsewhere.

Notes

1. "Informe Defensorial sobre Desplazamiento Forzado por la Violencia en Colombia," *Defensoría del Pueblo,* https://www.defensoria.gov.co/attachment/48/El%20Desplazamiento%20Forzado%20por%20la%20Violencia%20en%20Colombia%20-.pdf.

2. Ibid.
3. "WHO Coronavirus Disease (COVID-19) Dashboard," *World Health* Organization, August 19, 2020, https://covid19.who.int/?gclid=CjwKCAjwm_P5BRAhEiwAwRzSO7uBTCELzkvRCbdaMHsgnAB8WJ2cJ7z-jLSOM3-QyXvihzOxnLjhXBoCTOcQAvD_BwE.
4. "WHO Coronavirus Disease (COVID-19) Dashboard," *World Health* Organization, May 4, 2021, https://covid19.who.int/table?tableChartType=heat.
5. "WHO Coronavirus Disease (COVID-19) Dashboard," *World Health* Organization, August 19, 2020, https://covid19.who.int/?gclid=CjwKCAjwm_P5BRAhEiwAwRzSO7uBTCELzkvRCbdaMHsgnAB8WJ2cJ7z-jLSOM3-QyXvihzOxnLjhXBoCTOcQAvD_BwE.
6. "WHO Coronavirus Disease (COVID-19) Dashboard," *World Health* Organization, May 4, 2021. https://covid19.who.int/table?tableChartType=heat.
7. Ibid.
8. "Empleo informal y seguridad social," *Departamento Nacional de Estadística,* September 10, 2020, https://www.dane.gov.co/index.php/estadisticas-por-tema/mercado-laboral/empleo-informal-y-seguridad-social#:~:text=La%20proporci%C3%B3n%20de%20ocupados%20informales,metropolitanas%20fue%2047%2C9%25.
9. Diego Noreña, "La informalidad peruana," *Gestion*, July 3, 2019, https://gestion.pe/blog/el-arte-de-emprender-y-fallar/2019/07/la-informalidad-peruana.html/#:~:text=De%20acuerdo%20con%20el%20Instituto,alrededor%20de%20190%20000%20personas.
10. "El desempleo cae al 11,9 por ciento en Brasil en 2019 y la informalidad sigue al alza," *Agencia EFE,* January 31, 2020, https://www.efe.com/efe/america/economia/el-desempleo-cae-al-11-9-por-ciento-en-brasil-2019-y-la-informalidad-sigue-alza/20000011-4163624#:~:text=El%20desempleo%20cae%20al%2011%2C9%20por%20ciento%20en%20Brasil,la%20informalidad%20sigue%20al%20alza&text=La.
11. Pierina Pighi Bel, "Cuarentena en Perú: 5 factores que explican por qué las medidas de confinamiento no impiden que sea el segundo país de América Latina con más casos de covid-19," *BBC,* May 22,

2020, https://www.bbc.com/mundo/noticias-america-latina-527 48764.
12. "Boletín Ranking 2019 de las 50 ciudades más violentas del mundo," *Seguridad, Justicia y Paz*, June 1, 2020, http://www.seguridadjusticiaypaz.org.mx/sala-de-prensa/1590-boletin-ran king-2019-de-las-50-ciudades-mas-violentas-del-mundo.
13. Max Roser, and Hannah Ritchie, "Homicides," *Our World in Data*, July 2013, https://ourworldindata.org/homicides.
14. Angela Olaya, and Josefina Salomon, "PCC and Brazil Government Engaged in Game of Chess," *Insight Crime*, July 22, 2020, https://www.insightcrime.org/news/analysis/bruno-paes-manso-brazil-pcc/.
15. Diosdado Cabello is the current head of the Constituent Assembly and has been appointed to several key political positions. He was remarkably close to Hugo Chavez and is one of the strongest politicians in Venezuela. Tareck el Aissami was the Vice President and is now the Minister of Petroleum, and Minister of Industries and National Production. Vladimir Padrino es the most powerful man in the military, as Minister of Defence.
16. Matteo Pazzona, "Coronavirus: crime cartels helping communities will extract a high price in years to come," *The Conversation,* May 15, 2020, https://theconversation.com/coronavirus-crime-cartels-helping-communities-will-extract-a-high-price-in-years-to-come-138592.
17. Parker Asmann, Chris Dalby, and Seth Robbins, "Six Ways Coronavirus Is Impacting Organized Crime in the Americas," *Insight Crime*, May 4, 2020, https://www.insightcrime.org/news/ana lysis/coronavirus-organized-crime-latin-america/.
18. Parker Asmann, "Implicaciones del coronavirus para la gobernanza criminal en América Latina," *Insight Crime*, March 31, 2020, https://es.insightcrime.org/noticias/analisis/coronavirus-gobernanza-criminal-america-latina/.
19. Richard Behar, "Organized Crime in the Time of Corona," *Forbes*, March 27, 2020, https://www.forbes.com/sites/richardbehar/2020/03/27/organized-crime-in-the-time-of-corona/#7988bb 1a150d.
20. Parker Asmann, "Implicaciones del coronavirus para la gobernanza criminal en América Latina," *Insight Crime*, March 31,

2020, https://es.insightcrime.org/noticias/analisis/coronavirus-gobernanza-criminal-america-latina/.

21. Matteo Pazzona, "Coronavirus: Crime Cartels Helping Communities Will Extract a High Price in Years to Come," *The Conversation*, May 15, 2020, https://theconversation.com/coronavirus-crime-cartels-helping-communities-will-extract-a-high-price-in-years-to-come-138592.
22. Parker Asmann, "Implicaciones del coronavirus para la gobernanza criminal en América Latina," *Insight Crime,* March 31, 2020, https://es.insightcrime.org/noticias/analisis/coronavirus-gobernanza-criminal-america-latina/.
23. Ibid.
24. Ibid.
25. Parker Asmann, Chris Dalby, and Seth Robbins, "Six Ways Coronavirus Is Impacting Organized Crime in the Americas," *Insight Crime*, May 4, 2020, https://www.insightcrime.org/news/analysis/coronavirus-organized-crime-latin-america/.
26. Luis Fajardo, "Coronavirus: Latin American Crime Gangs Adapt to Pandemic," *BBC*, April 21, 2020, https://www.bbc.com/news/world-latin-america-52367898.
27. Victoria Dittmar, "Grupos criminales en México presumen apoyo social durante coronavirus," *Insight Crime,* April 28, 2020, https://es.insightcrime.org/noticias/analisis/criminales-mexico-viveres-coronavirus/.
28. Ibid.
29. Joaquin Guzman, alias "El Chapo" was the former boss of Sinaloa Cartel, and the most powerful kingpin in Mexico. He was captured and is now imprisoned in the United States; The Organized Crime and Corruption Reporting Project (OCCRP), "Cuál cuarentena? Eso es lo de menos para el tráfico global de cocaína," *Insight Crime*, May 26, 2020, https://es.insightcrime.org/noticias/analisis/trafico-cocaina-cuarentena/; Emily Hancock, "Coronavirus Profiteers: The Pandemic and Organized Crime," *The Organization for World Peace*, April 29, 2020, https://theowp.org/coronavirus-profiteers-the-pandemic-and-organised-crime/.
30. Parker Asmann, "Implicaciones del coronavirus para la gobernanza criminal en América Latina," *Insight Crime,* March 31, 2020, https://es.insightcrime.org/noticias/analisis/coronavirus-

gobernanza-criminal-america-latina/; Matteo Pazzona, "Coronavirus: Crime Cartels Helping Communities Will Extract a High Price in Years to Come," *The Conversation*, May 15, 2020, https://theconversation.com/coronavirus-crime-cartels-helping-communities-will-extract-a-high-price-in-years-to-come-138592.
31. Ibid., Asmann.
32. "The Pandemic Is Creating Fresh Opportunities for Organized Crime," *The Economist*, May 16, 2020, https://www.economist.com/international/2020/05/16/the-pandemic-is-creating-fresh-opportunities-for-organised-crime.
33. Richard Behar, "Organized Crime in the Time of Corona," *Forbes*, March 27, 2020, https://www.forbes.com/sites/richardbehar/2020/03/27/organized-crime-in-the-time-of-corona/#7988bb1a150d.
34. Matteo Pazzona, "Coronavirus: Crime Cartels Helping Communities Will Extract a High Price in Years to Come," *The Conversation*, May 15, 2020, https://theconversation.com/coronavirus-crime-cartels-helping-communities-will-extract-a-high-price-in-years-to-come-138592.
35. "The Pandemic Is Creating Fresh Opportunities for Organized Crime," *The Economist,* May 16, 2020, https://www.economist.com/international/2020/05/16/the-pandemic-is-creating-fresh-opportunities-for-organised-crime.
36. Daniel Brinks, Steven Levistky, and Maria Victoria Murillo, *The Politics of Institutional Weakness in Latin America* (Cambridge: Cambridge University Press, 2020).
37. Mariano Aguirre, "Failed States or Weak Democracies? The State in Latin America," *TNI*, January 17, 2006, https://www.tni.org/es/node/13912.
38. Luis Fajardo, "Coronavirus: Latin American Crime Gangs Adapt to Pandemic," *BBC,* April 21, 2020, https://www.bbc.com/news/world-latin-america-52367898.
39. Matteo Pazzona, "Coronavirus: Crime Cartels Helping Communities Will Extract a High Price in Years to Come," *The Conversation,* May 15, 2020, https://theconversation.com/coronavirus-crime-cartels-helping-communities-will-extract-a-high-price-in-years-to-come-138592.
40. The Organized Crime and Corruption Reporting Project (OCCRP), "Cuál cuarentena? Eso es lo de menos para el tráfico

global de cocaína," *Insight Crime*, May 26, 2020, https://es.insightcrime.org/noticias/analisis/trafico-cocaina-cuarentena/.

41. Parker Asmann, Chris Dalby, and Seth Robbins, "Six Ways Coronavirus Is Impacting Organized Crime in the Americas," *Insight Crime*, May 4, 2020, https://www.insightcrime.org/news/analysis/coronavirus-organized-crime-latin-america/.
42. Ibid.
43. "The Pandemic Is Creating Fresh Opportunities for Organized Crime," *The Economist*, May 16, 2020, https://www.economist.com/international/2020/05/16/the-pandemic-is-creating-fresh-opportunities-for-organised-crime.
44. Ibid.
45. María Alejandra Navarrete, "Robo de implementos médicos crece en Latinoamérica por coronavirus," *Insight Crime,* April 22, 2020, https://es.insightcrime.org/noticias/noticias-del-dia/robos-implementos-medicos-coronavirus/.; Anastasia Austin, "Coronavirus genera mercado negro de equipos médicos en Cuba," *Insight Crime,* April 21, 2020, https://es.insightcrime.org/noticias/noticias-del-dia/coronavirus-mercado-negro-medicos-cuba/; Richard Behar, "Organized Crime in the Time of Corona," *Forbes*, March 27, 2020, https://www.forbes.com/sites/richardbehar/2020/03/27/organized-crime-in-the-time-of-corona/#7988bb1a150d; Parker Asmann, Chris Dalby, and Seth Robbins, "Six Ways Coronavirus Is Impacting Organized Crime in the Americas," *Insight Crime*, May 4, 2020, https://www.insightcrime.org/news/analysis/coronavirus-organized-crime-latin-america/.
46. Emanuele Ottolenghi, "COVID-19 in Latin America: Organized Crime Gains and States Weaken," *Foundation for Defense of Democracies*, May 22, 2020, https://www.fdd.org/analysis/2020/05/22/covid-19-in-latin-america:-organized-crime-gains-and-states-weaken/.
47. Robert Muggah, "The Pandemic Has Triggered Dramatic Shifts in the Global Criminal Underworld," *Foreign Policy,* May 8, 2020, https://foreignpolicy.com/2020/05/08/coronavirus-drug-cartels-violence-smuggling/.
48. Ruth A Butler, "The Top 10 Most Biodiverse Countries," *Mongabay,* May 21, 2016, https://news.mongabay.com/2016/05/top-10-biodiverse-countries/.

49. Ministerio de Defensa Nacional, "Política de Defensa y Seguridad PDS," *Política de Defensa y Seguridad PDS,* January 2019, https://www.mindefensa.gov.co/irj/go/km/docs/Mindefensa/Documentos/descargas/Prensa/Documentos/politica_defensa_deguridad2019.pdf.
50. "2020 State of Malware Report," *Malwarebytes Labs*, February 2020, https://resources.malwarebytes.com/files/2020/02/2020_State-of-Malware-Report.pdf.
51. Richard Behar, "Organized Crime in the Time of Corona," *Forbes*, March 27, 2020, https://www.forbes.com/sites/richardbehar/2020/03/27/organized-crime-in-the-time-of-corona/#7988bb1a150d.
52. "Latinoamérica, en mayor riesgo de ciberataques durante cuarentena," *La Voz de Michoacán,* April 10, 2020, https://www.lavozdemichoacan.com.mx/mundo/sin-fronteras/latinoamerica-en-mayor-riesgo-de-ciberataques-durante-cuarentena/.
53. Ibid.
54. "Corruption Perceptions Index 2019," *Transparency International New Zealand,* https://www.transparency.org.nz/corruption-perceptions-index/.
55. Parker Asmann, Chris Dalby, and Seth Robbins, "Six Ways Coronavirus Is Impacting Organized Crime in the Americas," *Insight Crime,* May 4, 2020, https://www.insightcrime.org/news/analysis/coronavirus-organized-crime-latin-america/.
56. Lourdes Romero, "La mafia que traficaba con medicamentos contra la COVID-19 en Ecuador," *Anadolu Agency,* July 13, 2020, https://www.aa.com.tr/es/mundo/la-mafia-que-traficaba-con-medicamentos-contra-la-covid-19-en-ecuador/1909220; Jorge Cantillo, "Corrupción y tráfico de medicamentos en medio de la pandemia en Colombia: investigan 56 contratos por USD 35 millones," *Infobae,* May 2, 2020, https://www.infobae.com/america/colombia/2020/05/02/corrupcion-y-trafico-de-medicamentos-en-medio-de-la-pandemia-en-colombia-investigan-56-contratos-por-usd-35-millones/.
57. Yurany Salamanca Arciniegas, "América Latina: la corrupción alcanza niveles alarmantes en medio de la crisis por el Covid-19," *France 24,* June 21, 2020, https://www.france24.com/es/20200620-corrupcion-america-latina-covid19-coronavirus-malversacion.

58. Richard Behar, "Organized Crime in the Time of Corona," *Forbes,* March 27, 2020, https://www.forbes.com/sites/richardbehar/2020/03/27/organized-crime-in-the-time-of-corona/#7988bb1a150d.
59. "The Pandemic Is Creating Fresh Opportunities for Organized Crime," *The Economist*, May 16, 2020, https://www.economist.com/international/2020/05/16/the-pandemic-is-creating-fresh-opportunities-for-organised-crime.
60. Roberto Saviano, "Why the Mafia Are Taking Care of Everyone's Business," *The Guardian*, April 25, 2020, https://www.theguardian.com/world/2020/apr/25/why-mafia-taking-care-of-everyones-business-in-pandemic.
61. "América Latina es la región en desarrollo más afectada en el mundo por la pandemia," *Noticias ONU*, March 4, 2021, https://news.un.org/es/story/2021/03/1489112.
62. Matteo Pazzona, "Coronavirus: Crime Cartels Helping Communities Will Extract a High Price in years to come," *The Conversation,* May 15, 2020, https://theconversation.com/coronavirus-crime-cartels-helping-communities-will-extract-a-high-price-in-years-to-come-138592.
63. César Niño, "Reclutamiento forzado y covid-19," *El Tiempo,* June 16, 2020, https://www.eltiempo.com/opinion/columnistas/otros-columnistas/reclutamiento-forzado-y-covid-19-cesar-nino-507602.
64. "The Pandemic Is Creating Fresh Opportunities for Organized Crime," *The Economist*, May 16, 2020, https://www.economist.com/international/2020/05/16/the-pandemic-is-creating-fresh-opportunities-for-organised-crime.
65. Ibid.
66. Parker Asmann, Chris Dalby, and Seth Robbins, "Six Ways Coronavirus is Impacting Organized Crime in the Americas," *Insight Crime,* May 4, 2020, https://www.insightcrime.org/news/analysis/coronavirus-organized-crime-latin-america/.
67. Jorge Mantilla, "¿El crimen se disparó con la reapertura?," *Razon Publica,* June 29, 2020, https://razonpublica.com/crimen-se-disparo-la-reapertura/.
68. Norma Fuller, "Repensando el Machismo Latinoamericano," *Masculinity and Social Change No.2* (2012):114–133, https://doi.org/10.17583/msc.2012.218.

69. "Feminicidios en América Latina: violencia machista que no cesa," *DW América Latina*, February 17, 2020, https://www.dw.com/es/feminicidios-en-am%C3%A9rica-latina-violencia-machista-que-no-cesa/a-52408153.
70. "Apoyo por violencia intrafamiliar a 4.385 mujeres, durante cuarentena," *Vicepresidencia de Colombia*, May 15, 2020, https://mlr.vicepresidencia.gov.co/Paginas/prensa/2020/Apoyo-por-violencia-intrafamiliar-a-4385-mujeres-durante-cuarentena.aspx.
71. Sandra Weiß, "Cuarentena por coronavirus dispara violencia contra las mujeres en América Latina," *DW América Latina*, April 27, 2020, https://www.dw.com/es/cuarentena-por-coronavirus-dispara-violencia-contra-las-mujeres-en-am%C3%A9rica-latina/a-53261868.
72. Ibid.
73. Luis Fajardo, "Coronavirus: Latin American Crime Gangs Adapt to Pandemic," *BBC*, April 21, 2020, https://www.bbc.com/news/world-latin-america-52367898.
74. "The Pandemic Is Creating Fresh Opportunities for Organized Crime," *The Economist*, May 16, 2020, https://www.economist.com/international/2020/05/16/the-pandemic-is-creating-fresh-opportunities-for-organised-crime.
75. "Asesinatos de líderes sociales: Colombia mata a quienes practican la democracia en las regiones," *Deutsche Welle*, January 14, 2021. https://www.dw.com/es/asesinatos-de-l%C3%ADderes-sociales-colombia-mata-a-quienes-practican-la-democracia-en-las-regiones/a-56218920
76. Rueda Bustamante, and Juan Pablo, "En 2020 han sido asesinados 37 líderes sociales: Gobierno," *El Tiempo*, July 9, 2020, https://www.eltiempo.com/politica/gobierno/cuantos-lideres-sociales-han-sido-asesinados-en-colombia-516050.
77. ONU Derechos Humanos Colombia (@ONUHumanRights), "Cumpliendo nuestro mandato, en lo que va de 2020, hemos documentado 33 masacres y restan 7 por documentar," Twitter, August 16, 2020, https://twitter.com/ONUHumanRights/status/1295093058552377346.

Bibliography

"2020 State of Malware Report." *Malwarebytes Labs*, February 2020. https://resources.malwarebytes.com/files/2020/02/2020_State-of-Malware-Report.pdf.

"Apoyo por violencia intrafamiliar a 4.385 mujeres, durante cuarentena." *Vicepresidencia de Colombia*, May 15, 2020. https://mlr.vicepresidencia.gov.co/Paginas/prensa/2020/Apoyo-por-violencia-intrafamiliar-a-4385-mujeres-durante-cuarentena.aspx

"Boletín Ranking 2019 de las 50 ciudades más violentas del mundo." *Seguridad, Justicia y Paz*, June 1, 2020. http://www.seguridadjusticiaypaz.org.mx/sala-de-prensa/1590-boletin-ranking-2019-de-las-50-ciudades-mas-violentas-del-mundo.

"Corruption Perceptions Index 2019." *Transparency International New Zealand*. https://www.transparency.org.nz/corruption-perceptions-index/.

"El desempleo cae al 11,9 por ciento en Brasil en 2019 y la informalidad sigue al alza." *Agencia EFE*, January 31, 2020. https://www.efe.com/efe/america/economia/el-desempleo-cae-al-11-9-por-ciento-en-brasil-2019-y-la-informalidad-sigue-alza/20000011-4163624#:~:text=El%20desempleo%20cae%20al%2011%2C9%20por%20ciento%20en%20Brasil,la%20informalidad%20sigue%20al%20alza&text=La.

"Empleo informal y seguridad social." *Departamento Nacional de Estadística*, September 10, 2020. https://www.dane.gov.co/index.php/estadisticas-por-tema/mercado-laboral/empleo-informal-y-seguridad-social#:~:text=La%20proporci%C3%B3n%20de%20ocupados%20informales,metropolitanas%20fue%2047%2C9%25.

"Feminicidios en América Latina: violencia machista que no cesa." *DW América Latina*, February 17, 2020. https://www.dw.com/es/feminicidios-en-am%C3%A9rica-latina-violencia-machista-que-no-cesa/a-52408153.

"Informe Defensorial sobre Desplazamiento Forzado por la Violencia en Colombia." *Defensoría del Pueblo*. https://www.defensoria.gov.co/attachment/48/El%20Desplazamiento%20Forzado%20por%20la%20Violencia%20en%20Colombia%20-.pdf.

"Latinoamérica, en mayor riesgo de ciberataques durante cuarentena." *La Voz de Michoacán*, April 10, 2020. https://www.lavozdemichoacan.com.mx/mundo/sin-fronteras/latinoamerica-en-mayor-riesgo-de-ciberataques-durante-cuarentena/.

"The Pandemic Is Creating Fresh Opportunities for Organised Crime." *The Economist*, May 16, 2020. https://www.economist.com/international/2020/05/16/the-pandemic-is-creating-fresh-opportunities-for-organised-crime.

"WHO Coronavirus Disease (COVID-19) Dashboard." *World Health Organization*, August 19, 2020. https://covid19.who.int/?gclid=CjwKCAjwm_P5BRAhEiwAwRzSO7uBTCELzkvRCbdaMHsgnAB8WJ2cJ7z-jLSOM3-QyXvihzOxnLjhXBoCTOcQAvD_BwE.

Aguirre, Mariano. "Failed States or Weak Democracies? The State in Latin America." *TNI*, January 17, 2006. https://www.tni.org/es/node/13912.

Arciniegas, Yurany Salamanca. "América Latina: la corrupción alcanza niveles alarmantes en medio de la crisis por el Covid-19." *France 24*, June 21, 2020. https://www.france24.com/es/20200620-corrupcion-america-latina-covid19-coronavirus-malveracion.

Asmann, Parker. "Implicaciones del coronavirus para la gobernanza criminal en América Latina." *Insight Crime*, March 31, 2020. https://es.insightcrime.org/noticias/analisis/coronavirus-gobernanza-criminal-america-latina/.

Asmann, Parker, Chris Dalby, and Seth Robbins. "Six Ways Coronavirus Is Impacting Organized Crime in the Americas." *Insight Crime*, May 4, 2020. https://www.insightcrime.org/news/analysis/coronavirus-organized-crime-latin-america/.

Austin, Anastasia. "Coronavirus genera mercado negro de equipos médicos en Cuba." *Insight Crime*, April 21, 2020. https://es.insightcrime.org/noticias/noticias-del-dia/coronavirus-mercado-negro-medicos-cuba/.

Behar, Richard. "Organized Crime in the Time of Corona." *Forbes*, March 27, 2020. https://www.forbes.com/sites/richardbehar/2020/03/27/organized-crime-in-the-time-of-corona/#7988bb1a150d.

Bustamante, Rueda, and Juan Pablo. "En 2020 han sido asesinados 37 líderes sociales: Gobierno." *El Tiempo,* July 9, 2020. https://www.eltiempo.com/politica/gobierno/cuantos-lideres-sociales-han-sido-asesinados-en-colombia-516050.

Butler, Ruth A. "The Top 10 Most Biodiverse Countries." *Mongabay,* May 21, 2016. https://news.mongabay.com/2016/05/top-10-biodiverse-countries/.

Cantillo, Jorge. "Corrupción y tráfico de medicamentos en medio de la pandemia en Colombia: investigan 56 contratos por USD 35 millones." *Infobae,* May 2, 2020. https://www.infobae.com/america/colombia/2020/05/02/corrupcion-y-trafico-de-medicamentos-en-medio-de-la-pandemia-en-colombia-investigan-56-contratos-por-usd-35-millones/.

Daniel Brinks, Steven Levistky, and Maria Victoria Murillo. *The Politics of Institutional Weakness in Latin America*. Cambridge: Cambridge University Press, 2020

Dittmar, Victoria. "Grupos criminales en México presumen apoyo social durante coronavirus." *Insight Crime*, April 28, 2020. https://es.insightcrime.org/noticias/analisis/criminales-mexico-viveres-coronavirus/.

Fajardo, Luis. "Coronavirus: Latin American Crime Gangs Adapt to Pandemic." *BBC,* April 21, 2020. https://www.bbc.com/news/world-latin-america-52367898.

Fuller, Norma. "Repensando el Machismo Latinoamericano." *Masculinity and Social Change No.2* (2012): 114–133. https://doi.org/10.17583/msc.2012.218.

Hancock, Emily. "Coronavirus Profiteers: The Pandemic and Organised Crime." *The Organization for World Peace,* April 29, 2020. https://theowp.org/coronavirus-profiteers-the-pandemic-and-organised-crime/.

Mantilla, Jorge. "¿El crimen se disparó con la reapertura?" *Razon Publica*, June 29, 2020. https://razonpublica.com/crimen-se-disparo-la-reapertura/.

Ministerio de Defensa Nacional. "Política de Defensa y Seguridad PDS." *Política de Defensa y Seguridad PDS*, January 2019. https://www.mindefensa.gov.co/irj/go/km/docs/Mindefensa/Documentos/descargas/Prensa/Documentos/politica_defensa_deguridad2019.pdf.

Muggah, Robert. "The Pandemic Has Triggered Dramatic Shifts in the Global Criminal Underworld." *Foreign Policy*, May 8, 2020. https://foreignpolicy.com/2020/05/08/coronavirus-drug-cartels-violence-smuggling/.

Navarrete, María Alejandra. "Robo de implementos médicos crece en Latinoamérica por coronavirus." *Insight Crime*, April 22, 2020. https://es.insightcrime.org/noticias/noticias-del-dia/robos-implementos-medicos-coronavirus/.

Niño, César. "Reclutamiento forzado y covid-19." *El Tiempo*, June 16, 2020. https://www.eltiempo.com/opinion/columnistas/otros-columnistas/reclutamiento-forzado-y-covid-19-cesar-nino-507602.

Noreña, Diego. "La informalidad peruana." *Gestion*, July 3, 2019. https://gestion.pe/blog/el-arte-de-emprender-y-fallar/2019/07/la-informalidad-peruana.html/#:~:text=De%20acuerdo%20con%20el%20Instituto,alrededor%20de%20190%20000%20personas.

Olaya, Angela, and Josefina Salomon. "PCC and Brazil Government Engaged in Game of Chess." *Insight Crime*, July 22, 2020. https://www.insightcrime.org/news/analysis/bruno-paes-manso-brazil-pcc/.

Ottolenghi, Emanuele. "COVID-19 in Latin America: Organized Crime Gains and States Weaken." *Foundation for Defense of Democracies*, May 22, 2020. https://www.fdd.org/analysis/2020/05/22/covid-19-in-latin-america:-organized-crime-gains-and-states-weaken/.

Pazzona, Matteo. "Coronavirus: Crime Cartels Helping Communities Will Extract a High Price in Years to Come." *The Conversation*, May 15, 2020. https://theconversation.com/coronavirus-crime-cartels-helping-communities-will-extract-a-high-price-in-years-to-come-138592.

Pighi Bel, Pierina. "Cuarentena en Perú: 5 factores que explican por qué las medidas de confinamiento no impiden que sea el segundo país de América Latina con más casos de covid-19." *BBC*, May 22, 2020. https://www.bbc.com/mundo/noticias-america-latina-52748764.

Romero, Lourdes. "La mafia que traficaba con medicamentos contra la COVID-19 en Ecuador." *Anadolu Agency*, July 13, 2020. https://www.aa.com.tr/es/mundo/la-mafia-que-traficaba-con-medicamentos-contra-la-covid-19-en-ecuador/1909220.

Roser, Max, and Hannah Ritchie. "Homicides." *Our World in Data,* July 2013. https://ourworldindata.org/homicides.

Saviano, Roberto. "Why the Mafia Are Taking Care of Everyone's Business." *The Guardian*, April 25, 2020. https://www.theguardian.com/world/2020/apr/25/why-mafia-taking-care-of-everyones-business-in-pandemic.

The Organized Crime and Corruption Reporting Project (OCCRP). "Cuál cuarentena? Eso es lo de menos para el tráfico global de cocaína." *Insight Crime*, May 26, 2020. https://es.insightcrime.org/noticias/analisis/trafico-cocaina-cuarentena/.

Weiß, Sandra. "Cuarentena por coronavirus dispara violencia contra las mujeres en América Latina." *DW América Latina*, April 27, 2020. https://www.dw.com/es/cuarentena-por-coronavirus-dispara-violencia-contra-las-mujeres-en-am%C3%A9rica-latina/a-53261868.

CHAPTER 3

The American Century in the Wake of COVID

Michael Stephens

Introduction

The United States has suffered a tumultuous 18 months, its reputation both at home and abroad is damaged, its prestige sullied, and its democracy pushed to the brink by a Presidency that has been quite unlike any other in US history. The Coronavirus certainly has not helped matters. Having suffered more COVID-related deaths than any other country in the G20, the United States struggled to respond effectively to the virus, leaving a deep stain on its leadership both at home and abroad.[1] Yet despite the paucity of its COVID response, and the chaotic events that accompanied the end of Donald J. Trump's term in the White House, the United States still stands alone as the most powerful nation on earth, and its democratic process the example for all other nations to follow. It has become popular these days to talk of the "end of the American era,"[2] an argument which posits that the United States no longer has the

M. Stephens (✉)
Foreign Policy Research Institute, Philadelphia, PA, USA
e-mail: michaels@rusi.org

C. Varin (ed.), *Global Security in Times of Covid-19*, New Security Challenges, https://doi.org/10.1007/978-3-030-82230-9_3

will to involve itself in the most problematic questions of the day, nor enforce an international world order that it has so long preserved. There is certainly a kernel of truth to this, the past four years have teased out the unwilling, isolationist side that has always existed in America. But if American decline is real, it is a result of faltering will, rather than a decline in American capacity, particularly its abundance of hard power.[3]

The election of President Joseph R. Biden heralded the return of America to the international stage, suggesting that some of this "faltering will" may have been both temporary, and not shared by many policy elites inside the Beltway. Nevertheless, the way in which the United States re-engages with its international commitments will define its legacy for decades to come. If one thing is for certain, it is that the United States will not return to a position of hegemony in the manner of years gone by. The American era might not be over just yet, but it will certainly be redefined. The rise of China and a resurgence of Russian influence in international affairs mean that the United States must contend with a multipolar order marked by state competition rather than cooperation. This requires the United States to answer some fundamental questions of grand strategy, that for the past four years it has largely shunned. The United States may choose to be a convenor, engaging this challenge multilaterally, using allies in Europe and Asia to box in Beijing and Moscow and seeking wide consensus to gradually bring diplomatic and military weight to bear upon its international rivals. Or Washington may choose to lead from the front, mobilizing hard power and coercive economic tools to face down its challengers, and then persuading, cajoling and even strong-arming its allies to fall in behind.

Whether Washington chooses one strategy or the other (or indeed some mixture of both), the first order of business will be to get its own house in order. The tools of American statecraft such as the State Department and USAID are in bad shape. Both have long suffered from institutional decline, much of which results from political decisions to systemically hollow their financial and human capital.[4] This would greatly enable the United States to refocus its attention on rebuilding what Malcolm Chalmers has termed the "Universal Security System" that Washington has been centrally involved in upholding across the world since 1945.[5] The key components of which include the right to self-determination for former colonies and the prohibition of aggression between states (including no change of borders without consent), alongside the creation of regimes for the prohibition of nuclear and other weapons of mass destruction. Although this system has not eroded completely, its edges have certainly frayed. Incidences in which states have impinged on the territory of others are numerous and have been increasing in number since Russia's *de-jure* annexation of Crimea in 2014, and *de-facto* annexation of Georgian land in 2008.[6] Additionally, issues of nuclear proliferation in North Korea,[7] and the use of chemical weapons by the Assad regime in Syria, (as well as Russia's use of chemical agents against political dissidents) have damaged international arms control norms. None of this has been helped by the Trump administration's approach to world affairs, which saw multilateralism as a constraint on US power. Accordingly, Washington withdrew from major international treaties, such as Open Skies and the International Arms Trade Treaty, as well as walking away from the Paris Climate accords, further eroding international consensus on several critical security issues that face the world today. It was not just Trump who eroded these norms, in the case of Syria it should be noted that President Barack Obama's failure to enforce his stated red lines against the usage of chemical weapons greatly damaged both US influence, and undermined the rules-based order.[8]

The increase in rule breaking and bad behaviour among states is not solely a consequence of US strategic retrenchment, although this has certainly not helped matters. Tectonic shifts in global order have brought both Russia and China to the fore, and have encouraged rule breaking and incentivized states to pursue their own interests, with less fear of censure or reprisal. Beijing's own questionable behaviours in the South-China Sea, combined with Russia's weaponization of the Security Council to effectively prevent any punishment against Assad for his use of chemical weapons, have set the tone for a world in which the Universal Security System is greatly weakened.[9]

Additionally, Moscow and Beijing have placed pressure on a third pillar of US foreign policy, which is the respect for human rights, and the promotion of democratic values. Both nations are "popularizing authoritarian governance, exporting their best practices, watering down human rights norms, backing each other up to defend strategic interests in multilateral forums, creating norms around cyber and internet sovereignty, and bolstering illiberal leaders and helping them stay in power."[10] If the Biden Administration wishes to affect some sort of return to the defence of rights across the world, then it will have little choice than to face down both Russia and China, neither of whom have displayed admirable track records. While the United States has bolstered a few illiberal leaders of its own over the years, most notably the authoritarian monarchs in the petrostates of the Gulf, it has broadly sought to encourage and support liberal values when it could, and certainly applied pressure upon those states which engaged in grievous human rights abuses. In wake of the storming of the US Capitol building by Trump supporters, many states scoffed at the notion that the United States is any sort of beacon for human rights and democracy. Yet, this has only strengthened the belief of many American Liberal Internationalists that the United States should double down on promoting values and democracy as a key part of repairing its image in the post-Trump era and pushing back against hypocritical authoritarians looking for any opportunity to take advantage of American weakness.[11] This sentiment finds welcome ears inside the Biden administration, a good example of which could be seen in the admonishment of Saudi Arabia by Biden's National Security Adviser Jake Sullivan for the detention of female activist Loujain al Hathloul.[12] This marked a clear break from the Trump days in which human rights violations were routinely overlooked.[13]

In the face of an eroding international system that the United States long sought to uphold, President Biden will need to quickly ascertain whether reasserting global norms is even possible, and if so, how much resource and energy the United States should dedicate to ensuring this is achieved. As alluded to above, Washington cannot turn the clock back to the moment of American primacy when Francis Fukayama declared "the End of History." The universal liberal order is a long-forgotten dream, and the United States must remove any aspirations it previously held to affect global change in its own image.[14]

So, what is to be done? For the United States to be "back" as Biden termed it, it must tackle the dual problems of Asian and European security, both of which were neglected by Trump. This requires deep and sustained engagement with allies, and a redoubled commitment to US force posture in both theatres, that will undoubtedly need to continue well after Biden has left office and his successor is in place. Such is the scale of the task ahead.

Beijing: The Global Challenger

And what of the Coronavirus? Although highly damaging to US prestige and influence, the virus has merely exacerbated the urgency of addressing the problems that the United States had long struggled with. On the key question facing Washington, that of the rise of China to Superpower status, the Coronavirus only emphasized the need to deal with a challenge that was already vitally important to Washington before COVID's global spread. The virus has brought many systemic problems of global order and competition into sharper focus, and the pandemic is likely to be "less of a turning point, than a way station along the road that the world has been travelling for the past few decades."[15] China's behaviour in the early stages of the pandemic—which involved covering up the severity and scale of the problem, and failing to adequately warn other countries of the ability of the virus to transmit between humans[16]—has led to further distrust and division between Washington and Beijing. Not only has this severely hampered global attempts to overcome the pandemic, but it has also sharply increased a sense of rivalry and competition between the two sides. China, for its part, has not benefited from its handling of the COVID outbreak: recent polling among Western democracies shows that negative opinions of China and Chinese intentions in the world are skyrocketing, and distrust of Beijing among states in its neighbourhood has similarly risen.[17] This has resulted in a tougher consensus on Chinese behaviour, encouraged by Republican hawks and amplified by repeated calls from business leaders and politicians across the world to urge businesses and nations alike to decouple their supply chains from Beijing's influence.[18,19] While this opinion has certainly gained traction in recent months, senior Biden administration officials shun the notion that fully decoupling from China is either possible, or indeed desirable.[20]

However, Washington's passive global role in preventing the spread of the Coronavirus, and aggressive accusatory behaviour particularly with regard to undermining the World Health Organization (to whom the United States remains the biggest donor) has been highly problematic. This has significantly damaged US attempts toward building a stronger consensus against China for the time being, particularly given that many nations do not regard the United States as speaking with any great authority on the matter, and if it is the aesthetic that matters, the United States and its COVID response does not look like the model any other country aspires to replicate.[21] Indeed, it is difficult to see how Washington can create a space for itself to lead the world in tackling the virus when the pandemic has been so costly at home. In the absence of US leadership for over a year, many smaller states have pursued COVID strategies that focus on their own narrow national concerns, and do not require Washington's input at this relatively late stage. Policy thinkers in the United States acknowledge that mobilizing Coronavirus rhetoric to build international consensus against China is unlikely to work at this point,[22] but the Coronavirus has been more of a wakeup call. In the words of one scholar.

> COVID really drove home the fact we [the US] let it get too far, China is too embedded into international markets and supply chains...what are we supposed to do? The conclusion is clearly that we need to be more present in Asia.[23]

The three major democracies and US allies in the region, South Korea, Japan and Taiwan have all handled the pandemic with relative distinction, in part owing to their experience dealing with the SARS outbreak in 2002. East Asian governments acted faster than the West, but they also benefited from "publics that saw masks as a social good while Western experts were busy wrongly arguing that they had little value."[24] As a result, the United States can have little to say on this matter, and it is highly unlikely that American allies in the East would listen anyway. Instead, what the three countries seek is simple; a renewed commitment to American defence and basing infrastructure in the region, coupled with a re-engagement on free trade mechanisms, such as existed under the Trans Pacific Partnership (TPP).[25] President Trump's withdrawal from the TPP and his trade war threats have done little to ingratiate Washington in the region in the past few years, this much is true.[26] That being said, US alliances and partnerships are in good shape—the result of a growing Indo-Pacific consensus on the existential economic and security threat China poses. Spurred on by distrust over the Coronavirus, regional states in the Chinese orbit are deeply concerned about Chinese behaviour, during and after the outbreak of the virus, suggesting that the Biden administration will not have to work too hard to repair US alliances and partnerships.[27] The pathway is therefore wide open for the United States to re-engage closely with partners and friends in the region, who would welcome a sustained engagement in the face of what is an ever growing threat, which the Coronavirus has only made more urgent.

Re-Engaging Europe: Repairing and Re-Energizing Old Relationships

The European theatre will also dominate US thinking in the years to come, but this will be an altogether trickier problem to solve than in Asia where the security imperative is more obvious. America's allies in Europe will be crucial to reinvigorating US power globally, but there is much work to be done. With the exception of the United Kingdom, US–European relations have reached their lowest point in decades. During Trump's Presidency, it became clear that he harboured a dislike for the EU and NATO that verged on disdain. In accusatory tones, he bullied and threatened other NATO allies,[28] and on more than one occasion openly discussed leaving the alliance altogether, undermining this most critical pillar of the Western order,[29] and arguably the single most important foreign policy initiative since the end of World War II. The scars run deep, and it will take some time to convince sceptical Europeans that America is indeed "back." It is important to note that the sentiments that drove Trump's ire did not emerge out of the blue, and to some extent American frustration with NATO is a common theme that runs through its foreign policy elite. The United States has historically shouldered 70% of the cost burden for the transatlantic alliance, and only four nations have consistently met the required 2% of GDP on defence spending. There is a genuine conversation to be had about alliance countries freeloading off American benevolence, and tough questions to be answered about what the United States receives in return for all its investment, given that many countries simply do not meet their obligations. However, as NATO was itself created at the behest of the United States, and served as the primary vector for US power projection for seven decades, enforcing a US-led order that benefitted US interests greatly, Trump's scornful treatment of an organization that has been an axiomatic component of US power was at best misguided, and at worse dangerously negligent.

It is difficult to know whether Trump's thinking on the alliance will continue to survive beyond his Presidency. There is little doubt that those seeking to carry on the Trumpian torch such as Senator Josh Hawley harbour a dislike for freeloading by NATO allies,[30] and that there are elements of the Republican Party that share Trump's dislike for both the EU and NATO. But the vast majority of GOP Congressmen and Senators have criticized Trump's approach toward the issue and noted their concerns to allies.[31] Indeed recent attempts to draw down on troops from Germany (a country with which Trump had particularly taken issue) met with fierce condemnation from party grandees such as former Presidential candidate Senator Mitt Romney who labelled the move a "grave error."[32] Given this contradiction within the Republican Party, and the near universal consensus among mainstream Democrats that European security is vital to the international standing of the United States, it is safe to assume that the majority of political elites in the United States still believe in a defence and security posture that is strongly Atlanticist. Indeed, senior Biden officials have made no secret of their desire to reintegrate the United States into the European security theatre[33] and re-engage NATO allies in conversations that should have existed on a continuum since 2014, following Russia's invasion and annexation of Ukrainian land.[34] Since that time, Russia has aimed to create a permissive political environment in western Europe through an opportunistic policy that seeks to exploit the growing fissures in western consensus wherever possible, and create new ones where it can. This is an approach, it should be noted, that is driven by strategic weakness as much as President Putin's own tactical cunning.[35]

But the United States will need to do more than simply reaffirm commitments to the Europeans if they are to bring them onside. With all Trump's talk of "America first," European leaders have begun to foment discussion about their own "Strategic Autonomy," a loosely defined phrase which as yet has little true meaning, but can range from defence integration, to agricultural protectionism, to increased self-reliance for medical supplies.[36] Much of this has been driven by the need to create a strategic environment (economically and militarily) in which the Europeans may better define and protect their interests, in the expectation of more divergence with the United States in the years ahead. The environment is therefore not permissive to an overly assertive US role in Europe; France and Germany in particular seek a working partnership with the United States, and both were quick to welcome news of Biden's election, but neither are in the mood to be pushed around after four years of tension.

It is worth mentioning that the Europeans (the EU, UK and Russia) have not dealt with the pandemic in a coordinated, or very successful manner. The UK's performance has been particularly dire, with France and Italy not far behind. Despite London's successful vaccination drive, the intra-European squabbling over vaccine allotments that subsequently emerged has only reinforced the impression that Europe's response has been weak and uncoordinated. Meanwhile, Russia has experienced far higher death tolls than its official pronouncements suggest, placing estimated casualties in the hundreds of thousands.[37] Most European nations have vacillated between trying to keep their economies in a functional state, and imposing a series of harsh lockdowns and travel bans, all of which have caused economic hardship across the continent. Due to the enormous expenditures that European states have incurred, there will inevitably be aspects of their foreign and security policy that suffer. Foreign aid budgets have been scaled back,[38] and there is likely to be a severe impact on the appetite of smaller European states to maintain defence expenditure at their current levels. This points to Europe being less of a player on the world stage in the years ahead. Yet this should not mean Europeans are ignored, as they too share a desire to see human rights promoted, advance a transition to a greener carbon-free future and are willing to invest in seeing that vision become a reality.

For all team Biden's charm offensive toward the Europeans, there is little to no real vision, or explanation of the role they wish the Europeans to play in global security outside of the European theatre. The pandemic has been a turning point in Europe's calculus regarding China. The Europeans have been just as concerned as the United States about the way in which the Chinese Communist Party has attempted to use the pandemic to advance its narrow interests, and Europe has grown more attuned to the "strategic challenge" China poses in the economic, technology and global governance realms as a result.[39] The United Kingdom is also extremely conscious of the threat, and has been particularly vocal about the need for European partners to do their part in facing down the threat of China in the post-pandemic world.[40] London's rapidly growing hostility to Beijing, triggered in part by the Chinese handling of the pandemic, and driven further by Britain's search for new trade markets and an urgent need to define a global role for itself post-Brexit, has produced the so-called "Indo-Pacific tilt."[41] As a result, the UK has raised defence spending in a manner that has not been seen for three decades, thereby maintaining expeditionary capabilities that it fully intends to use in the Pacific theatre in the coming years.

This provides Washington with options, should it wish to take advantage of them. The United States would do well to see the Europeans as a force multiplier in world affairs, and not simply an arena to be fixed so that more time can be freed up to deal with bigger problems in Asia. The

European and Asian security theatres need not be bifurcated, and if Washington is able to identify what it wants from Europe, it is likely to find more willing partners who are able to assist with the realization of Washington's security and policy goals than US policy makers may previously have thought.

The Iranian Question, a Chance to Reinforce Arms Control?

The Europeans will also be crucial to solving the key arms control question facing the United States in the coming years, that of the Islamic Republic of Iran, and its nuclear enrichment program. The Trump administration's unilateral withdrawal from the Joint Comprehensive Plan of Action (JCPoA) or nuclear deal with Iran in May 2018, and re-imposition of crippling sanctions on its oil exports was a source of deep frustration for the E3 powers, France, Germany and the UK. None of whom supported the Trump administration's position, and who all believed the deal was the right approach to preventing Iran from obtaining enough enriched Uranium to build a nuclear weapon.[42] As tensions between the United States and Iran increased, the Europeans attempted to keep the deal alive, while maintaining a modicum of deterrence vis-à-vis Tehran, who had responded to US pressure by acting in a highly destabilizing manner, mining ships, seizing oil tankers, attacking civil infrastructure across the Gulf.[43] The result has been a highly combustible mix, which has threatened at times to spill over into outright conflict.[44] Iran, for its part, slowly but surely walked back on a number of commitments it made in the JCPoA regarding its stockpiles of both low and high enriched uranium.[45] The result is that the Biden administration—which is composed of many Obama Administration officials who engaged with Iran in 2015—must now reassess the nuclear deal, albeit from a position where trust on both sides is low.

Tensions between the US, Europe and Iran over its nuclear program predated the outbreak of the Coronavirus by some fifteen years and have continued to simmer in the background in relative isolation from it. Tehran has struggled to cope with the COVID outbreak inside its borders, suffering tens of thousands of deaths (although the actual figure is suspected to be even higher). This may have provided some extra impetus to Tehran's desire to lift the punitive sanctions placed upon it, but in truth the Iranian economy was struggling long before COVID ever arrived.[46] The virus only made things worse.[47] This may provide Biden's negotiators with the extra leverage they need to persuade Iran to come back into compliance with the terms of the deal, although this is by no means guaranteed. The United States for its part has been undeterred from pushing forward on signalling to the Iranians that it wishes to talk, quite separate from the severe domestic effects of the pandemic within its own borders. For Biden's team, re-engaging successfully with Iran looks to be the first step toward re-establishing a baseline of arms control norms, which will eventually extend to Iranian missile development.

The logic to this approach is relatively sound. The Middle East remains important to the United States from a security perspective but is not central to US interests in the way it was at the turn of the century. Driven by the US' increasing energy independence, which now requires little to no oil from the Middle East region, the rationale for engaging with the Middle East is greatly diminished. In addition, as a consequence of the largely failed intervention in Iraq in 2003, the US public has tired of endless conflict. In recent times there has been no shortage of commentaries; American commentators bemoaning the Middle East's lack of stability, and urging the United States to draw back from the region.[48] Military-focused scholarship has similarly viewed "aspirational changes, such as catalyzing democracy and halting intrastate conflict" as falling "outside the scope of change that the United States can readily bring about in a region that is beset by authoritarian legacies and seemingly chronic conflict."[49] In the words of Jake Sullivan's former Whitehouse colleague Rhodes, "The 9/11 era is over"[50] and Washington has no desire to occupy or invade countries as it once did. At the very most, light footprint interventions involving small numbers of troops to deal with highly specific security threats such as Operation Inherent Resolve, Operation Freedom's Sentinel and Operation Enduring Freedom-Philippines are the new norm.[51]

With this in mind, US engagement with Iran over its nuclear program would potentially remove the last major strategic threat to the United States that emanates from the region. If the mistakes of the past can be avoided, whereby US regional allies such as Saudi Arabia and UAE were not consulted and their concerns about Iran largely ignored, then there is a much better chance of getting a second iteration of the JCPoA to hold. This would free up more of time for Washington to focus on regional prosperity questions, and also to dedicate time to security challenges elsewhere in Asia. This is especially important given that the Coronavirus has not just affected Iran's economy, but all oil producing states in the region. Washington will need to assist with helping nations (such as Iraq, Saudi Arabia, Kuwait, Oman and the UAE), whose economies rely on oil for the lion's share of their government spending to diversify in the coming years before the arrival peak oil permanently damages their economies, raising the prospect of instability in an already volatile part of the world, and potentially inviting in China as a potential benefactor. An outcome that the United States would not view as being in its interests.

Conclusion

This chapter has sought to outline the major challenges for the United States as it prepares to tackle a world greatly affected by the global pandemic, and still in a state of deep uncertainty. As nations slowly emerge from their respective lockdowns, and the COVID vaccine becomes more widely distributed, it will be possible for the United States to survey the landscape better and understand how and in what ways it needs to assert itself on the global stage in order to protect its interests. The problems that have resulted from the COVID-19 pandemic have merely underscored the need for a globally active and engaged US. The challenges of 2019 did not simply fade away because the world became ill. If anything, problematic trends for the US, such as the rise of China, the misbehaviour of Russia, the sense of frustration among historical allies, and the problems of Iran's nuclear proliferation only increased in severity and scale. The United States has faced difficult social and political challenges as a result of badly handling the pandemic within its borders, but the need to address challenges in its foreign and security policy has not diminished. If the United States wishes to reassert its interests and reinforce the Universal Security System that it spent seventy years trying to build, then, as the Biden Administration rightly concludes, it must go back out into the world, fix fractured relationships with its allies, reassure doubting partners and reassert international rules and norms. Multilateralism need not be a constraint on American power. On the contrary in many cases, it advances US interests; events such as the US-led launch to replenish the Gavi/COVAX advanced market commitment in April 2021 are a perfect example of where US leadership on the global stage benefits the United States, and its allies by mobilizing resources to return the world to some sort of normality.

Four years of President Trump have left a bitter taste in the mouth for some of America's traditional allies. Yet, for all the ups and downs of the past administration, the United States will find a world that is largely welcoming of its influence during a time of great turmoil. After all, there remains something utterly captivating about America that holds the world's attention. American politics, ideas, fashions and personalities flow beyond borders, impacting the world in a manner that makes America's problems almost seem like our own. Most of us across the world can identify with America in some way, everyone has seen the movies, and everyone has a view on what America "should" look like. Whether America likes it or not, it remains the shining city on a hill, the place people around the world aspire to, no matter how much they despise its politics, its materialism and its quasi-imperialist arrogance. The attack on the Capitol by Trump loyalists was not just an assault on US democracy, but on all democracies, serving as a warning to all those who value liberal freedoms of the dangers of political division. It is in this light that the United States steps back into the world, a flawed and scarred polity of diminished stature, but still with the requisite power and stature to rebuild a global order that it had so nearly left to ruin.

Notes

1. Edward Luce, "Inside Trump's Coronavirus Meltdown," *The Financial Times*, May 14, 2020, https://www.ft.com/content/97dc7de6-940b-11ea-abcd-371e24b679ed.
2. Stephen Walt, "The End of the American Era," *The National Interest*, October 25, 2011, https://nationalinterest.org/article/the-end-the-american-era-6037.
3. Richard Haass, "The Pandemic Will Accelerate History Rather Than Reshape It," *Foreign Affairs*, April 7, 2020, https://www.foreignaffairs.com/articles/united-states/2020-04-07/pandemic-will-accelerate-history-rather-reshape-it.
4. William J. Burns and Linda Thomas-Greenfield, "The Transformation of Diplomacy, How to Save the State Department," *Foreign Affairs*, November/December 2020, https://www.foreignaffairs.com/articles/united-states/2020-09-23/diplomacy-transformation.

5. Malcolm Chalmers, "Which Rules? Why There is No Single 'Rules-Based International System,'" *RUSI Occasional Papers* (April 2019): 7–8.
6. Recent examples include renewed conflicts and territorial change Nagorno-Karabakh; Turkish de-facto occupation of northern Syria, and frequent military interventions into the Kurdistan Region of Iraq outside of the agreed "hot pursuit" parameters; renewed conflict and territorial change in Western Sahara between Morocco and the Polisario Front; and Chinese encroachment on Indian controlled territory in Aksai Chin.
7. North Korea has detonated six nuclear devices to date, the first being in October 2006, and the latest in September 2017.
8. Jeffery Goldberg, "The Obama Doctrine," *The Atlantic*, March 10, 2016, https://www.theatlantic.com/magazine/archive/2016/04/the-obama-doctrine/471525/.
9. Edith Lederer, "Russia and West Clash Over Syria Chemical Weapons Sanctions," *Associated Press*, January 6, 2021, https://news.yahoo.com/russia-west-clash-over-syria-044901792.html.
10. Andrea Kendall-Taylor, and David Shullman, "Navigating the Deepening Russia–China Partnership," *Centre for New American Security*, January 14, 2020, https://www.cnas.org/publications/reports/navigating-the-deepening-russia-china-partnership.
11. Thomas Wright, "The US Must Now Repair Democracy at Home and Abroad," *The Brookings Institute*, January 11, 2021, https://www.brookings.edu/blog/order-from-chaos/2021/01/11/the-us-must-now-repair-democracy-at-home-and-abroad/.
12. Jake Sullivan (@jakejsullivan), "Saudi Arabia's Sentencing..," Twitter, December 28, 2020, https://twitter.com/jakejsullivan/status/1343610818814992386?s=20.
13. Josie Ensor, "Trump told Bob Woodward: 'I saved Mohammed bin Salman's a–' After Jamal Khashoggi Murder," *The Telegraph*, September 10, 2020, https://www.telegraph.co.uk/news/2020/09/10/trump-told-bob-woodward-saved-mohammed-bin-salmans-ass-jamal/.
14. Stephen Walt, "The Pandemic Is How to Ruin a Superpower," *Foreign Policy Magazine*, July 23, 2020, https://foreignpolicy.com/2020/07/23/how-to-ruin-a-superpower/.
15. Richard Haass, "The Pandemic Will Accelerate History Rather Than Reshape It," *Foreign Affairs*, April 7, 2020. https://www.

foreignaffairs.com/articles/united-states/2020-04-07/pandemic-will-accelerate-history-rather-reshape-it.

16. Sharri Markson, "Global Dossier into China's COVID-19 Deception Highlights a Deliberate Cover Up," *The Daily Telegraph*, May 4, 2020, https://www.dailytelegraph.com.au/coronavirus/bombshell-dossier-lays-out-case-against-chinese-bat-virus-program/news-story/55add857058731c9c71c0e96ad17da60.
17. Laura Silver, Kat Devling and Christine Huang, "Unfavorable Views of China Reach Historic Highs in Many Countries," *Pew Research Centre*, October 6, 2020, https://www.pewresearch.org/global/2020/10/06/unfavorable-views-of-china-reach-historic-highs-in-many-countries/?fbclid=IwAR12bzWCMH9l_ZBIBzdfLAHWwRIstSSolDVM9EqpfSsT11L7PvcLubM-5Xo.
18. Michael Schumann, "Think It's Too Hard to Decouple From China? Think Again," *Bloomberg*, July 15, 2020, https://www.bloomberg.com/opinion/articles/2020-07-15/u-s-companies-can-and-will-decouple-from-china.
19. Sebastian Whale, "The End of a Golden Era? The Growing Calls for Decoupling from China," *Politics Home*, May 11, 2020, https://www.politicshome.com/thehouse/article/end-of-the-golden-era-the-growing-calls-for-a-decoupling-from-china.
20. Andrea Shalal, "Biden Adviser Says Unrealistic to 'Fully Decouple' from China," *Reuters*, September 22, 2020, https://www.reuters.com/article/uk-usa-trade-china-biden-idUKKCN26D1SC?edition-redirect=uk.
21. Tom McTague, "The Decline of the American World," *The Atlantic*, June 24, 2020, https://www.theatlantic.com/international/archive/2020/06/america-image-power-trump/613228/.
22. Dr Kenneth Pollack, American Enterprise Institute, September 2020.
23. Dr Aaron Stein, Foreign Policy Research Institute, September 2020.
24. Hilton Yip, et al., "East Asia Takes a Cautious Coronavirus Victory Lap," *Foreign Policy Magazine*, December 29, 2020, https://foreignpolicy.com/2020/12/29/east-asia-coronavirus-cautious-victory-lap/.
25. Kazuhito Yamashita, "Biden Should Look to Obama's Asia–Pacific trade strategies," *The Japan Times*, December 18, 2020, https://www.japantimes.co.jp/opinion/2020/12/18/commen

tary/world-commentary/biden-look-obamas-asia-pacific-trade-strategies/.

26. Derek Grossman, "Biden Will Inherit Healthy Indo-Pacific Alliances," *RAND*, January 11, 2021, https://www.rand.org/blog/2021/01/biden-will-inherit-healthy-indo-pacific-alliances.html.
27. Derek Grossman, "Biden Will Inherit Healthy Indo-Pacific Alliances," *RAND*, January 11, 2021, https://www.rand.org/blog/2021/01/biden-will-inherit-healthy-indo-pacific-alliances.html.
28. "WATCH: Trump BLASTS Leaders @ NATO, Tells Them They Need to Pay Their Share (FULL SPEECH) – FNN," *YouTube*, May 25, 2017, https://www.youtube.com/watch?v=W_KrwW1Knms.
29. Julian E. Barnes and Helene Cooper, "Trump Discussed Pulling U.S. From NATO, Aides Say Amid New Concerns Over Russia," *The New York Times*, January 14, 2019, https://www.nytimes.com/2019/01/14/us/politics/nato-president-trump.html.
30. Josh Hawley (@HawleyMO), "This is Dereliction of Duty by Germany. Serious Miscalculation. We Need & Expect Our NATO Allies to do MORE, Not Less," *Twitter*, March 19, 2019, https://twitter.com/HawleyMO/status/1108079176295333888?s=20.
31. Kim Darroch, *Collateral Damage: Britain, America and Europe in the Age of Trump* (Glasgow, William Collins, 2020), 212.
32. Phil Stewart and Idrees Ali, "U.S. to Withdraw About 12,000 Troops from Germany but Nearly Half to Stay in Europe," *Reuters*, July 29, 2020, https://www.reuters.com/article/us-usa-trump-germany-military-idUSKCN24U20L.
33. Walter Russell Mead, "Dialogues on American Foreign Policy and World Affairs: A Conversation with Former Deputy Secretary of State Antony Blinken," *The Hudson Institute*, July 9, 2020, https://www.hudson.org/research/16210-transcript-dialogues-on-american-foreign-policy-and-world-affairs-a-conversation-with-former-deputy-secretary-of-state-antony-blinken.
34. Hillary Clinton, "Statement From Jake Sullivan On Trump's NATO Comments Online by Gerhard Peters and John T. Woolley," *The American Presidency Project*, July 22, 2016, https://www.presidency.ucsb.edu/documents/statement-from-jake-sullivan-trumps-nato-comments.

35. Michael Clarke, "The Foreign Policy Landscape in the Post-Brexit Era," in *What's next for Britain in the Middle East?*, ed. Michael Stephens and Christopher Phillips (Bloomsbury: 2021), 38.
36. Paola Tamma, "Europe Wants 'Strategic Autonomy'—It Just Has to Decide What That Means," *Politico*, October 15, 2020, https://www.politico.eu/article/europe-trade-wants-strategic-autonomy-decide-what-means/.
37. "Russian COVID Deaths Three Times the Official Toll," *BBC*, December 29, 2020, https://www.bbc.co.uk/news/world-europe-55474028.
38. "Coronavirus: UK Foreign Aid Spending Cut by £2.9bn amid economic downturn," *BBC*, July 23, 2020, https://www.bbc.co.uk/news/uk-politics-53508933.
39. Carisa Nietsche, "Broadening the Transatlantic Partnership to Address the China Challenge," *Instituto Affari Internazionali* 20|97 (December 2020), https://www.iai.it/en/pubblicazioni/broadening-transatlantic-partnership-address-china-challenge.
40. Tom Tugendhat, "China's Rulers Aren't Those We Partnered with a Decade Ago': Foreign Affairs Committee Chairman TOM TUGENDHAT Says It's Time to Confront the Reality We've Ignored for Too Long," *The Daily Mail*, January 9, 2021, https://www.dailymail.co.uk/debate/article-9129891/Chinas-rulers-arent-partnered-decade-ago-says-TOM-TUGENDHAT.html.
41. "A Very British Tilt, Towards a New UK Strategy in the Indo-Pacific Region," *Policy Exchange*, November 22, 2020, https://policyexchange.org.uk/publication/a-very-british-tilt/.
42. Dominic Green, "Leaked Letter: Boris Johnson Rejects Trump on Iran Sanctions," *The Spectator*, August 27, 2020, https://spectator.us/topic/leaked-letter-boris-johnson-rejects-trump-iran-sanctions/.; The UK is siding with France and Germany at the UN.
43. Michael Stephens, "Whether It Likes It or Not Europe Is Being Pushed and Pulled into America's Iran Policy," *War on the Rocks*, August 1, 2019, https://warontherocks.com/2019/08/whether-it-likes-it-or-not-europe-is-being-pushed-and-pulled-into-americas-iran-policy/.
44. Michael Stephens, "Iran's First Response to Soleimani's Death, and Tehran's Future Moves," *RUSI Commentary*, January 8, 2020, https://www.rusi.org/commentary/iran%E2%80%99s-

first-response-soleimani%E2%80%99s-death-and-tehran%E2%80%99s-future-moves.
45. "Iran Resumes Enriching Uranium to 20% Purity at Fordo Facility," *BBC*, January 4, 2020, https://www.bbc.co.uk/news/world-middle-east-55530366.
46. Krishnadev Calamur, "Iran's Economy Was Struggling, Even Without US sanctions," *The Atlantic,* August 6, 2018, https://www.theatlantic.com/international/archive/2018/08/iran-economy/566708/.
47. Amin Mohseni-Cheraghlou, "Iran and the Economic Fallout of COVID-19," *The Middle East Institute*, April 14, 2020, https://www.mei.edu/publications/iran-and-economic-fallout-COVID-19.
48. Daniel R. DePetris, "Americans Are Tired of Middle East Mayhem," *The National Interest*, January 17, 2019, https://news.yahoo.com/americans-tired-middle-east-mayhem-135400967.html.; Mara Karlin and Tamara Cofman Wittes, "Ending America's Middle East Purgatory: The Case for Doing less," *Foreign Affairs*, January/February, 2019, https://www.foreignaffairs.com/articles/middle-east/2018-12-11/americas-middle-east-purgatory.
49. Karl P. Mueller, et al., "U.S. Strategic Interests in the Middle East and Implications for the Army," *RAND Perspective* (2017), 8.
50. Ben Rhodes, "The 9/11 Era Is Over," *The Atlantic*, April 6, 2020, https://www.theatlantic.com/ideas/archive/2020/04/its-not-september-12-anymore/609502/.
51. Karl P. Mueller, et al., "U.S. Strategic Interests in the Middle East and Implications for the Army," *RAND Perspective* (2017), 9.

Bibliography

"A Very British Tilt, Towards a New UK Strategy in the Indo-Pacific Region." *Policy Exchange*, November 22, 2020. https://policyexchange.org.uk/publication/a-very-british-tilt/.

"Coronavirus: UK Foreign Aid Spending Cut by £2.9bn Amid Economic Downturn." *BBC*, July 23, 2020. https://www.bbc.co.uk/news/uk-politics-53508933.

"Iran Resumes Enriching Uranium to 20% Purity at Fordo Facility." *BBC*, January 4, 2020. https://www.bbc.co.uk/news/world-middle-east-55530366.

"Russian COVID Deaths Three Times the Official Toll." *BBC*, December 29, 2020. https://www.bbc.co.uk/news/world-europe-55474028.

"WATCH: Trump BLASTS Leaders @ NATO, Tells Them They Need to Pay Their Share (FULL SPEECH) – FNN." *YouTube*, May 25, 2017. https://www.youtube.com/watch?v=W_KrwW1Knms.

Barnes, Julian E., and Helene Cooper. "Trump Discussed Pulling U.S. From NATO, Aides Say Amid New Concerns Over Russia." *The New York Times*, January 14, 2019. https://www.nytimes.com/2019/01/14/us/politics/nato-president-trump.html.

Burns, William J., and Linda Thomas-Greenfield. "The Transformation of Diplomacy, How to Save the State Department." *Foreign Affairs*, November/December 2020. https://www.foreignaffairs.com/articles/united-states/2020-09-23/diplomacy-transformation.

Calamur, Krishnadev. "Iran's Economy Was Struggling, Even Without U.S. Sanctions." *The Atlantic*, August 6, 2018. https://www.theatlantic.com/international/archive/2018/08/iran-economy/566708/.

Chalmers, Malcolm. "Which Rules? Why There Is No Single 'Rules-Based International System'." *RUSI Occasional Papers*, April, 2019.

Clarke, Michael. "The Foreign Policy Landscape in the Post-Brexit Era." In *What's Next for Britain in the Middle East?* edited by Michael Stephens and Christopher Phillips, 38. Bloomsbury, 2021.

Clinton, Hillary. "Statement from Jake Sullivan on Trump's NATO Comments Online by Gerhard Peters and John T. Woolley." *The American Presidency Project*, July 22, 2016, https://www.presidency.ucsb.edu/documents/statement-from-jake-sullivan-trumps-nato-comments.

Darroch, Kim. *Collateral Damage: Britain, America and Europe in the Age of Trump*. Glasgow: William Collins, 2020.

DePetris, Daniel R. "Americans Are Tired of Middle East Mayhem." *The National Interest*, January 17, 2019. https://news.yahoo.com/americans-tired-middle-east-mayhem-135400967.html.

Ensor, Josie. "Trump told Bob Woodward: 'I saved Mohammed bin Salman's a—' after Jamal Khashoggi murder." *The Telegraph*, September 10, 2020. https://www.telegraph.co.uk/news/2020/09/10/trump-told-bob-woodward-saved-mohammed-bin-salmans-ass-jamal/.

Goldberg, Jeffery. "The Obama Doctrine." *The Atlantic*, March 10, 2016. https://www.theatlantic.com/magazine/archive/2016/04/the-obama-doctrine/471525/.

Green, Dominic. "Leaked Letter: Boris Johnson Rejects Trump on Iran Sanctions." *The Spectator*, August 27, 2020. https://spectator.us/topic/leaked-letter-boris-johnson-rejects-trump-iran-sanctions/.

Grossman, Derek. "Biden Will Inherit Healthy Indo-Pacific Alliances." *RAND*, January 11, 2021. https://www.rand.org/blog/2021/01/biden-will-inherit-healthy-indo-pacific-alliances.html.

Haass, Richard. "The Pandemic Will Accelerate History Rather Than Reshape It." *Foreign Affairs*, April 7, 2020. https://www.foreignaffairs.com/articles/united-states/2020-04-07/pandemic-will-accelerate-history-rather-reshape-it.

Hawley, Josh. "This Is Dereliction of Duty by Germany. Serious Miscalculation. We Need & Expect Our NATO Allies to do MORE, Not Less." *Twitter*, March 19, 2019. https://twitter.com/HawleyMO/status/1108079176295333888?s=20.

Karlin, Mara, and Tamara Cofman Wittes. "Ending America's Middle East Purgatory: The Case for doing less." *Foreign Affairs*, January/February, 2019. https://www.foreignaffairs.com/articles/middle-east/2018-12-11/americas-middle-east-purgatory.

Kendall-Taylor, Andrea, and David Shullman. "Navigating the Deepening Russia-China Partnership." *Centre for New American Security*, January 14, 2020. https://www.cnas.org/publications/reports/navigating-the-deepening-russia-china-partnership.

Lederer, Edith. "Russia and West Clash Over Syria Chemical Weapons Sanctions." *Associated Press*, January 6, 2021. https://news.yahoo.com/russia-west-clash-over-syria-044901792.html.

Luce, Edward. "Inside Trump's Coronavirus Meltdown." *The Financial Times*, May 14, 2020. https://www.ft.com/content/97dc7de6-940b-11ea-abcd-371e24b679ed.

Markson, Sharri. "Global Dossier into China's COVID-19 Deception Highlights a Deliberate Cover Up." *The Daily Telegraph*, May 4, 2020. https://www.dailytelegraph.com.au/coronavirus/bombshell-dossier-lays-out-case-against-chinese-bat-virus-program/news-story/55add857058731c9c71c0e96ad17da60.

McTague, Tom. "The Decline of the American World." *The Atlantic*, June 24, 2020. https://www.theatlantic.com/international/archive/2020/06/america-image-power-trump/613228/.

Mohseni-Cheraghlou, Amin. "Iran and the Economic Fallout of COVID-19." *The Middle East Institute*, April 14, 2020. https://www.mei.edu/publications/iran-and-economic-fallout-COVID-19.

Mueller, Karl P., Becca Wasser, Jeffrey Martini, and Stephen Watts. "U.S. Strategic Interests in the Middle East and Implications for the Army." *RAND Perspective*, 2017. https://www.rand.org/pubs/perspectives/PE265.html

Nietsche, Carisa. "Broadening the Transatlantic Partnership to Address the China Challenge." *Instituto Affari Internazionali*, December, 2020. https://www.

iai.it/en/pubblicazioni/broadening-transatlantic-partnership-address-china-challenge.

Pollack, Dr Kenneth. American Enterprise Institute. Interview September 2020.

Rhodes, Ben. "The 9/11 Era Is Over." *The Atlantic*, April 6, 2020. https://www.theatlantic.com/ideas/archive/2020/04/its-not-september-12-anymore/609502/.

Russell Mead, Walter. "Dialogues on American Foreign Policy and World Affairs: A Conversation with Former Deputy Secretary of State Antony Blinken." *The Hudson Institute*, July 9, 2020. https://www.hudson.org/research/16210-transcript-dialogues-on-american-foreign-policy-and-world-affairs-a-conversation-with-former-deputy-secretary-of-state-antony-blinken.

Schumann, Michael. "Think It's Too Hard to Decouple From China? Think Again." *Bloomberg*, July 15, 2020. https://www.bloomberg.com/opinion/articles/2020-07-15/u-s-companies-can-and-will-decouple-from-china.

Shalal, Andrea. "Biden Adviser Says Unrealistic to 'Fully Decouple' from China." *Reuters*, September 22, 2020. https://www.reuters.com/article/uk-usa-trade-china-biden-idUKKCN26D1SC?edition-redirect=uk.

Silver, Laura, Kat Devling, and Christine Huang. "Unfavorable Views of China Reach Historic Highs in Many Countries." *Pew Research Centre*, October 6, 2020. https://www.pewresearch.org/global/2020/10/06/unfavorable-views-of-china-reach-historic-highs-in-many-countries/?fbclid=IwAR12bzWCMH9l_ZBIBzdfLAHWwRIstSSolDVM9EqpfSsT11L7PvcLubM-5Xo.

Stein, Dr Aaron. Foreign Policy Research Institute. Interview September 2020.

Stephens, Michael. "Iran's First Response to Soleimani's Death, and Tehran's Future Moves." *RUSI Commentary*, January 8, 2020. https://www.rusi.org/commentary/iran%E2%80%99s-first-response-soleimani%E2%80%99s-death-and-tehran%E2%80%99s-future-moves.

Stephens, Michael. "Whether It Likes It or Not Europe Is Being Pushed and Pulled into America's Iran Policy." *War on the Rocks*, August 1, 2019. https://warontherocks.com/2019/08/whether-it-likes-it-or-not-europe-is-being-pushed-and-pulled-into-americas-iran-policy/.

Stewart, Phil, and Idrees Ali. "U.S. to Withdraw About 12,000 Troops from Germany But Nearly Half to Stay in Europe." *Reuters*, July 29, 2020. https://www.reuters.com/article/us-usa-trump-germany-military-idUSKCN24U20L.

Sullivan, Jake. "Saudi Arabia's Sentencing…" Twitter, December 28, 2020. https://twitter.com/jakejsullivan/status/1343610818814992386?s=20.

Tamma, Paola. "Europe Wants 'Strategic Autonomy' — It Just Has to Decide What That Means." *Politico*, October 15, 2020. https://www.politico.eu/article/europe-trade-wants-strategic-autonomy-decide-what-means/.

Tugendhat, Tom. "China's Rulers Aren't Those We Partnered with a Decade Ago': Foreign Affairs Committee Chairman TOM TUGENDHAT Says It's

Time to Confront the Reality We've Ignored for Too Long." *The Daily Mail*, January 9, 2021. https://www.dailymail.co.uk/debate/article-9129891/Chinas-rulers-arent-partnered-decade-ago-says-TOM-TUGENDHAT.html.

Walt, Stephen. "The End of the American Era." *The National Interest*, October 25, 2011. https://nationalinterest.org/article/the-end-the-american-era-6037.

Walt, Stephen. "The Pandemic Is How to Ruin a Superpower." *Foreign Policy Magazine*, July 23, 2020. https://foreignpolicy.com/2020/07/23/how-to-ruin-a-superpower/.

Whale, Sebastian. "The End of a Golden Era? The Growing Calls for Decoupling from China." *Politics Home*, May 11, 2020. https://www.politicshome.com/thehouse/article/end-of-the-golden-era-the-growing-calls-for-a-decoupling-from-china.

Wright, Thomas. "The US Must Now Repair Democracy at Home and Abroad." *The Brookings Institute*, January 11, 2021. https://www.brookings.edu/blog/order-from-chaos/2021/01/11/the-us-must-now-repair-democracy-at-home-and-abroad/.

Yamashita, Kazuhito. "Biden Should Look to Obama's Asia-Pacific Trade Strategies." *The Japan Times*, December 18, 2020. https://www.japantimes.co.jp/opinion/2020/12/18/commentary/world-commentary/biden-look-obamas-asia-pacific-trade-strategies/.

Yip, Hilton, William Sposato, Kirsten Han, S. Nathan Park and David Volodzko. "East Asia Takes a Cautious Coronavirus Victory Lap." *Foreign Policy Magazine*, December 29, 2020. https://foreignpolicy.com/2020/12/29/east-asia-corona.

CHAPTER 4

Europe: A Geographical Expression or Unity of Purpose?

Arthur de Liedekerke and Matthew Robinson

Introduction

In a speech to the Reichstag on 14 May 1872, the first Chancellor of the German Empire, Otto von Bismarck remarked, "Whoever speaks of Europe is wrong, it is a geographical expression."[1]

While Europe has evolved by leaps and bounds since, from the creation of the European Coal and Steel Community following World War II, to the formation of the present-day European Union, a unity of purpose as it relates to a common European security and defense identity is still a matter of prodigious contention. Compounded with Brexit, the coronavirus pandemic could spark unforeseen security challenges or crystallize pre-existing trends. This chapter fleshes out two opposite but equally plausible, scenarios for Europe's collective security architecture.

A. de Liedekerke (✉)
Rasmussen Global, Brussels, Belgium

M. Robinson
Euro-Gulf Information Centre, Rome, Italy

C. Varin (ed.), *Global Security in Times of Covid-19*, New Security Challenges, https://doi.org/10.1007/978-3-030-82230-9_4

There is a danger that the strategic uncertainty brought about by COVID-19 will torpedo any sort of ambitious European Union–United Kingdom security and defense relationship in the years post-Brexit. Indeed, it is hard to be very optimistic about wide-ranging cooperation on these matters in light of the near-absence of foreign policy, external security and defense matters emerging from the EU–UK Trade and Cooperation Agreement (TCA),[2] a departure from the October 2019 Political Declaration. Unexpectedly however, the virus could provide much-needed momentum to build a lasting and meaningful alliance. With the world likely headed for a recession that will dwarf the economic downturn following the 2008 financial crisis and confronted with a reshuffle in the international power structure, the EU and UK should reaffirm their readiness to act together in tackling future crises and shoring up Europe's security.

Stuck Between a Rock and a Hard Place: Great Power Competition

The pandemic has accelerated two pre-existing geopolitical trends, which will have a lasting impact on Europe's place in the world: Firstly, the US remains in retreat from its position as global leader and, secondly, China continues its assertive global rise. The former implies that European states—including the UK—may not be able to rely blindly on transatlantic cooperation and US leadership and the security umbrella it provided that reinforced the liberal, rules-based international order that have persisted since the end of World War II. The Trump Administration's America First policies, exemplified during the pandemic by the US's withdrawal from the World Health Organization and its antagonism to multilateralism, have severely eroded trust in Washington. And, the so-called "special relationship" that the UK once prided itself on has also taken a hit: London and Washington are at loggerheads on topics ranging from digital service taxes to chlorinated chicken. The Biden administration will seek to reinvigorate ties with Britain and the EU; but it is unlikely to prioritize them over the "pivot" to Asia, which Joe Biden championed as Obama's Vice-President.

On the other hand, the ascendancy of China may signal that a new era of great power competition is unfolding. The current health crisis has been a painful reminder of Europe's (and global) dependency on Chinese production and Beijing has capitalized on this unique situation to launch an unprecedentedly aggressive propaganda (and charm) offensives—including so-called "mask" diplomacy. It has even traded barbs with Washington to rewrite the narrative concerning the origins of the virus. The new security law on Hong Kong, deadly clashes along the disputed China–India border, a surge in flybys over Taiwan and Japan are provocative actions designed to bolster Beijing's position on the world stage and are a clear signal of its ambitions.[3] Increasingly, China is attempting to carve out a role as "a systemic rival promoting alternative models of governance"[4] to the US-led order. The pandemic has created more political, diplomatic and even operational space for contenders, including Russia and Turkey, to assert themselves.

Common Security Concerns in the MENA Region

Western democracies are finding themselves increasingly isolated, with the values and systems they have long championed at risk—one that is compounded by a number of external threats. Despite its insular nature, the "UK and the countries of the EU share the same strategic environment and, by default, the same threats to their peace and security."[5] As stated in the 2018 British National Security Capability Review: "Europe's security is our security."[6] Among the main converging external security interests are: curbing the terrorist threat emanating from the Middle East and North Africa (MENA) region, deterring Muscovite meddling as well as breathing new life into the Iranian nuclear deal. COVID-19 has temporarily overshadowed some of these preoccupying developments yet, there too, the virus will undoubtedly further degrade the security environment.

Indeed in its *Risk 2020* report, Frontex, the European Border and Coast Guard Agency, warns that due to the pandemic, "some regimes may be unable to maintain order and the outbreak of internal and interstate conflict could occur, potentially creating new displaced populations or irregular migration, possibly also moving towards Europe."[7] The European Council on Foreign Relations paints an even grimmer picture, describing the EU's southern neighborhood as "heading for a perfect storm of pandemic, famine and collapsing oil revenues."[8] Millions of refugees stranded in Turkey, Jordan and Libya are packed into camps and particularly vulnerable to an explosion of infections. With limited access to water, sanitation systems and health facilities, refugees and other displaced people are at increased risk due to overcrowding and unhygienic living conditions. These refugees are for the most part hosted in low- to middle-income countries, and COVID-19 has hit these developing economies particularly hard, exacerbating long-standing structural deficiencies. As a result, a 2020 Arab Youth Survey has found that "nearly one third of Arab youth are more likely to emigrate due to the impact of the coronavirus.".[9]

In parallel, Daesh has been taking advantage of the mayhem to step up its attacks in Iraq: with the withdrawal of US-led coalition troops in early 2020 and the local government too absorbed in tackling the coronavirus outbreak, there are well-founded concerns that the terrorist organization could rebound: By August 2020, the Middle East Institute reported 126 attacks by ISIS across Syria—compared to 144 in all of 2019.[10] COVID-19 has also served as material for jihadi propaganda, spinning the virus as a punishment of God for their foes, and urging their Europe-based followers to carry out attacks.[11] Recent events, notably the November 2020 shooting in Vienna at the hands of a Daesh sympathizer, have shown that the group remains a very real threat to the European continent.

Russia

COVID-19 may have changed many things but, from the Ukraine to the Baltic Sea, Russia has not relented in its quest to aggressively further its strategic objectives. NATO fighter jets are regularly scrambled to intercept Russian military aircraft flying close to Allied airspace, with around 350 such incidents happening over the course of 2020.[12] The "latest flash-points in Europe's relationship with Russia—the crisis in Belarus and the attack on Navalny—illustrate the challenge facing Western leaders"[13]; the Kremlin displaying its traditionally dismissive attitude to the international outcry.

Significant Russian disinformation operations revolving around the coronavirus have targeted the UK and EU alike with the aim of sowing division and hampering response efforts. In an April 2020 report by The University of Calgary's School of Public Policy, the author notes "COVID-19 is seen as an ideal way for Russia to deal a powerful blow not only to the EU, but to inflict damage on the ties between Europe and its North American allies."[14] Shortly after, in July 2020, the UK's National Cyber Security Centre (NCSC) said, in a shared assessment with US and Canada intelligence agencies, that drug companies and research groups involved in developing a vaccine for COVID-19 were being targeted by Russian state-sponsored hackers.[15] Just like China, Russia is using the pandemic to take advantage of a "perceived opportunity" to weaken Western societies, while the world's attention is focused elsewhere.[16]

Saving the Iran Nuclear Deal

The change in administration in the US signals a possible return of Washington to the negotiating table with Iran. The governments of France, Germany and the United Kingdom (the "E3"), with the support of the European External Action Service, have worked tirelessly to preserve the Joint Comprehensive Plan of Action (JCPoA) despite the US's withdrawal from the framework under Donald Trump and Iranian non-compliance with the terms of the agreement.

Deep divisions have become entrenched in the past four years, not least with the US drone strike that killed prominent military leader Qassem Suleimani in January 2020. Not only will a Biden presidency likely lead to a thawing of relations between the two countries but COVID-19, which has ravaged Iran with fatality rates among the highest in the world, means Tehran will be looking to resume negotiations to get sanctions relief.[17] The E3 may be able to play a crucial role in revitalizing this process.

The UK and EU will have to work closely to leverage their combined clout—diplomacy, technical cooperation, military operations or peacekeeping missions, humanitarian aid—and deter malicious actors, from terrorist groups to rival states and blocs, from further exploiting the pandemic.

Shrinking Military Might: Putting the Emphasis on Multinational Cooperation

The economic cost of the coronavirus is equally pressing. Countries of the EU were set to face a contraction of 7.8% of their economic activity in 2020, while the OECD predicted that the UK would likely suffer from the deepest recession of any nation in the developed world.[18]

The boost in defense spending, an extra 16.5 billion pounds over the four years, represents a welcome boon to the UK's military credibility, after several rounds of deep cuts in its armed forces initiated in 2010. Since 2015, it has dropped from having the world's fourth defense budget to the eighth.[19] As an analysis by the Director of Military Sciences for the Royal United Services Institute underlines:

> While the British Armed Forces continue to be a much-respected military with friends, the decades-long hollowing out of capabilities and reducing numbers mean they are not the dreaded foe they once were. Rebuilding that reputation with adversaries, not allies, will take some time, and will need to consist of actions rather than words.[20]

France, the other major military power of the continent, is only marginally more advanced and despite a hike in spending over the past three years, it lacks a number of strategic capabilities, including sufficient transport helicopters. And, it is highly reliant on US Reaper drones, which prevents it from being fully autonomous in many of its operations abroad.

More generally, with the recent agreement on the 2021–2027 Multiannual Financial Framework (MFF), the EU budget saw funds allocated to defense drop from €13 billion to €7.014 billion.[21] This figure, representing roughly a 40% drop from the initial ambition, is the result of intense negotiations in Brussels where the response to COVID-19 prevailed over the strengthening of European defense. The ECFR Coalition Explorer, presenting the results of a survey conducted in the 27 EU member states shows that "defense" as a policy area is ranked 14th in terms of priority, well behind "Migration," "Digital" or "Western Balkans."[22] In a positive development for cooperation however, the European Council agreed on 5 November 2020 on the rules to allow third-country entities to participate in capability projects falling within the European Union's Permanent Structured Cooperation (PESCO) agreement. This means the UK could, conditional on the unanimous support from project members, take part in some of these initiatives.

At the same time, around the world, states are re-arming. The latest Stockholm Institute Peace Research Institute (SIPRI) report reveals that global military expenditure has seen its largest annual increase in a decade, reaching $1,917 billion in 2019.[23] According to their research, Europe accounts for around 19% of this (it is worth noting these numbers include Russia) making it the third-largest spending region after the Americas and Asia and Oceania. To avoid a further decline of Europe's military might, the EU and the UK would do well to stick together.

Preserving the Defense Industry

From an industrial point of view, the British and European defense industries are deeply intertwined: British "companies have been acquired by continental groups (helicopters and electronics, for example). In others,

British firms have taken the lead—the prime example is MBDA, a pan-European missile house in which Britain and France predominate."[24] Airbus is another European-wide success story. The Eurofighter Typhoon multirole fighter jet perfectly embodies the interweaving of industries. Approximately 75 companies from across Europe are involved in its production and the plane is in service in five European militaries: the UK, Austria, Germany, Italy and Spain.

When the COVID-19 outbreak hit, aerospace companies that were already nervously following Brexit-related discussions regarding a Free-Trade Agreement (FTA) had to add shrinking home markets and the shutdown of international traffic and transportation to their list of grievances.[25] Indeed, not only does the military share civilian infrastructure to some degree but some of the biggest European defense players are also civil aerospace companies (Airbus, BAE Systems, Thales.) Moreover, for an "industry which hitherto has become increasingly internationalized, the disruption of global value chains is particularly devastating for small and medium-sized and niched companies."[26] Immediate negative effects were felt on the supply-side with deliveries delayed or cancelled.

Despite a number of prominent rival projects—such as the Franco-German Future Combat Aircraft System (FCAS) and the British-led Tempest fighter project—an absence of cooperation post-Brexit, and *a fortiori* post-COVID, would be a "disaster" as the head of Saab, Britain's partner in the Tempest programme, Micael Johansson warned in an interview with *Financial Times*.[27] As in many other sectors, the defense supply chain is an international one. If some of the negative ramifications of Brexit have been avoided (notably additional tariffs), the existence of two separate markets, distinct regulatory and legal spaces will create barriers to trade as well as possible erosion of trust in this sensitive field. Such disincentives to industrial collaboration can only benefit adversaries.

Deal or no Deal: A Rocky But Long-Standing Partnership

A final reason, which one hopes could, in the long run, facilitate an ambitious external security arrangement between the UK and its continental counterparts, is the successful and long-standing cooperation between them in times of crisis. The relationship between London and Brussels may not be easy and Brexit has certainly hardened attitudes on both sides of the Channel, however, cooperation in times of trouble has, generally, superseded parochial views. At the height of the first wave of COVID-19, Britain obtained EU support to help cover the costs of repatriation flights from Japan, the US and Peru, while in May 2020 some 1.5 million medical masks were delivered to 17 Member States and the UK to protect healthcare workers against coronavirus.[28]

These examples do not overshadow many of the difficulties encountered by the EU in coordinating their responses when the crisis hit or some of the clashes between the Commission and the UK over the British share of the COVID-19 fund. However, they serve as a reminder that, when faced with common hardships, the two often do come together. The latest row over access to limited coronavirus vaccine supplies is a case in point: for all the acrimony and threat of trade wars, Brussels and London have been trying to smooth things over and issued a common statement on 24 March 2021 promising to cooperate and continue their discussions to ensure a reciprocally beneficial relationship.

A lot of political goodwill has already been squandered in endless rounds of Brexit talks. Governments on both sides of the Channel would do well to remember that, for all their differences and disagreements, they have a long, shared history of trust and cooperation as well as tangible, mutual interests that endure. The very fact that an accord was concluded on 24 December 2020, a mere seven days before the UK was due to crash out, is evidence that both sides needed an agreement for economic and political reasons.

COVID-19 is dramatically altering the world we live in and offering up one of "multipolar disorder."[29] One thing COVID-19 will not change however, is geography and the fact that London and Brussels are embedded in the same and increasingly tumultuous strategic environment. Defense and external security cooperation is one of the areas in the EU–UK relationship still facing an uncertain future. There is little chance a comprehensive and binding arrangement will see the light of day in the near future. But too much divergence between both parties, an entirely ad-hoc and unstructured relationship would inevitably undermine their collective security.

Mind the Gap—Britain and Europe's Security Interests May Drift Apart

On 29 March 2019, Members of the UK Parliament (MPs) cast their vote on Prime Minister Theresa May's third and final ill-fated "meaningful vote" on the United Kingdom's Withdrawal from the European Union.[30] With its rejection, the Prime Minister's own vision of a "deep and special partnership with the European Union," as she articulated in her autumn 2017 Florence speech,[31] was effectively dead and her premiership ended shortly thereafter. Her successor, Boris Johnson, despite his numerous stints in Brussels both as a child and adult, would prove far less amenable to the continental European culture of compromise in the Brexit negotiations. This set the scene for a drift apart in the relationship, a somewhat more divergent path between the UK and the EU than previously envisaged.

While the political and commentariat class remained primarily focused on the minutiae of the future economic and trading partnership, the specifics of what the future security partnership between the UK and EU will resemble should not be overlooked. Even with the TCA now concluded and being applied since 1 January 2021, future cooperation in this area is still very much uncertain, and perhaps even more so once Europe emerges from the post-pandemic fog that is COVID-19. This uncertainty exists despite the initial positive tone in the "Political Declaration," which set out the framework for the future UK–EU relationship covering a comprehensive list of areas including: Law enforcement and judicial cooperation in criminal matters, foreign policy, security and defense, thematic cooperation and classified and sensitive non-classified information.[32] While the text is ambitious, further scrutiny shows that the *juris lingua* is drafted to allow for maximum flexibility for either side to chart their path if their own strategic interests diverge. Note that: "The Parties will shape and pursue their foreign policies according to their respective strategic and security interests, and their respective legal orders."[33]

The Political Declaration continues by emphasizing,

> [t]he Parties should design flexible and scalable cooperation [...] and flexible consultation between the Parties at different levels [...][34]

An example of how truly scalable the security relationship between both sides will be is being tested with regards to how the new framework on law enforcement and now judicial cooperation will develop Britain's membership in the EU Agency for Law Enforcement Cooperation (Europol), EU Agency for Criminal Justice Cooperation (Eurojust), and the European Arrest Warrant has ended. While the TCA builds new operational capabilities, taking account of the fact that the UK is no longer a member of the aforementioned agencies, it will not have the same facilities as before. Britain does retain access to some critical security databases, namely "Passenger Name Records" (PNR) and the DNA information exchange (Prüm), however, its access to the EU's criminal records exchange (ECRIS) and instant operational alerts on the movement of people and objects on mandated crime areas, including terrorism through the Schengen Information System II (SIS II) has ceased. Furthermore, the UK can no longer submit a legally binding request to have investigative measures to gather or use evidence in criminal matters carried out in another EU country by a specific deadline, known as a "European Investigation Order." The British must now send its European neighbors a "Letter Rogatory," an internationally recognized diplomatic request for assistance, which historically tends to be slow, and are at times ignored entirely.

All this marks a dramatic shift, especially considering that the UK, until recently, played a leading role in Europe's security architecture, holding key positions such as the Director of Europol under Rob Wainwright (2009–2018) and European Commissioner for the Security Union under Sir Julian King (2016–2019). In an interview with Dick Roche, the former Minister of State for European Affairs in the Irish Government who was involved in the negotiations that led to the Treaty of Lisbon and who headed both of the Irish referendum campaigns on its ratification, he made the following assessment:

> The low priority the British government paid to the question of post-Brexit security relations with Europe is surprising and unsurprising in equal measure. Surprising, if one considers security issues was given little prominence during the withdrawal negotiations and attracted little space in the Withdrawal Agreement and TCA, […] and unsurprising considering the dominance of trade during the Brexit negotiations and the scant attention to the UK's service sector […] if services that account for 70% of GDP, got only passing attention, Europol, Eurojust and access to SIS were always destined to be down the political priority list.[35]

He continues,

> […] as with so much else, the challenges posed by *the coronavirus* pandemic has drawn focus away from the reality that Brexit has brought real challenges. It is only a matter of time before those begin to show, and one of the areas where tensions will arise is when gaps in security arrangements come to be filled.[36]

Rule Britannia—The Impact of Boris Johnson

The revisions to the final Political Declaration as renegotiated and agreed between Prime Minister Boris Johnson, President of the European Council Donald Tusk and President of the European Council Jean-Claude Juncker (17 October 2019) mark an evolution in thinking when compared to the previous text negotiated by Prime Minister May on 25 November 2018.[37] In the "Foreign policy, security and defense" chapter additional text was inserted to stress that UK involvement in Common Security and Defense Policy (CSDP) operations

> [...] would be without prejudice to the decision-making autonomy of the Union or the sovereignty of the United Kingdom, and the United Kingdom will maintain the right to determine how it would respond to any invitation or option to participate in operations or missions.[38]

This new tougher language reflects a pre-existing "Rule Britannia" sentiment in the British Conservative Party that Brussels needs London far more than the other way around with regards to security. This was aptly articulated by a backbench Conservative MP in a May 2019 parliamentary debate on leaving the EU as it relates to security:

> [...] the Bundesnachrichtendienst has already made it absolutely clear that the United Kingdom is one of the biggest intelligence services in the world, is a member of Five Eyes, and that Europe is dependent on the United Kingdom for intelligence.[39]

This Eurosceptic sentiment was crystallized with Boris Johnson's sweeping majority in the December 2019 General Election.[40] With the Prime Minister's commanding majority, he brought 107 newly elected Conservative MPs, all of which are pro-Brexit and champions of the UK Government's "Global Britain" foreign policy strategy, with the British "[...] leading by example as a force for good in the world."[41]

The potential for a future drift as a result of this strategy can clearly be seen. UK Foreign Secretary, Dominic Raab, repeatedly stressed that Britain would prioritize the use of international rather than regional fora, namely the United Nations (UN) and the North Atlantic Treaty Organization (NATO) to "reinforce Britain's role in the world as a good global citizen."[42] The tone of his past remarks on this subject has very much underlined the foreign policy opportunities for the UK on leaving the

EU, perhaps even hinting to the effect that the EU has held Britain back to lead as it should, with the Foreign Secretary stating that,

> [w]hen we leave the EU, we will also reinforce our sanctions legislation to hold those who commit serious abuses of human rights to account [...] [w]hen we leave the EU, there will be enormous opportunities across the world.[43]

From the view of the UK government, Brexit has afforded global opportunities that were perhaps frustrated during its 47 years of EU membership.

The impact of Johnson's premiership has been further felt with his decision to promote Brexit talks *sherpa*, Lord Frost to Minister of State (and full member of the Cabinet)[44] and the UK Chairman of the EU–UK Partnership Council, is highly significant. With a devoted Brexiteer and Eurosceptic like Frost rooted both at the heart of the UK Government and as the British representative responsible for issues relating to the implementation, application and interpretation of the TCA, there is little to suggest the UK will deviate from its globalist mantra as it seeks more autonomy in security and defense.

The Future of the JCPoA

The JCPoA is another potential fault-line for drift between the EU and the UK. Federica Mogherini lauded the Iran nuclear deal as one of the EU's hard fought and crowning foreign policy achievements during her tenure as High Representative of the EU for Foreign Affairs and Security Policy and in the wake of the United States (US) withdrawal from the agreement under President Donald Trump in May 2018.[45] She was quick to stress the EU's "[...] commitment to ensuring that [the JCPoA] can continue to be delivered."[46] Her successor as High Representative, Josep Borrell has since reaffirmed the EU's commitment by noting that:

> The JCPoA is an historic achievement for global nuclear non-proliferation contributing to regional and global security. I remain determined to continue working with the participants of the JCPoA and the international community to preserve it.[47]

The EU's continued enthusiastic endorsement of the JCPoA is in contrast to a more measured tone struck by the UK Government, with the British Foreign Office responding to the aforementioned Borrell statement with a firm qualification of its support for the JCPoA, "[t]he UK remains committed [...], but it is being put at risk by systematic Iranian non-compliance."[48] This follows previous critical remarks from the British Foreign Secretary in January 2020 in which he warned, "[...] the regime in Tehran is at a crossroads. It can slip further and further into political and economic isolation."[49]

While COVID-19 has afforded Boris Johnson some breathing room to take stock of the British position on the Iranian nuclear deal, it is clear the UK Government is rapidly approaching a critical juncture. It can either lean into its long-standing "Special Relationship" with the US, and distance, perhaps even withdraw itself from the JCPoA depending on the course of action from the new Biden administration, or alternatively halt this apparent diplomatic drift in its tracks and double-down on its past European solidarity with Brussels on this issue. The rhetoric over the past 12 months from Downing Street and Whitehall points to the fact that the former proposition is very much on the table for the British in response to Iran's flagrant disregard to the terms of the JCPoA.

China and the "Special Relationship"

> It will not be any European statesman who will unite Europe, Europe will be united by the Chinese.[50]

To the contrary of Charles de Gaulle's forecast, a potential geopolitical wedge for drift on either side of the Channel could in fact be the People's Republic of China. To the surprise of some, on 20 July 2020 the European Council issued a press release in which it announced that it has adopted decisions on the signature of an agreement between the EU and China on "geographical indications" (GIs).[51] The first significant bilateral trade agreement between the two trading blocs. The following day, US Secretary of State Mike Pompeo landed in London to meet with his British counterpart, Dominic Raab, and he continued to pressure the UK to take a tougher line on Beijing.[52] Pompeo's efforts in this regard were further underscored when ahead of his meeting with the Foreign

Secretary, he met with a cross-party group of backbench British MPs, the majority of whom are China hawks.

While European Commission President Ursula von der Leyen in June 2020 warned China of severe consequences in light of their new wide-ranging security law for Hong Kong, the EU was slow to act materially. German Chancellor Angela Merkel cautioned against severing dialogue with China, stating "[i]t is important that EU member states are trying to find a common policy toward China and a common answer, [but] this is no reason not to remain in dialogue with China."[53] The joint position eventually agreed by EU Member States in late July 2020 did include measures for export restrictions to Hong Kong but it fell short of sanctions and was silent on how the restrictions could be implemented. Brussels is clearly eager not to inflame tensions with Beijing and thus distanced itself from the hard line adopted by President Trump.

This has been somewhat in contrast to the British response, which has growingly signaled a subtle nod to the "Special Relationship." In quick succession, frustrated with Beijing's apparent exploitation of the coronavirus pandemic for its own strategic interests, the UK suspended its extradition treaty with Hong Kong and extended its arms embargo on China to Hong Kong.[54] These moves were duly lauded by Pompeo on this visit, "I want to take this opportunity to congratulate the British Government for its principled responses to these challenges. [...] We support those sovereign choices; we think, well done."[55]

A further divergence in strategy between the UK and Brussels can be seen in cybersecurity with regards to the evolution of the British position on Huawei in line with the US, with Prime Minister Johnson's decision on 14 July 2020 to order British telecommunication operators to remove the Chinese technology giant from their fifth-generation of mobile networks (5G) by 2027.[56] In contrast, the European Commission refused to expressly exclude any specific telecommunication supplier, in the unveiling of its "EU toolbox" of mitigating measures to address security risks related to the rollout of 5G.[57] This move was warmly welcomed by Huawei in a statement following the Commission's announcement:

> Huawei welcomes Europe's decision, which enables Huawei to contin-ueparticipating in Europe's 5G roll-out. This non-biased and fact-based approach towards 5G security allows Europe to have a more secure and faster 5G network.[58]

The apparent British drift to the way of American thinking on China has not gone unnoticed, with the Foreign Secretary subsequently challenged by a member of the press on this point: "how do you respond to critics who say the UK is being strong-armed [...] into its China position by [US] officials."[59]

Conclusion

By the end of the first quarter in 2021, the relationship between the UK and the EU had already run into a number of stumbling blocks, from the disruption of trade, to the Northern Ireland Protocol, to the vaccine tussle. While there is undoubtedly a recognition and a need for continued strong cooperation between the UK and the EU on security and defense policy, as prescribed in the TCA, it is now on a looser footing to reflect Britain's lack of appetite for a formal institutional framework with its continental partners.

Collaboration will be challenging. It will, more likely than not, be flexible, rooted in pragmatic mutual interest and an ad-hoc approach rather than formal commitments or shared values. Nonetheless, it will be necessary, as evidenced in the UK Government's 2021 "Integrated Review":

> [A]s a European nation, we will enjoy constructive and productive relationships with our neighbors in the [EU], based on mutual respect for sovereignty and the UK's freedom to do things differently, economically and politically, where that suits our interests.[60]

When looking at the big picture, there are clear reasons for both sides to figure out a blueprint for cooperative and enduring security and defense ties. There is a history after all, over 40 years of partnership in these matters. The UK and Europe have the same "operational backyard."[61] Many of the aforementioned threats in this chapter—assaults on multilateralism, Russian sabre rattling, the deteriorating MENA environment, the future of the JCPoA, cyberattacks, migration and a global epidemic—are of shared concern.

The COVID-19 pandemic has been a timely and painful reminder of the fact that geography is unavoidable; Britain and the EU are condemned to work together, in some form at least. Whether that reality is embraced or resisted, remains to be seen.

Notes

1. Otto von Bismarck, "Speech to Reichstag, 14 May 1872," in *Bismarck's Speeches and Letters*, ed. Otto Bismarck (Berlin: Reclam, 1986), 301.
2. "The EU–UK Trade and Cooperation Agreement," signed on December 30, 2020, *EUR-Lex*, https://eur-lex.europa.eu/legal-content/EN/TXT/?uri=uriserv%3AOJ.L_.2020.444.01.0014.01.ENG.
3. Sam Bresnick and Paul Haenle, "Amid Coronavirus Pandemic, China Seeks Larger Role on World Stage," *Carnegie Endowment for International Peace*, April 9, 2020, https://carnegieendowment.org/2020/04/09/amid-coronavirus-pandemic-china-seeks-larger-role-on-world-stage-pub-81515.
4. "EU–China—A Strategic Outlook," *European Commission*, March 12, 2019, https://ec.europa.eu/info/sites/info/files/communication-eu-china-a-strategic-outlook.pdf.
5. Tania Latici, "What Role in European Defence for a Post-Brexit United Kingdom?," *European Parliamentary Research Service*, April 2019, https://www.europarl.europa.eu/RegData/etudes/BRIE/2019/637941/EPRS_BRI(2019)637941_EN.pdf.
6. Cabinet Office, "National Security Capability Review," *HM Government*, March 2018, https://assets.publishing.service.gov.uk/government/uploads/system/uploads/attachment_data/file/705347/6.4391_CO_National-Security-Review_web.pdf.
7. European Border and Coast Guard Agency, "Risk Analysis for 2020," *Frontex*, March 2020, 58, https://frontex.europa.eu/assets/Publications/Risk_Analysis/Risk_Analysis/Annual_Risk_Analysis_2020.pdf.
8. "Written Evidence Submitted by Nick Witney," *UK Parliament*, May 2020, https://committees.parliament.uk/writtenevidence/4534/pdf/.
9. "Arab Youth Survey 12th Annual Edition 2020," *ASDA'A BCW*, https://www.arabyouthsurvey.com/.
10. Elizabeth Dent, "US Policy and the Resurgence of ISIS in Iraq and Syria," *Middle Eastern Institute*, October 21, 2020, https://www.mei.edu/publications/us-policy-and-resurgence-isis-iraq-and-syria.

11. Joseph Hincks, "With the World Busy Fighting COVID-19, Could ISIS Mount a Resurgence?," *Time*, April 29, 2020, https://time.com/5828630/isis-coronavirus/.
12. Ivan Bedrov, "NATO Official Says Jets Intercepted Russian Aircraft In European Airspace Nearly 300 Times In 2019," *Radio Free Europe/Radio Liberty*, May 23, 2020, https://www.rferl.org/a/nato-official-says-jets-intercepted-russian-aircraft-in-european-airspace-nearly-300-times-in-2019/30630161.html.
13. Andrew S. Weiss, "Russia and Europe: Stuck on Autopilot," *Carnegie Endowment for International Peace*, September 24, 2020, https://carnegieendowment.org/2020/09/24/russia-and-europe-stuck-on-autopilot-pub-82773.
14. Sergey Sukhankin, "COVID-19 as a Tool of Information Confrontation: Russia's Approach," *The School of Public Policy Publications—University of Calgary*, April 2020, https://www.policyschool.ca/wp-content/uploads/2020/03/COVID-19-Tool-of-Information-Sukhankin.pdf.
15. Chris Fox, and Leo Kelion, "Russian Spies Target COVID-19 Vaccine Research," *BBC*, July 16, 2020, https://www.bbc.com/news/technology-53429506.
16. Imogen Braddick, "Foreign Secretary Dominic Raab Accuses Russia of Trying to 'Exploit' Coronavirus Pandemic," *Evening Standard*, June 18, 2020, https://www.standard.co.uk/news/politics/dominic-raab-russia-exploit-pandemic-a4472421.html.
17. "Top US Diplomat Says Iran Desperate to Negotiate Ending Sanctions," *Voice of America*, December 4, 2020, https://www.voanews.com/middle-east/top-us-diplomat-says-iran-desperate-negotiate-ending-sanctions.
18. "Autumn 2020 Economic Forecast: Rebound Interrupted as Resurgence of Pandemic Deepens Uncertainty," *European Commission*, November 5, 2020, https://ec.europa.eu/commission/presscorner/detail/en/ip_20_2021.
19. George Allison, "UK Ranks 8th Globally for Defence Spending Say SIPRI," *UK Defence Journal*, April 27, 2020, https://ukdefencejournal.org.uk/uk-ranks-8th-globally-for-defence-spending-say-sipri/.
20. Peter Roberts, "Britain's Defences: The Biggest Spending Boost Since the Cold War," *Royal United Services Institute*, November 19, 2020, https://rusi.org/commentary/britain-defences-biggest-spending-boost-cold-war.

21. Niklas Novaky, "The Budget Deal and EU Defence Cooperation: What Are the Implications?," *Euractiv*, July 23, 2020, https://www.euractiv.com/section/defence-and-security/opinion/the-budget-deal-and-eu-defence-cooperation-what-are-the-implications/.
22. Claire Busse et al., "EU Coalition Explorer," *European Council on Foreign Relations*, July 8, 2020, https://ecfr.eu/special/eucoalitionexplorer/.
23. Nan Tian, et al., "Trends in World Military Expenditure, 2019," *SIPRI,* April 2020, https://www.sipri.org/publications/2020/sipri-fact-sheets/trends-world-military-expenditure-2019.
24. Nick Witney, "The Brexit Threat to Britain's Defence Industry," *European Council on Foreign Relations*, February 1, 2018, https://ecfr.eu/article/commentary_the_brexit_threat_to_britains_defence_industry/
25. "Brexit and COVID-19 Combination Threatening European Aerospace Firms," *Aviation Week*, July 17, 2020, https://aviationweek.com/aerospace/manufacturing-supply-chain/brexit-COVID-19-combination-threatening-european-aerospace.
26. Johan Eriksson and Giampiero Giacomello, "Doom, Boom or Hibernation? COVID-19 and the Defense Industry," *E-International Relations*, July 7, 2020, https://www.e-ir.info/pdf/86019.
27. Peggy Hollinger and Richard Milne, "Saab Chief Urges UK and EU to Avoid Defence Co-operation Disaster," *Financial Times*, July 15, 2020, https://www.ft.com/content/7cd97593-b3f7-4b2a-afaf-c00f7da57fbb.
28. Hélène De Pooter, "The Civil Protection Mechanism of the European Union: A Solidary Tool at Test by the COVID-19 Pandemic," *The American Society of International Law*, May 1, 2020, https://www.asil.org/insights/volume/24/issue/7/civil-protection-mechanism-european-union-solidarity-tool-test-COVID-19.
29. Beatriz Rios, "Borrell: COVID-19 Outbreak 'Has Ended Up Blowing Up' the Global Order," *Euractiv*, May 7, 2020, https://www.euractiv.com/section/global-europe/news/borrell-COVID-19-outbreak-has-ended-blowing-up-the-global-order/.

30. "United Kingdom's Withdrawal from the European Union Division 395," *UK Parliament*, March 29, 2019, https://hansard.parliament.uk/Commons/2019-03-29/division/B6052BBD-43BE-4A30-8365-E3A8B108009E/UnitedKingdom%E2%80%99SWithdrawalFromTheEuropeanUnion?outputType=Names.
31. Theresa May MP, "PM's Florence Speech: A New Era of Cooperation and Partnership Between the UK and the EU," *UK Government*, September 22, 2017, https://www.gov.uk/government/speeches/pms-florence-speech-a-new-era-of-cooperation-and-partnership-between-the-uk-and-the-eu.
32. "Revised Text of the Political Declaration Setting Out the Framework for the Future Relationship Between the European Union and the United Kingdom," *European Commission*, October 17, 2019, https://ec.europa.eu/info/sites/info/files/revised_political_declaration.pdf.
33. Ibid., 18, para 92.
34. Ibid., 18, para 92.
35. Dick Roche, telephone interview with the author, Matthew Robinson, March 10, 2020.
36. Ibid.
37. General Secretariat of the Council, "Political Declaration Setting Out the Framework for the Future Relationship Between the European Union and the United Kingdom," *Council of the European Union*, November 22, 2018, https://www.consilium.europa.eu/media/37059/20181121-cover-political-declaration.pdf.
38. Ibid, note 33, para 99.
39. "Leaving the EU: Security Volume 660: Debated on Thursday 16 May 2019," *House of Commons*, https://hansard.parliament.uk/Commons/2019-05-16/debates/822A3895-0FDE-4E68-AC1C-29DCF37BA171/LeavingTheEUSecurity EUSecurity.
40. Carl Baker, Elise Uberoi, and Richard Cracknell, "General Election 2019: Full Results and Analysis," *House of Commons*, January 28, 2020, https://commonslibrary.parliament.uk/research-briefings/cbp-8749/.
41. Dominic Raab, "Global Britain Is Leading the World as a Force for Good," *The Telegraph*, September 21, 2019, https://www.telegraph.co.uk/politics/2019/09/21/global-britain-leading-world-force-good/.
42. Ibid.

43. Ibid.
44. "Lord Frost CMG Appointed as a Minister of State in the Cabinet Office," *Cabinet Office Press Release*, February 17, 2021, https://www.gov.uk/government/news/lord-frost-cmg-appointed-as-a-minister-of-state-in-the-cabinet-office.
45. "President Donald J. Trump is Ending United States Participation in an Unacceptable Iran Deal," *Trump White House Archives*, May 8, 2018, https://trumpwhitehouse.archives.gov/briefings-statements/president-donald-j-trump-ending-united-states-participation-unacceptable-iran-deal/.
46. "Declaration by the High Representative on Behalf of the EU Following US President Trump's Announcement on the Iran Nuclear Deal (JCPOA)," *European Council Press Release*, May 9, 2018, https://www.consilium.europa.eu/en/press/press-releases/2018/05/09/declaration-by-the-high-representative-on-behalf-of-the-eu-following-us-president-trump-s-announcement-on-the-iran-nuclear-deal-jcpoa/.
47. "JCPOA: Statement by the High Representative Josep Borrell as Coordinator of the Joint Commission of the Joint Comprehensive Plan of Action on the Dispute Resolution Mechanism," *European Union External Action Service*, July 3, 2020, https://eeas.europa.eu/headquarters/headquarters-homepage/82059/jcpoa-statement-high-representative-josep-borrell-coordinator-joint-commission-joint_en.
48. "JCPoA Implementation: UK Government Statement, 4 July 2020," *Foreign & Commonwealth Office Press Release,* July 4, 2020, https://www.gov.uk/government/news/uk-statement-on-jcpoa-implementation-04-july.
49. "Iran Volume 669: Debated on Monday 13 January 2020," *House of Commons,* https://hansard.parliament.uk/Commons/2020-01-13/debates/44B1EA65-94AE-4167-A2B3-CFA6720DF31F/Iran?highlight=foreign%20secretary#contribution-B7A8B86A-66C9-4018-9461-4C95A3E1F086.
50. Charles de Gaulle, "Charles de Gaulle, quote 1089," in *The Wordsworth Book of Humorous Quotations*, ed. Connie Robertson (London: Bibliophile Books, 1993), 51.
51. "EU–China: Council Authorises Signature of the Agreement on Geographical Indications," *European Council Press Release*, July 20, 2020, https://www.consilium.europa.eu/en/press/press-releases/2020/07/20/eu-china-council-authorises-signature-of-the-agreement-on-geographical-indications/.

52. "Secretary Michael R. Pompeo and British Foreign Secretary Dominic Raab at a Press Availability," *US Department of State Archives*, July 21, 2020, https://2017-2021.state.gov/secretary-michael-r-pompeo-and-british-foreign-secretary-dominic-raab-at-a-press-availability/index.html.
53. Robin Emmott, "EU Preparing Measures Aainst China over Hong Kong," *Reuters*, July 13 2020, https://www.reuters.com/article/us-hongkong-security-eu/sweden-joins-france-germany-in-weighing-measures-against-china-over-hong-kong-idUSKCN24E17P.
54. "China Volume 678: Debated on Monday 20, 2020," *House of Commons*, https://hansard.parliament.uk/Commons/2020-07-20/debates/E0E37EC2-FB95-4FA6-86A7-76F82D2118C3/China?highlight = foreign%20secretary#contribution-0A705BD8-CC45-4A49-98D1-FA1304CDDAFB.
55. Ibid, note 56.
56. "UK Telecommunications Volume 678: Debated on Tuesday 14 July 2020," *House of Commons*, https://hansard.parliament.uk/Commons/2020-07-14/debates/9467A1F1-B87B-4E16-AD0C-DFF02A51981A/UKTelecommunications?highlight=secretary#contribution-8548AC01-3C2B-454A-86EC-9BF841EFDB57.
57. "Secure 5G Networks: Commission Endorses EU Toolbox and Sets Out Next Step," *European Commission Press Release*, January 29, 2020, https://ec.europa.eu/commission/presscorner/detail/en/IP_20_123.
58. "Huawei Media Statement Following the Publication of the European Commission's 5G Security Toolbox," *Huawei Press Release*, January 29, 2020, https://huawei.eu/press-release/huawei-media-statement-following-publication-european-commissions-5g-security-toolbox.
59. Ibid., note 56.
60. "Global Britain in a Competitive Age: the Integrated Review of Security, Defence, Development and Foreign Policy," *Cabinet Office*, https://www.gov.uk/government/publications/global-britain-in-a-competitive-age-the-integrated-review-of-security-defence-development-and-foreign-policy/global-britain-in-a-competitive-age-the-integrated-review-of-security-defence-development-and-foreign-policy.

61. Julian King and John Scarlett, "The Future of UK–EU Security Cooperation", *Royal United Services Institute*, January 18, 2021, https://rusi.org/commentary/future-uk-eu-security-cooperation.

Bibliography

"Arab Youth Survey 12th Annual Edition 2020." *ASDA'A BCW*. https://www.arabyouthsurvey.com/.

"Autumn 2020 Economic Forecast: Rebound Interrupted as Resurgence of Pandemic Deepens Uncertainty." *European Commission*, November 5, 2020. https://ec.europa.eu/commission/presscorner/detail/en/ip_20_2021.

"Brexit and COVID-19 Combination Threatening European Aerospace Firms." *Aviation Week*, July 17, 2020. https://aviationweek.com/aerospace/manufacturing-supply-chain/brexit-COVID-19-combination-threatening-european-aerospace.

"China Volume 678: Debated on Monday 20, 2020." *House of Commons*. https://hansard.parliament.uk/Commons/2020-07-20/debates/E0E37EC2-FB95-4FA6-86A7-76F82D2118C3/China?highlight=foreign%20secretary#contribution-0A705BD8-CC45-4A49-98D1-FA1304CDDAFB.

"Declaration by the High Representative on Behalf of the EU Following US President Trump's Announcement on the Iran Nuclear Deal (JCPOA)." *European Council Press Release*, May 9, 2018. https://www.consilium.europa.eu/en/press/press-releases/2018/05/09/declaration-by-the-high-representative-on-behalf-of-the-eu-following-us-president-trump-s-announcement-on-the-iran-nuclear-deal-jcpoa/.

"EU-China—A Strategic Outlook." *European Commission*, March 12, 2019. https://ec.europa.eu/info/sites/info/files/communication-eu-china-a-strategic-outlook.pdf.

"EU-China: Council Authorises Signature of the Agreement on Geographical Indications." *European Council Press Release*, July 20, 2020. https://www.consilium.europa.eu/en/press/press-releases/2020/07/20/eu-china-council-authorises-signature-of-the-agreement-on-geographical-indications/.

"Huawei Media Statement Following the Publication of the European Commission's 5G Security Toolbox." *Huawei Press Release*, January 29, 2020. https://huawei.eu/press-release/huawei-media-statement-following-publication-european-commissions-5g-security-toolbox.

"Iran Volume 669: Debated on Monday 13 January 2020." *House of Commons*. https://hansard.parliament.uk/Commons/2020-01-13/debates/44B1EA65-94AE-4167-A2B3-CFA6720DF31F/Iran?highlight=foreign%20secretary#contribution-B7A8B86A-66C9-4018-9461-4C95A3E1F086.

"JCPoA Implementation: UK Government Statement, 4 July 2020." *Foreign & Commonwealth Office Press Release*, July 4, 2020. https://www.gov.uk/government/news/uk-statement-on-jcpoa-implementation-04-july.

"JCPOA: Statement by the High Representative Josep Borrell as Coordinator of the Joint Commission of the Joint Comprehensive Plan of Action on the Dispute Resolution Mechanism." *European Union External Action Service,* July 3, 2020. https://eeas.europa.eu/headquarters/headquarters-homepage/82059/jcpoa-statement-high-representative-josep-borrell-coordinator-joint-commission-joint_en.

"Leaving the EU: Security Volume 660: Debated on Thursday 16 May 2019." *House of Commons*. https://hansard.parliament.uk/Commons/2019-05-16/debates/822A3895-0FDE-4E68-AC1C-29DCF37BA171/LeavingTheEUSecurity.

"Lord Frost CMG Appointed as a Minister of State in the Cabinet Office." *Cabinet Office Press Release*, February 17, 2021. https://www.gov.uk/government/news/lord-frost-cmg-appointed-as-a-minister-of-state-in-the-cabinet-office.

"President Donald J. Trump Is Ending United States Participation in an Unacceptable Iran Deal." *Trump White House Archives*, May 8, 2018. https://trumpwhitehouse.archives.gov/briefings-statements/president-donald-j-trump-ending-united-states-participation-unacceptable-iran-deal/.

"Revised Text of the Political Declaration Setting Out the Framework for the Future Relationship Between the European Union and the United Kingdom." *European Commission*, October 17, 2019. https://ec.europa.eu/info/sites/info/files/revised_political_declaration.pdf.

"Secretary Michael R. Pompeo and British Foreign Secretary Dominic Raab at a Press Availability." *US Department of State Archives*, July 21, 2020. https://2017-2021.state.gov/secretary-michael-r-pompeo-and-british-foreign-secretary-dominic-raab-at-a-press-availability/index.html.

"Secure 5G Networks: Commission Endorses EU Toolbox and Sets Out Next Step." *European Commission Press Release*, January 29, 2020. https://ec.europa.eu/commission/presscorner/detail/en/IP_20_123.

"The EU-UK Trade and Cooperation Agreement." signed on December 30, 2020. *EUR-Lex*. https://eur-lex.europa.eu/legal-content/EN/TXT/?uri=uriserv%3AOJ.L_.2020.444.01.0014.01.ENG.

"Top US Diplomat Says Iran Desperate to Negotiate Ending Sanctions." *Voice of America*, December 4, 2020. https://www.voanews.com/middle-east/top-us-diplomat-says-iran-desperate-negotiate-ending-sanctions.

"UK Government to Acquire Cutting-Edge Satellite Network." *Department for Business, Energy & Industrial Strategy Press Release*, July 3, 2020. https://www.gov.uk/government/news/uk-government-to-acquire-cutting-edge-satellite-network.

"UK Telecommunications Volume 678: Debated on Tuesday 14 July 2020." *House of Commons*. https://hansard.parliament.uk/Commons/2020-07-14/debates/9467A1F1-B87B-4E16-AD0C-DFF02A51981A/UKTelecommunications?highlight=secretary#contribution-8548AC01-3C2B-454A-86EC-9BF841EFDB57.

"UK to Tell EU it Will no Longer Seek Access to Secure Aspects of Galileo." *UK Government Press Release*, December 1, 2018. https://www.gov.uk/government/news/uk-to-tell-eu-it-will-no-longer-seek-access-to-secure-aspects-of-galileo.

"United Kingdom's Withdrawal from the European Union Division 395." *UK Parliament*, March 29, 2019. https://hansard.parliament.uk/Commons/2019-03-29/division/B6052BBD-43BE-4A30-8365-E3A8B108009E/UnitedKingdom%E2%80%99SWithdrawalFromTheEuropeanUnion?outputType=Names.

"Written Evidence Submitted by Nick Witney." *UK Parliament,* May 2020. https://committees.parliament.uk/writtenevidence/4534/pdf/.

Allison, George. "UK ranks 8th Globally for Defence Spending Say SIPRI." *UK Defence Journal*, April 27, 2020. https://ukdefencejournal.org.uk/uk-ranks-8th-globally-for-defence-spending-say-sipri/.

Baker, Carl, Elise Uberoi, and Richard Cracknell. "General Election 2019: Full Results and Analysis." *House of Commons*, January 28, 2020. https://commonslibrary.parliament.uk/research-briefings/cbp-8749/.

Bedrov, Ivan. "NATO Official Says Jets Intercepted Russian Aircraft In European Airspace Nearly 300 Times In 2019." *Radio Free Europe/Radio Liberty*, May 23, 2020. https://www.rferl.org/a/nato-official-says-jets-intercepted-russian-aircraft-in-european-airspace-nearly-300-times-in-2019/30630161.html.

Bismarck, Otto von. "Speech to Reichstag, 14 May 1872." In *Bismarck's Speeches and Letters*, edited by Otto Bismarck. Berlin: Reclam, 1986.

Braddick, Imogen. "Foreign Secretary Dominic Raab accuses Russia of Trying to 'Exploit' Coronavirus Pandemic." *Evening Standard*, June 18, 2020. https://www.standard.co.uk/news/politics/dominic-raab-russia-exploit-pandemic-a4472421.html.

Bresnick, Sam, and Paul Haenle. "Amid Coronavirus Pandemic, China Seeks Larger Role on World Stage." *Carnegie Endowment for International Peace*, April 9, 2020. https://carnegieendowment.org/2020/04/09/amid-coronavirus-pandemic-china-seeks-larger-role-on-world-stage-pub-81515.

Busse, Claire, Ulrike Franke, Rafael Loss, Jana Puglierin, Marlene Riedel, and Pawel Zerka. "EU Coalition Explorer." *European Council on Foreign Relations*, July 8, 2020. https://ecfr.eu/special/eucoalitionexplorer/.

Cabinet Office. "National Security Capability Review." *HM Government*, March 2018. https://assets.publishing.service.gov.uk/government/uploads/sys

tem/uploads/attachment_data/file/705347/6.4391_CO_National-Security-Review_web.pdf.

Coleman, Judie. "The Impact of Coronavirus on Terrorism in the Sahel." *International Centre for Counter-Terrorism*, April 16, 2020. https://icct.nl/publication/the-impact-of-coronavirus-on-terrorism-in-the-sahel/.

De Pooter, Hélène. "The Civil Protection Mechanism of the European Union: A Solidary Tool at Test by the COVID-19 Pandemic." *The American Society of International Law*, May 1, 2020. https://www.asil.org/insights/volume/24/issue/7/civil-protection-mechanism-european-union-solidarity-tool-test-COVID-19.

Dent, Elizabeth. "US Policy and the Resurgence of ISIS in Iraq and Syria." *Middle Eastern Institute*, October 21, 2020. https://www.mei.edu/publications/us-policy-and-resurgence-isis-iraq-and-syria.

Emmott, Robin. "EU Preparing Measures Against China over Hong Kong." *Reuters*, July 13, 2020. https://www.reuters.com/article/us-hongkong-security-eu/sweden-joins-france-germany-in-weighing-measures-against-china-over-hong-kong-idUSKCN24E17P.

Eriksson, Johan, and Giampiero Giacomello. "Doom, Boom or Hibernation? COVID-19 and the Defense Industry." *E-International Relations*, July 7, 2020. https://www.e-ir.info/pdf/86019.

European Border and Coast Guard Agency. "Risk Analysis for 2020." *Frontex*, March 2020. https://frontex.europa.eu/assets/Publications/Risk_Analysis/Risk_Analysis/Annual_Risk_Analysis_2020.pdf.

Fox, Chris, and Leo Kelion. "Russian Spies Target COVID-19 Vaccine Research." *BBC*, July 16, 2020. https://www.bbc.com/news/technology-53429506.

Gaulle, Charles de. "Charles de Gaulle, quote 1089." In *The Wordsworth Book of Humorous Quotations*, edited by Connie Robertson, London: Bibliophile Books, 1993.

General Secretariat of the Council. "Political Declaration Setting Out the Framework for the Future Relationship Between the European Union and the United Kingdom." *Council of the European Union*, November 22, 2018. https://www.consilium.europa.eu/media/37059/20181121-cover-political-declaration.pdf.

Hincks, Joseph. "With the World Busy Fighting COVID-19, Could ISIS Mount a Resurgence?." *Time*, April 29, 2020. https://time.com/5828630/isis-coronavirus/.

Hollinger, Peggy, and Richard Milne. "Saab Chief Urges UK and EU to Avoid Defence Co-operation Disaster." *Financial Times*, July 15, 2020. https://www.ft.com/content/7cd97593-b3f7-4b2a-afaf-c00f7da57fbb.

King, Julian, and John Scarlett. "The Future of UK–EU Security Cooperation." *Royal United Services Institute*, January 18, 2021. https://rusi.org/commentary/future-uk-eu-security-cooperation.

Latici, Tania. "What Role in European Defence for a Post-Brexit United Kingdom?." *European Parliamentary Research Service*, April 2019. https://www.europarl.europa.eu/RegData/etudes/BRIE/2019/637941/EPRS_BRI(2019)637941_EN.pdf.

May MP, Theresa. "PM's Florence Speech: A New Era of Cooperation and Partnership Between the UK and the EU." *UK Government*, September 22, 2017. https://www.gov.uk/government/speeches/pms-florence-speech-a-new-era-of-cooperation-and-partnership-between-the-uk-and-the-eu.

Novaky, Niklas. "The Budget Deal and EU Defence Cooperation: What Are the Implications?." *Euractiv*, July 23, 2020. https://www.euractiv.com/section/defence-and-security/opinion/the-budget-deal-and-eu-defence-cooperation-what-are-the-implications/.

Raab, Dominic. "Global Britain Is Leading the World as a Force for Good." *The Telegraph*, September 21, 2019. https://www.telegraph.co.uk/politics/2019/09/21/global-britain-leading-world-force-good/.

Rios, Beatriz. "Borrell: COVID-19 Outbreak 'Has Ended Up Blowing Up' the Global Order." *Euractiv*, May 7, 2020. https://www.euractiv.com/section/global-europe/news/borrell-COVID-19-outbreak-has-ended-blowing-up-the-global-order/.

Roberts, Peter. "Britain's Defences: The Biggest Spending Boost Since the Cold War." *Royal United Services Institute*, November 19, 2020. https://rusi.org/commentary/britain-defences-biggest-spending-boost-cold-war.

Speech by Michel Barnier at the EU Institute for Security Studies conference. "The Future of the EU Foreign, Security and Defence Policy Post Brexit." *European Commission*, May 14, 2018. https://ec.europa.eu/commission/presscorner/detail/en/SPEECH_18_3785.

Sukhankin, Sergey. "COVID-19 as a Tool of Information Confrontation: Russia's Approach." *The School of Public Policy Publications—University of Calgary*, April 2020. https://www.policyschool.ca/wp-content/uploads/2020/03/COVID-19-Tool-of-Information-Sukhankin.pdf.

Tian, Nan, Alexandra Kuimova, Diego Lopes da Silva, Pieter D. Wezeman, and Siemon T. Wezeman. "Trends in World Military Expenditure, 2019," *SIPRI*, April, 2020. https://www.sipri.org/publications/2020/sipri-fact-sheets/trends-world-military-expenditure-2019.

Weiss, Andrew S. "Russia and Europe: Stuck on Autopilot." *Carnegie Endowment for International Peace*, September 24, 2020. https://carnegieendowment.org/2020/09/24/russia-and-europe-stuck-on-autopilot-pub-82773.

Witney, Nick. "The Brexit Threat to Britain's Defence Industry." *European Council on Foreign Relations*, February 1, 2018. https://ecfr.eu/article/commentary_the_brexit_threat_to_britains_defence_industry/.

CHAPTER 5

Africa, Virus and Vulnerability: COVID-19 Pandemic in Africa

Freedom Chukwudi Onuoha and Casmir Chukwuka Mbaegbu

Introduction

Since the novel coronavirus (COVID-19) first emerged in Wuhan, in China's Hubei province, in December 2019, its rapid transmissibility and lethality has nearly brought the world to a standstill. The pandemic has generated unprecedented effects on the social, economic, health, political and security structures of states and communities around the world.[1] As the COVID-19 crisis unfolds, individuals, households, organizations and states are feeling its effects and reacting in extraordinary ways: many individuals and households have adopted restrictive measures in social relations to reduce their exposure to the virus; industry leaders are dealing with massive transformations of their sectors to be able to stay afloat in

F. C. Onuoha (✉) · C. C. Mbaegbu
Department of Political Science, University of Nigeria, Nsukka, Nigeria
e-mail: freedom.onuoha@unn.edu.ng

C. C. Mbaegbu
e-mail: casmir.mbaegbu@unn.edu.ng

C. Varin (ed.), *Global Security in Times of Covid-19*, New Security Challenges, https://doi.org/10.1007/978-3-030-82230-9_5

an extremely volatile economy; and, most importantly, governments have restricted movement, closed borders and frozen economic activity in a desperate attempt to curb the spread of the virus.

These efforts have partly contributed to the suppression of its global spread, but transmissibility and mortality have been uneven across the continents. As of January 2021, figures from the World Health Organization (WHO) showed that Africa had the second lowest number of cases (1,961,234) and deaths with (43,592) compared to the Americas with the highest numbers of cases (36,674,670) and deaths (876,031). This was closely followed by Europe with 26,881,446 cases and 588,479 deaths; South-East Asia with 12,077,882 cases and 184,941 deaths. Eastern Mediterranean with 5,000,203 cases 122,472 deaths; and Western Pacific with 1,119,437 cases and 20,373 deaths.[2]

Since the first case was confirmed in Africa on 14 February 2020, in Egypt, the virus has spread to almost all the states in the continent.[3] While the rate of contagion is much lower in Africa than other continents, there are fears that Africa will be worst hit by COVID-19. At the outset of the pandemic, the Director General of the WHO Tedros Adhanom Ghebreyesus, issued a chilling warning to African countries: “The best advice for Africa is to prepare for the worst.”[4] With a high debt burden, pervasive poverty, widespread infectious diseases, fragile health systems, overcrowded informal settlements and poor governance, Africa faces a preponderance of risk factors that threaten to exacerbate the pandemic on the continent.[5] Aware of this reality, most African countries imposed strict measures such as travel restrictions, frontier closures, lockdowns, mask-wearing, curfews and social distancing, including banning public gatherings in worship centres. Notwithstanding these emergency moves, there is a worrying rise in the number of infections recorded from early June 2020 across the continent.

It is against this backdrop that this chapter investigates COVID-19 in Africa. It seeks to examine the diverse perspectives and theories on the manifestation of the pandemic with a view to highlight the impact on security and stability. This chapter is organized into six parts. Following this introduction, the work discusses the two dominant perspectives on COVID-19 in Africa—alarmist and optimist—while outlining some of the contending explanations for the low rate of COVID-19 transmission and lethality in Africa., The third section provides an overview of pre-existing vulnerabilities in Africa. The fourth section turns to highlighting some of the key measures taken by governments to stem COVID-19. The fifth section assesses some of the impacts of the pandemic on the continent, with greater emphasis on security and stability. Finally, this work concludes with some lessons learned by Africa countries in their effort to preserve security and stability.

Competing Narratives on COVID 19 and Africa's Future

There are two broad competing perspectives or narratives regarding the nature of the Covid-19 pandemic and the fate of the continent: alarmist and optimist. It is pertinent to briefly reflect on these viewpoints.

Alarmist Perspective

The alarmist perspective paints an apocalyptic view of a continent that would largely be decimated by the virus. The major proponents of this perspective include the United Nations Economic Commission for Africa

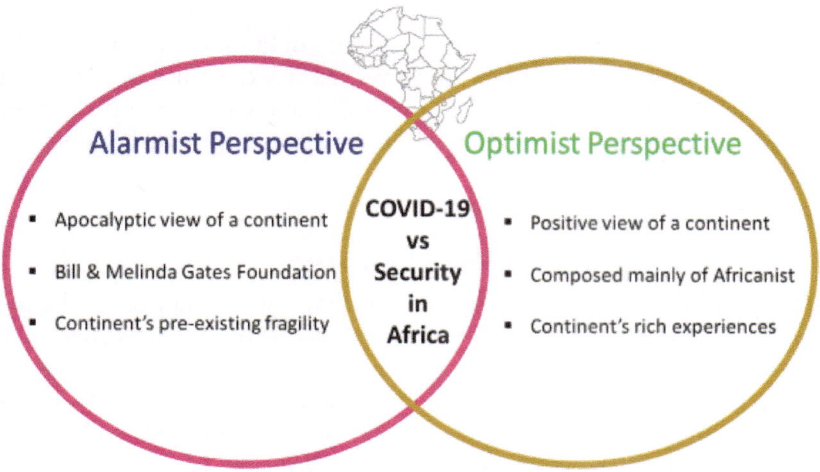

Fig. 5.1 Competing Securitization of COVID-19 and Africa's Future (*Source* Onuoha, F.C. "Civil Military Relations in the Context of Policing COVID-19 Pandemic in Nigeria" presented at the "Virtual Accountability Forum on Civil-Military Relations during the COVID-19 Pandemic in Nigeria," organized by the CLEEN Foundation, Abuja, Nigeria, 31 August 2020)

(UNECA), the WHO and the Bill & Melinda Gates Foundation, among others. For instance, the UNECA (2020) warned that even with intense containment measures, the continent of 1.3 billion people could have nearly 123 million cases in the first year, and 300,000 people could die of the disease. A similar sombre prediction was made by the WHO[6] when it warned African countries to "prepare for the worst." If predictions of UNECA and WHO are troubling, the alarm bell sounded by Melinda Gates in an interview with the CNN is, perhaps, the scariest:

> It's going to be horrible in the developing world. And part of the reason you're seeing that case numbers don't look very bad is because they don't have access to very many tests...Look at Ecuador. Look at what's going on in Ecuador. They're putting bodies out on the street. You're going to see that in countries in Africa.[7]

Given Africa's pre-existing fragility—evidenced by decayed health infrastructure, pervasive poverty and a large number of people lacking access to sanitation and safe water, among other things—those behind this narrative contend that the continent will experience a coronavirus catastrophe. The strength of this perspective lies in the recognition of certain vulnerabilities such as the fragile health system that could make yet another viral outbreak seriously challenging. However, its weakness lies in the failure to recognize the rich experience Africa, especially West African countries, have acquired while dealing with infectious diseases or innovating its way out of similar problems.

Optimist Perspective

The optimist perspective is, at best, a riposte to the assumptions and arguments of the alarmist perspective. The core narrative of this perspective is that swift aggressive measures adopted by African countries in preparation for the anticipated pandemic coupled with greater coordination across African Union (AU) member states served as critical speed bumps in slowing the coronavirus infection. Composed mainly of African analysts, they countered that:

> If the low numbers are only a result of the lack of testing, African countries would be seeing increased rates of hospitalizations and even deaths, which has not been the case so far. Predictions of mass deaths in Africa are

> problematic for reasons beyond inaccuracy. They assume that nothing that African countries do can mitigate the spread of the disease and prevent high death tolls.[8]

This perspective dismisses the alarmist view as Eurocentric, suggesting that its analytic optic is deeply rooted in colonial ideology that sees Africa as inherently backward, dysfunctional and incapable of addressing major challenges without outside help. While the optimists acknowledge that low testing may have blurred the true picture of the spread of the virus in Africa, they emphasize that the absence of mass deaths or hospitalization proves that something is ticking favourably for the continent.[9]

The utility of this perspective lies in its appreciation of the contributions of Africa's response in containing an explosive outbreak of the virus so far. However, its weakness borders on the tendency to over-amplify Africa's success story, thereby encouraging complacency that may prove tragic eventually. Critics of the optimists warn that the "comparatively low numbers of coronavirus infection and fatality rates may ultimately indicate that the continent is basking in the calm before an impending storm."[10]

Although cases on the continent are increasing, many African countries are not experiencing the exponential daily growth in confirmed cases, nor in mortality, that has been happening in the United States and Western Europe. This reality has birthed several theories seeking to explain the low transmissibility and lethality of the virus in the continent.

The demographic theory is one of the most compelling explanations about the slower rate of infections and deaths in the continent. The underlying assumption is that many countries that have escaped mass epidemics have relatively younger populations. Proponents argue that COVID-19 is a disease that is often asymptomatic or mild in youths. Therefore, Africa's young population is a strong mitigating factor, since over 70 percent of its population is under the age of thirty (see Fig. 5.1).

Because the virus afflicts the generations differently, it is possible that Africa's experience of coronavirus may vary greatly from that of the ageing American, Western and Asian worlds.[12] For instance, it has also been argued that in one of the hardest hit countries, Italy, 23.1% of the population is over age 65, versus 5% in Africa.[13] With the median age of Africa at 18 years, it is expected that the continent's population will better withstand the physiological impact of the virus. The fact that Africa has not been overwhelmed by the spread and lethality of the virus given obvious fragilities in its health and economic sectors point to the fact that its

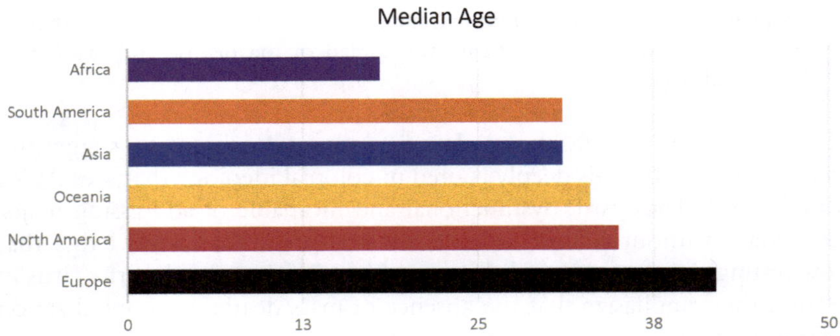

Fig. 5.2 Median Ages by Continent, February 2019 (*Source* World Economic Forum[11])

demographic advantage over other continents may well be the major mitigating factor.

Population density is another theory used to explain the low rate of transmission of the virus in Africa. With the exception of a few countries like Algeria, Egypt, Morocco and South Africa, and certain large metropolitan areas, population density is lower in Africa on average than in other parts of the world—Western Europe and North America—where the coronavirus has been the most devastating.[14] Africa has an average of 42.5 inhabitants per square kilometre, compared to 207 in Italy and 275 in the United Kingdom. In Nigerian cities like Lagos and Kano with very high population density, the infection rate has been very high compared to other less populous cities like Enugu and Port Harcourt.

Africa's experience with combating infectious diseases such as cholera, tuberculosis, HIV/AIDS and Ebola, has equally been used as explanation for the low infection rate. The most recent being the way African countries contained the 2014 Ebola outbreak. With the advent of the coronavirus, many African countries leveraged previous experiences in containing virus outbreaks to act swiftly in instituting temperature checks, cancelling international flights and imposing isolation measures on those who appear ill.[15, 16, 17]African governments were also quick to establish special COVID-19 task forces, enabling experts to guide or coordinate the national response. Health officials swiftly repurposed Ebola protocols and health infrastructure to meet the exigencies of the coronavirus spread.

The contention is that while Western Europe and North American countries have better healthcare infrastructure, they lag behind Africa in terms of rich hands-on experience in handling infectious diseases. Recent experiences with such infectious diseases have led to changes to social interactions, including moving away from touching people to greeting them and the way dead bodies are treated. Such socio-cultural adaptations are more noticeable where there is a recent experience of death and trauma linked to infectious diseases in Africa.

There are other less compelling theories behind Africa's low infection rates, anchored on assumptions such as enhanced cross-border cooperation, better use of masks and low rate of travels in Africa. For instance, a breakdown by region of the distribution of airline passenger traffic worldwide in 2019, reveals that Asia–Pacific reported the highest passenger traffic share (34%), compared to Europe (23%), North America (23%), Middle East (9%), Latin America (5%) and Africa (2%).[18] Thus, Africa's very low level of travels and inter-continental movement may have protected it from the quick spread of the virus.

Underlying Vulnerability of Africa to COVID-19

Some of the major factors behind Africa's heightened vulnerability to coronavirus include a high debt burden, dependence on primary commodity export, decrepit health system, economic marginality and poor governance. It is useful to examine these individually to better understand how they affect the African experience with COVID-19.

High Debt Burden

While debt is a global issue, Africa's past debt crises have been choking, constricting the ability of states to effectively respond to the pandemic. Concerns about an impending debt crisis in Africa are rising alongside the region's growing debt levels. As of 2017, 19 African countries have exceeded the 60% debt-to-gross domestic product (GDP) threshold set by the African Monetary Co-operation Program for developing economies, while 24 countries have surpassed the 55% debt-to-GDP ratio suggested by the International Monetary Fund (see Fig. 5.2). Surpassing this threshold means that these countries are highly vulnerable to economic changes and their governments have a reduced ability to provide support to the economy in the event of a recession or complex emergencies (pandemic). In Africa, the average debt-to-GDP ratio has increased from 39.5% in 2011, to 61.3% in 2019.[19]

Heavy debt burdens are partly due to commercial borrowing to finance the continent's large annual infrastructure financing gap of US$68 billion to US$108 billion—equivalent to about 3 to 5 percent of the continent's GDP.[20] The high debt burden in Africa is also a reflection of low domestic saving rates, low levels of domestic resource mobilization, high illicit financial outflows, capital flight, volatile commodity prices and stagnating foreign direct investment flows.[21] Thus, Africa's capacity to weather the COVID-19 storm is made worse by the fact that debt sustainability in low-income countries was deteriorating amidst the urgent need for them to support public health needs and the economy.[22]

Dependence on Commodity Export

The risks associated with the COVID-19 pandemic in Africa are amplified by the continent's heavy dependence on primary commodity export. The unequal trade relations existing between the developed and African countries have resulted in economic dependency. For instance, African countries specialize in the production of primary goods or raw materials like cocoa, groundnut, crude oil and palm oil, among others, which usually have elastic demand, while the developed countries focus on the industrial manufacturing of finished goods like machinery, cars, computers, equipment and pharmaceuticals, among others, which have inelastic demand.

African countries are thus faced with the challenge of a deficit balance of payment, since the value of exports is less than imports. In addition, Africa is a net importer of agricultural and food products, with ten basic foods making up 66% (US$46 billion) of total African food imports.[23] The implication of the above is that Africa's external economic relations reinforce its structural dependence on international finance capital, making it extremely vulnerable to incessant fluctuations of global prices of primary commodities and the supply chain of finished products. This situation becomes even more challenging in periods of global uncertainties such as the current pandemic.

Decrepit Health System

The decrepit state of Africa's health system is one of the most serious underlying conditions that heightens the continent's vulnerability to the pandemic. Africa's health systems are generally under-resourced in personnel, funding, equipment and facilities. Many African states lack adequate health workers to effectively respond to health challenges.[24] Overall access to quality services is low, especially in rural areas. Across the continent, there is less than one intensive care bed per 100,000 people. Africa's three most populous countries—Nigeria, Ethiopia and Egypt—only have 1,920 intensive care beds to service more than 400 million people between them.[25] As of 17 April 2020, some 10 countries in Africa did not possess any ventilators at all. In addition, just 2,000 ventilators were available across 41 countries home to hundreds of millions of people.[26] As the data in Fig. 5.3 reveal, there is a huge gap between available ventilators and the quantity needed at the projected peak of the pandemic in most of the African countries.

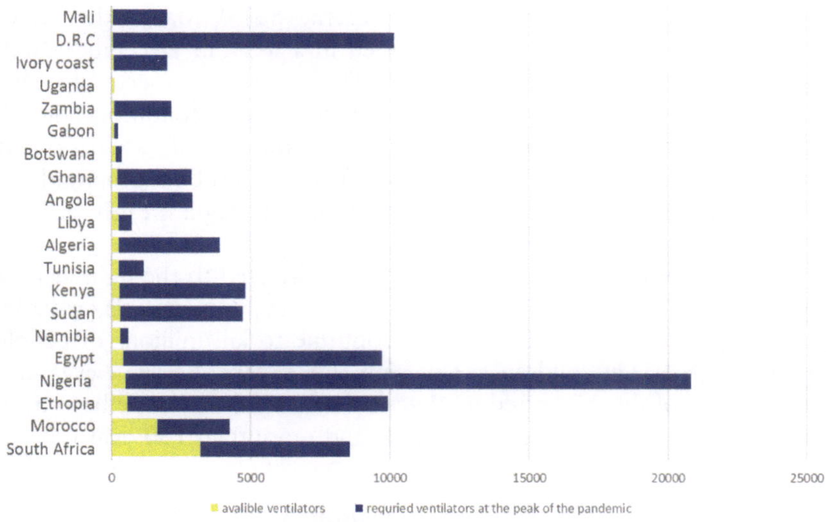

Fig. 5.3 Ventilators Gap in the Health Sector of 20 Africa's countries (*Source* Houreld, Lewis, McNeill and Granados [2020][27])

In many Africa countries like Nigeria, South Sudan and Zimbabwe, electricity is extremely unreliable and most hospitals depend on diesel-powered generators. In addition, there is an acute shortage of critical healthcare workers—doctors, nurses, anaesthesiologists and biotechnicians—essential for critical health provisioning and equipment maintenance. Meanwhile, there are many people with underlying health problems such as HIV/AIDS, heart diseases, stroke, hepatitis, tuberculosis, malaria and malnutrition.[28] Weak health systems and the prevalence of these underlying health conditions, render a significant segment of the continent's population particularly susceptible to the contagion.[29] Worst still, African healthcare is largely being funded by foreign donors, who in most cases determine priority areas of interests that may not align with the health needs of recipient communities. Limited access to personal protective equipment coupled with weak infection prevention measures has heightened the risk of health workers contracting the virus. As at July 2020, more than 10,000 health workers in 40 African countries had been infected with COVID-19. The African countries with the highest estimated numbers of health workers who died from COVID-19 include South Africa (240), Egypt (159) and Algeria (84).[30] Many others have died since then, as some 10 doctors died in a week in December 2020 in Nigeria after contracting the virus.[31] The number is expected to keep climbing in the continent due partly to unsafe working conditions, dearth of personal protective equipment (PPE) and low rate of vaccination. It was feared that the COVID-19 explosion could lead to thousands of hospitalizations, which would overwhelm already fragile health facilities in Africa.[32]

As resources and attention are devoted or diverted to the fight against COVID-19, other deadly diseases such as HIV, tuberculosis, malaria, measles, pneumonia and Lassa fever, continue to kill millions of people in Africa, especially children. At present, for instance, Lassa Fever kills about 17.8% of those infected in Nigeria. In 2020 alone, there have been nearly 4,000 suspected Lassa fever cases and more than 160 deaths.[33]

Economic Marginality

The number of unemployed young people on the continent is estimated at nearly 60%, while more than 70% of the world's poorest people live in Africa. It is estimated that some 85% of Africans live on less than \$5.50 per day.[34]

The state of economic marginality further undermines the ability for most of Africa's population to meet the basic necessities of life—food, clothing, water and sanitation. The COVID-19 pandemic began to impact African economies negatively well before it reached the shores of the continent. COVID-19 exacerbated the continent's weak economic base in at least three ways: the loss of an estimated $69 billion in the first six months of 2020 following imposition of lockdown, a drop in the growth forecast and a deepening of poverty. Among the factors were: falling demand for Africa's commodities; capital flight from Africa; a virtual collapse of tourism and air transport associated with lockdowns and border closures; and depreciation of local currencies as a result of a deterioration in the current account balance.[35]

The UNECA forecasts that economic growth in Africa will fall from 3.2% to 1.8% in 2020 as a result of COVID-19 pandemic.[36] The pandemic has equally resulted in a delay in the July 2020 start date of regional trade under the African Continental Free Trade Area (AFCFTA), thereby stalling opportunities for new exports, jobs, investments in infrastructure and financing for Africa's development.[37] Measures taken to contain the virus' spread such as lockdowns, border closure and travel restrictions further compounded disruption in productivity, forcing firms and industries to lay off staff in a bid to minimize costs. This in turn makes the risk of debt distress, poverty, unemployment and hunger even greater now and in the coming years. In Mali, for instance, "some retail traders who sold only at night saw their businesses close, as was the case with coffee vendors at the bus stations in the main cities. Managers of nightclubs and bars, and even sex workers, have felt the consequences of COVID-19."[38] Groundswell of frustration at the governments' policies and incompetence further exacerbates the risk of civil unrest.

Responses of African States to COVID-19 Pandemic

The weaknesses highlighted above perhaps partly informed the sombre predictions that Africa will be worse off in terms of the spread and severity of the virus. In the early stages of the virus' contagion, African states adopted a number of measures to curb its spread. Experts believe that these measures may have contributed to the successful slowing down of the virus' spread.[39]

One of the earliest and swiftest measures was instituting or scaling-up screening for temperature at almost all entry ports—land ports, airports and seaports. This precautionary airport health check was to ensure timely detection of possible carriers of the virus to prevent or minimize importation into the continent. By early March 2020, some 25 African countries including Egypt, Ethiopia, Ghana, Kenya, Morocco, Nigeria and South Africa had already imposed health checks at their airports, travel restriction and quarantine measures.[40] Most travellers entering or exiting Africa, especially through international airports, were subjected to enhanced screening with thermal cameras or by health agents deployed to maintain a high level of surveillance.

The swift response was partly a function of the lessons learned by many African countries from the Ebola virus disease (EVD) outbreaks in West Africa and DRC, in the area of enhanced screening and the logistical strengthening of epidemic response capacity. Many African nations have equally battled with, and learned from, other public health diseases such as Lassa fever, yellow fever, cholera and measles, among others. This expertise makes these countries more alert and willing to deploy scarce resources to stop outbreaks before they become widespread.[41] In addition, Africa CDC through its Regional Collaborating Centres supported information sharing and preparedness by Member States, by leveraging lessons from disease outbreaks to influence the continent's early response and resilience to COVID-19.[42,43]

Airport health checks and quarantine were followed-up with travel restrictions. For instance, while President Donald Trump was assuring Americans in January 2020 that the few known cases would soon drop to zero,[44] African countries such as Senegal were closing their borders, initiating contact tracing and scaling up hospital facilities to accommodate COVID-19 patients. In early March 2020, Ghana and Kenya announced new measures prohibiting travellers from countries affected by COVID-19, the first two African nations to put in place blanket travel bans. The Democratic Republic of Congo imposed quarantine measures on travellers from Italy, France, China and Germany.[45] Many other African countries followed suit in a bid to arrest the virus penetration of their territories.

As the spread of the virus gathered momentum globally, the majority of African countries almost simultaneously closed their air, land and sea borders to contain the spread of the virus. It is pertinent to note that the restrictions of movement across the borders, however, has had considerable economic impact on the economies, contributing to fears of a new food crisis, poverty and a delay in continental free trade agreements.

With the continent recording many confirmed cases who came from abroad, most African governments further ramped up restrictive measures including implementing lockdowns in some areas and the shutting down of schools, markets and worship centres. By late March 2020, dozens of African nations had imposed restrictions ranging from night-time curfews to total lockdowns or shutdowns. These included, Ghana, Gabon, Kenya, Nigeria, Uganda, Senegal, South Africa and Zimbabwe, among others. This intervention did not necessarily improve the overall security situation, as security forces reportedly exploited the movement restrictions by taking bribes from defaulters in exchange for free passage.[46]

Experts believe that social distancing, mask wearing and other public health measures are crucial for reducing the virus contagion. Social distancing and infection control were used in earlier efforts to contain tuberculosis and Ebola in Africa. In the wake of the pandemic, most African states and civil society groups intensified efforts in awareness creation on the need for people to maintain social distancing and wear masks, as directed by the government. Town criers were used in villages and rural areas to ensure impactful and penetrative reach, using local languages and dialects in promoting awareness on social distancing or communicating the ban or suspension of burial ceremonies by government.

There are certainly several challenges to the practice and effectiveness of social distancing in Africa. Africa's communal way of life, ubiquity of slums and overcrowded settlements in major cities and limited public transport infrastructure, among others, meant that practising social (physical) distancing in many African states was difficult, if not entirely impossible. Nonetheless, ongoing sensitization efforts by African governments and other non-state actors have encouraged some citizens to embrace it especially during religious, cultural, socio-economic and political activities.

Since the onset of the pandemic in the continent, African countries have responded in creative and innovative ways. At the continental level, the Africa Centres for Disease Control and Prevention (Africa CDC) established the Africa Task Force for Novel Coronavirus (AFCOR) in February 2020 to oversee Africa's preparedness and response to the pandemic. At the national level, most states equally established presidential task forces to provide expert guidance on national response to the virus.

Impact of COVID-19 Pandemic on Security and Stability in Africa

The outbreak of COVID-19 and measures adopted to contain it have impacted severely on almost every facet of life in Africa. Beyond the health and economic implications, there are growing concerns that COVID-19 will almost certainly exacerbate existing insecurity or create new problems in Africa.

The pandemic is taking place at a time when several countries in the region are engrossed in managing protracted political and security challenges. The outbreak of the virus has compounded challenges related to governance and democratization in some African states, on account of sudden deaths of some key political figures, postponement of planned elections and manipulation of the political processes, among others. For instance, the death of President Pierre Nkurunziza of Burundi on 8 June 2020 of suspected complications from COVID-19 generated political apprehension. If not properly managed, unexpected developments such as this have the potential to derail electoral and political transition processes in fragile states, leading to descent into authoritarianism or instability.

COVID-19 related disruption on elections further strained Africa's security and political fragility. At least 22 countries in Africa were to hold presidential, parliamentary or municipal elections in 2020; namely, Burkina Faso, Burundi, Cameroon, Central African Republic, Chad, Comoros, Côte d'Ivoire, Egypt, Ethiopia, Gabon, Ghana, Guinea, Liberia, Malawi, Mali, Mauritius, Namibia, Niger, Seychelles, Somalia, Tanzania and Togo. By June 2020, countries such as Ethiopia, Gambia and Zimbabwe had decided to postpone polls.[47] But such postponement was not without political and security consequences in some states, in particular Ethiopia. For instance, the northern region of Tigray in Ethiopia defied Prime Minister Abiy Ahmed to hold local elections on 9 September. The election was considered illegal by the central government, who postponed general elections earlier in the year because of the COVID-19 pandemic. This escalated longstanding tensions between Ethiopia's central government and the Tigray region, culminating in the launch of a military operation against the region. Thousands of people have reportedly been killed and more than 40,000 people have fled Ethiopia since the escalation of the conflict.[48]

Some other countries like Burundi, Côte d'Ivoire, Ghana, Guinea, Malawi, Mali, Mauritius, Seychelles, Tanzania and Togo, among others, held planned elections amidst tension and violence. Meanwhile, concerns persist over gradual descent to authoritarianism in Africa, as some African leaders have used the pretext of the pandemic to re-enforce their powers. The pandemic provided some leaders with the opportunity to weaken democratic institutions and political processes. This played out in West Africa, where said leaders were running for controversial third terms. Democratic regression in Guinea, for example, shows how the coronavirus has been dangerously used to serve political interests and strengthen leaders' holds on power.[49]

Furthermore, political imposition of restrictions and lockdowns have impacted negatively on human security across Africa, given weak mechanisms for accountability and oversight of the security sector. The use of state security forces—military, police and paramilitary outfits—to enforce frontier closures, lockdowns and curfew has resulted in significant incidents of human rights abuses, including extrajudicial killings. Cases of excessive use of force when enforcing COVID-19 measures have been documented in several African states such as Angola, Morocco, Mozambique, Nigeria, South Africa and Tunisia (Onuoha et al., 2021).[50] In April 2020, Nigeria's National Human Rights Commission reported that security agents had killed 18 people in the first two weeks of the lockdown. This was more than the number of national COVID-19 fatalities at that time.[51] In South Africa, security forces enforcing stay-at-homes killed at least 10 people; in Kenya, security forces had killed 15 people in lockdown-related incidents; and Ugandan security have killed at least six people while enforcing COVID guidelines by June 2020.[52,53]

One of the most dramatic consequences of the coronavirus pandemic is the increase in sexual and gender-based violence (SGBV).[54] As with past epidemics, the COVID-19 pandemic heightened the vulnerability of women and girls to domestic and sexual violence globally. As families are forced to stay at home, women and girls are at a heightened risk of SGBV largely caused by psychological stress and economic hardship exacerbated by COVID-19 disruption of patterns of daily lives. The result was the increase in incidence of ***rapedemic*** or what the UN aptly described as the "shadow pandemic."[55] Liberia, for instance, recorded a 50% increase in gender-based violence between January and June 2020, with more than 600 reported rape cases.[56] The reports of SGBV in Liberia are following a similar trend elsewhere in the continent. Nigeria recorded a monthly increase of 149% in reports of SGBV following the introduction of lockdowns at the end of March. Some 3,600 rape cases were reported between March and July 2020 during lockdown.[57] Almost 4,000 schoolgirls became pregnant in Kenya when schools were closed during the COVID-19 lockdown. In most cases they had allegedly been raped by relatives or police officers.[58]

As with the increase in SGBV, the lockdown also exacerbated poverty in the continent with implications for peace and security. Over 700 million people worldwide are currently estimated to be living in extreme poverty, with Africa accounting for over 70% of global poverty.[59] As the pandemic and measures to control it weakened African economies, the African Development Bank projected that up to 37.5 million additional people in Africa would slide into extreme poverty in 2020[60] and that this number could reach 49.2 million by the end 2021. African countries that are likely to experience the highest increases in extreme poverty in the years ahead include Nigeria, Democratic Republic of the Congo (DRC), Sudan and Angola, among others.

The pandemic is equally exacerbating food insecurity in the continent where 239 million people were undernourished as of 2018.[61] The state of food insecurity was already alarming before the pandemic, and supply disruptions caused by COVID-19 is further aggravating the hunger crisis. Thus, rising poverty, inflation and food shortages are undermining peace and security in the continent by contributing to protests, violence and civil unrest. For instance, when preventive measures in the form of national lockdowns were instituted across African countries beginning from March 2020, some protest action took place in a number of countries by people who were frustrated with these restrictions, as it compromised their lives and livelihoods.[62] At least six people were killed in Guinea during violent protests against coronavirus restrictions in May 2020.[63] Similar protests across several cities in Senegal in June 2020 over a government-implemented coronavirus curfew resulted in the destruction of three police vehicles, an ambulance and a coronavirus treatment centre.[64] Meanwhile, thousands of people took to the streets of Mali's capital city, Bamako, in June 2020 to demand the resignation of President Ibrahim Boubacar Keita. The protest was underpinned by a convergence of frustrations as a result of the regime's poor governance—faltering economy, weak coronavirus response, and allegations of corruption.[65] These protests reflect pre-existing frustrations with socio-economic and political conditions that have now been further exacerbated by COVID-19 restrictions.

Besides protest, people severely impacted by these harsh economic realities cope or react in different ways. Some may take to criminality or fall prey to violent extremist recruitment incentives while others may migrate to new areas in search of better livelihood prospects. Already, some COVID-19-specific criminal scams have emerged. For example, Kenyan police in early April warned of criminal gangs impersonating COVID-19 surveillance teams on door-to-door testing to conduct robberies. South Africa's first levels of lockdown substantially reduced violent crime, making it one of the few countries in the world to record fewer deaths overall because of the COVID-19 pandemic in that period. Nonetheless, criminals have also posed as workers from the Department of Health to gain access to business and residences.[66]

Rising poverty and economic stress in Africa due to COVID-19 undermine national, regional and international security. Some individuals whose lives and livelihood have worsened due to the pandemic have migrated to other areas in search of greener pasture, potentially adding to pressure on existing scarce resources. Migration has remained a significant political, security and humanitarian issue during the COVID-19 pandemic, as migrants are stuck in transit and rescue operations are being frustrated or ignored by some countries.[67] Data from 35 key transit points across West and Central Africa indicate that regional migration has dropped by nearly 50% during the first half of 2020 (compared with 2019) due to government travel restrictions to prevent the spread of COVID-19.[68] However, prohibitive responses to irregular migration by states has led to deaths as irregular migrants and migrant smuggling networks resort to dangerous routes.[69] African migrants and trafficking networks have switched to the dangerous route between western Africa to Spain's Islands in the Atlantic instead of across the Mediterranean to the southern coast of the country's mainland. As of August 2020, there had been a 520% rise in migrant arrivals to the Canary Islands (Spain) compared with the same period in 2019, with 3,448 migrants reaching the islands. Between January and mid-August 2020, a total of 239 migrants died trying to reach the Canaries, compared to 210 in the whole of 2019 and 43 in 2018.[70]

Furthermore, the coronavirus pandemic undermines the security situation in the continent by limiting or disrupting African states' capacity to combat evolving offshore and onshore threats. One evidential impact of COVID-19 offshore is the way it has disrupted or limited cooperation between international partners and African forces in promoting maritime security. Since the onset of COVID-19, external partners have systematically withdrawn their navies or scaled-down the support they provide to African partner nations in order to concentrate their attention on containing the spread of COVID-19 at home.[71] A good number of these projects in the Gulf of Guinea, for instance, are from partners in the West. For instance, the French Navy suspended its Mission Corymbe in March 2020. In the same month, the United States Africa Command (AFRICOM) cancelled the annual Obangame Express exercise designed to improve the collective capabilities of participating nations to combat maritime threats and crime. Similarly, the European Union Critical Maritime Route equally suspended the GOGIN and the EUWeCA projects designed to promote maritime security in West and Central Africa. Criminal elements such as pirates, smugglers and traffickers have exploited the gaps occasioned by COVID-19-related disruptions to sustain, if not increase, their nefarious activities. The International Maritime Bureau's latest global piracy report details 132 attacks since the start of 2020, up from 119 incidents in the same period last year.[72] Of the 85 seafarers kidnapped from their vessels and held for ransom, 80 were taken in the Gulf of Guinea—in 14 attacks reported off Nigeria, Benin, Gabon, Equatorial Guinea and Ghana.

The pandemic compounds Africa's security challenges onshore. As the governments of African countries such as Burkina Faso, Chad, Côte d'Ivoire, Niger, Mali, Nigeria and Togo struggle to implement measures to contain the virus, they are also having to contend with an ever-present and mounting threat posed by domestic armed groups. For instance, the Nigerian military struggled to balance its role in countering unconventional threats with maintaining COVID-19 lockdown. The negative consequences were most evident in ongoing military operations against the Boko Haram terrorists in the northeast.[73]

Military capability to respond to evolving security challenges was further hampered by unprecedented disruption in global supply chains caused by COVID-19, further heightening the strategic vulnerability of Nigeria's defence sector. In August 2020, President Buhari noted that the COVID-19 pandemic has not only made scarce resources even scarcer, but severely affected the supply chain of military equipment and spare parts needed to counter security threats. In the face of these and other setbacks, the military has underperformed. Suboptimal performance of the military amidst policing the pandemic led to a decline of civilian trust and confidence in the military.[74]

Elsewhere in Mali, army detachments that were deployed in several communes, including Dialloubé, Sendeguee and Togguere Coumbe in the areas of Mopti and Tenenkou, abandoned their positions during the COVID-19 period. This move enabled the extremist groups to consolidate, re-establish themselves in some of these areas and to make new inroads towards the west of the country despite the presence of several international forces like the United Nations Multidimensional Integrated Stabilization Mission in Mali (MINUSMA), a French force (Barkhane), the G5 Sahel force, two European Union (EU) training missions and a new European special force operation known as Takouba.[75]

The pandemic constrained operational flexibility of international peacekeeping and stabilization missions in Mali and elsewhere in Africa. There are currently seven United Nations peacekeeping operations based in Africa and 17 special political missions working on African issues.[76] Despite preventive measures by these missions to stop the spread of the virus, operational readiness and capability have been impacted. As an example, 73 members of the MINUSMA and 6 UN staffers tested positive and two peacekeepers died from the virus in June 2020.[77] Although they have tried to maintain essential operations, overall, their presence has been reduced.

In addition, the pandemic has significantly disrupted peacebuilding. Mediators and local peacemakers have postponed meetings and community dialogues, cancelled key diplomatic events and suspended confidence building measures. For countries such as Liberia, Guinea-Bissau, Mali and The Gambia, local conflict dynamics and structural challenges emanating from the temporal halt or cancellation of peacebuilding programmes and dialogues have generated grievances that can be exploited by extremist groups and spoilers.[78] National and global responses to COVID-19 in the African countries affected by conflict is hampering the movement of international and national peacebuilders. These professionals have been unable to travel to conflict zones to meet with partners on the ground, or to make assessments, conduct trainings and implement programmes.[79]

The COVID-19 pandemic has added another layer of complexity to how the UN is adapting its peace operations such as in Sudan. Although the UN initially committed to establishing a successor mission to the African Union (AU)–UN Hybrid Operation in Darfur (UNAMID) by 31 March in Sudan, the pandemic made this deadline impossible to meet. Virtual working methods adopted by the UNSC in mid-March to ensure minimum levels of business continuity could not compensate for the valuable, in-person discussions that had brokered previous diplomatic impasses on Sudan.[80] The pandemic has equally contributed to multiple delays in the Juba peace process between the Sudanese transitional government and some of the country's armed movements. In South Sudan too, COVID-19 has affected the 2018 Revitalized Agreement on the Resolution of the Conflict in the Republic of South Sudan (R-ARCSS). When the first vice president, two vice presidents and a few national ministers tested positive for COVID-19 in May 2020, the meetings of the Presidency and the Council of Ministers had to be suspended for months, putting further strain on the fragile political process and security situation in the country.[81]

With the rapid spread of COVID-19, the likelihood of a worsening security situation in Africa is a possibility. At least 22 African countries are experiencing political violence. Countries like Nigeria, Cameroon, Somalia, Libya, South Sudan and DR Congo are experiencing high intensity armed conflicts between armed opposition groups and national governments. Violent non-state actors in Africa have sought to exploit the pandemic to sustain or increase their operations—recruitment, radicalization and smuggling. There are examples of attempts made by terrorist and extremist groups to exploit the pandemic to undermine state authority, destabilize governments and attack targets—military, humanitarian and civilians. In the Sahel region, for example, armed groups are directly targeting schools, forcing health centres to close and depriving communities of critical services. According to the United Nations Office for the Coordination of Humanitarian Affairs (OCHA), more than 3,600 schools and 241 health centres are closed or non-operational due to insecurity in Burkina Faso, Mali, and in the regions of Tahoua and Tillaberi in western Niger. In Burkina Faso, Mali and Niger, attacks have continued unabated during the pandemic.

The experience of the Lake Chad region, where Boko Haram and its splinter faction, Islamic State West Africa Province (ISWAP) have long threatened regional stability, is quite telling. The Abubakar Shekau's faction released recordings claiming non-Muslims and their Muslim puppets are using COVID-19 to attack Islam by stopping Muslims from practicing their faith, while encouraging people to keep taking part in group prayers and other religious activities. Also, ISWAP had boasted that the virus and subsequent economic downturn would divert government attention, offering it an opportunity to step up efforts and expand activities.[82] Attacks against African Union Mission in Somalia (AMISOM) and the civilian population by Al-Shabaab have also been sustained despite COVID-19.[83] What these terrorist organizations are doing is taking advantage of the pandemic and the lacklustre government responses to it to sustain attacks as well as recruit from the impressionable local population.

Conclusion

The unprecedented impact of COVID-19 on Africa has led to a series of extraordinary responses by governments across the continent. COVID-19 has affected all dimensions of human security on the continent. As the pandemic evolves, African governments have been faced with having to balance the threat to life by the virus with the increasing threat to livelihoods following restrictive measures put in place to contain it. For the foreseeable future, individuals, organizations and states will continue to grapple with the tremendous challenges and changes occasioned by the pandemic.

Some observers contend that Africa's strong response might not be able to hold on for much longer. Notwithstanding, the continent's response thus far has provided valuable lessons for the rest of the world. The adaptation of intersectoral task forces composed of experts and practitioners has created a mechanism to harness Africa's unique experience in combating public health crises. In addition, most African countries moved fast to deepen regional coordination, deploy health workers and enforce travel restrictions, lockdowns and border closures. Governments and health authorities also drew on the experience of past epidemics to repurpose health facilities to quickly adapt to the crisis. The issue of local innovations is one that can be leveraged in promoting production capacity across Africa to minimize huge dependence on foreign countries for some medical and pharmaceutical products.

As of writing, the full impact of the pandemic on Africa may be difficult to thoroughly assess, and the effectiveness of existing responses challenging to gauge. What seems clear, nonetheless, is that the pandemic has severely impacted the health, economic, political and social stability of many African states, and these changes are likely to have long-term consequences for a continent that is known for its fragility. Thus, sustained vigilance and robust adaptive responses are critical as the virus remains a threat to life and livelihoods across the continent.

Notes

1. Mukesh Kumar Mishra, "The World After COVID-19 and its impact on Global Economy," *ZBW—Leibniz Information Centre for Economics*, 2020, https://www.econstor.eu/bitstream/10419/215931/1/MKM%20PAPER%20FOR%20COVID.pdf.
2. "WHO Coronavirus Disease (COVID-19) Dashboard," *World Health Organization*, 2021, https://COVID19.who.int/.
3. AbdulAzeez A. Anjorin, "The Coronavirus Disease 2019 (COVID-19) Pandemic: A Review and an Update on Cases in Africa," *Asian Pacific Journal of Tropical Medicine* 13, no. 5 (April 2020) https://doi.org/10.4103/1995-7645.281612, p. 200.
4. Samira Sawlani, "COVID-19: Africa Told to Prepare for Worst: What's the Response?," *Aljazeera*, March 19, 2020, https://www.aljazeera.com/news/2020/03/COVID-19-africa-told-prepare-worst-response-200319085112877.html.
5. "African Adaptations to the COVID-19 Response," *Africa Center for Strategic Studies,* April 15, 2020, https://africacenter.org/spotlight/african-adaptations-to-the-COVID-19-response/.
6. "New WHO Estimates: Up to 190 000 People Could die of COVID-19 in Africa if Not Controlled," *World Health Organization Regional Office for Africa*, May 7, 2020, https://www.afro.who.int/news/new-who-estimates-190-000-people-could-die-COVID-19-africa-if-not-controlled.
7. "Exclusive: Melinda Gates on Fighting COVID-19, Searching for Vaccines," *YouTube*, April 10, 2020, https://www.youtube.com/watch?v=qSVse07y2O4.
8. Caleb Okereke, and Kelsey Nielsen, "The Problem with Predicting Coronavirus Apocalypse in Africa," *Aljazeera*, May 7, 2020, https://www.aljazeera.com/indepth/opinion/problem-predicting-coronavirus-apocalypse-africa-200505103847843.html.
9. Chukwuma Muanya, "Why Africa Is Least Affected by Deaths from COVID-19," *The Guardian*, May 19, 2020, https://guardian.ng/news/why-africa-is-least-affected-by-deaths-from-COVID-19/.
10. Ryan Cummings, "The Calm Before a Spike in Coronavirus Cases in Africa," *IPI Global Observatory*, May 7, 2020, https://theglobalobservatory.org/2020/05/calm-before-spike-coronavirus-cases-africa/.

11. Jeff Desjardins, "Mapped: The Median Age of the Population on Every Continent," *World Economic Forum*, February 20, 2019, https://www.weforum.org/agenda/2019/02/mapped-the-median-age-of-the-population-on-every-continent/.
12. Bronwyn Bruton "What Does the Coronavirus Mean for Africa?," *Atlantic Council*, March 24, 2020, https://www.atlanticcouncil.org/blogs/africasource/what-does-the-coronavirus-mean-for-africa/.
13. Olivier Marbot, "Coronavirus: Unpacking the Theories Behind Africa's Low Infection Rate," *The Africa Report*, May 5, 2020, https://www.theafricareport.com/27470/coronavirus-unpacking-the-theories-behind-africas-low-infection-rate/.
14. Ibid.
15. Ryan Cummings, "The Calm Before a Spike in Coronavirus Cases in Africa," *IPI Global Observatory*, May 7, 2020, https://theglobalobservatory.org/2020/05/calm-before-spike-coronavirus-cases-africa/.
16. Olivier Marbot, "Coronavirus: Unpacking the Theories Behind Africa's Low Infection Rate," *The Africa Report*, May 5, 2020, https://www.theafricareport.com/27470/coronavirus-unpacking-the-theories-behind-africas-low-infection-rate/.
17. Bronwyn Bruton "What Does the Coronavirus Mean for Africa?," *Atlantic Council*, March 24, 2020, https://www.atlanticcouncil.org/blogs/africasource/what-does-the-coronavirus-mean-for-africa/.
18. E. Mazareanu, "Worldwide Air Passenger Traffic Share by Region 2019," *Statista*, November 19, 2020, https://www.statista.com/statistics/619777/air-passenger-traffic-by-region/.
19. Chukwuka Onyekwena, and Mma Amara Ekeruche, "Is a Debt Crisis Looming in Africa?," April 10, 2019, https://www.brookings.edu/blog/africa-in-focus/2019/04/10/is-a-debt-crisis-looming-in-africa/.
20. Ayodele Odusola, "Investing in Africa Is Sound Business and a Sustainable Corporate Strategy," *United Nations Africa Renewal*, 2018, https://www.un.org/africarenewal/web-features/investing-africa-sound-business-and-sustainable-corporate-strategy.
21. "Policy Brief: Impact of COVID-19 in Africa," *United Nations*, May 20, 2020, https://unsdg.un.org/resources/policy-brief-impact-COVID-19-africa.

22. Nick Wilkinson, "Debt Relief for Pain Relief: Public Finances and COVID-19 in Low-Income Countries," *International Growth Centre*, April 3, 2020, https://www.theigc.org/blog/debt-relief-for-pain-relief-public-finances-and-COVID-19-in-low-income-countries/.
23. "Policy Brief: Impact of COVID-19 in Africa," *United Nations*, May 20, 2020, https://unsdg.un.org/resources/policy-brief-impact-COVID-19-africa.
24. Ibid.
25. Felix Tih, "WHO Calls for Clinical Trial of Madagascar's Virus Cure," *Anadolu Agency*, May 7, 2020, https://www.aa.com.tr/en/africa/who-calls-for-clinical-trial-of-madagascars-virus-cure/1832600.
26. "New WHO Estimates: Up to 190 000 People Could Die of COVID-19 in Africa if Not Controlled," *World Health Organization Regional Office for Africa*, May 7, 2020, https://www.afro.who.int/news/new-who-estimates-190-000-people-could-die-COVID-19-africa-if-not-controlled.
27. Katharine Houreld, David Lewis, Ryan McNeill and Samuel Granados, "Understanding COVID-19: Virus Exposes Gaping Holes in Africa's Health Systems," *Reuters*, May 7, 2020, https://graphics.reuters.com/HEALTH-CORONAVIRUS/AFRICA/yzdpxoqbdvx/.
28. Abdinor Hassan Dahir, "Africa and the Coronavirus Pandemic: Responses, Challenges and Consequences," *TRT World Research Centre*, April 3, 2020, https://researchcentre.trtworld.com/publications/info-packs/africa-and-the-coronavirus-pandemic-responses-challenges-and-consequences.
29. "Policy Brief: Impact of COVID-19 in Africa," *United Nations*, May 20, 2020, https://unsdg.un.org/resources/policy-brief-impact-COVID-19-africa.
30. "Global: Amnesty Analysis reveals over 7,000 Health Workers have Died from COVID-19," *Amnesty International*, September 3, 2020, https://www.amnesty.org/en/latest/news/2020/09/amnesty-analysis-7000-health-workers-have-died-from-COVID19/.
31. Anadolu Agency, "20 Nigerian Doctors Die in One Week from COVID-19," *AA, December 26, 2020*, https://www.aa.com.tr/en/africa/20-nigerian-doctors-die-in-one-week-from-COVID-19/2089037.

32. "New WHO Estimates: Up to 190 000 People Could Die of COVID-19 in Africa if Not Controlled," *World Health Organization Regional Office for Africa*, May 7, 2020, https://www.afro.who.int/news/new-who-estimates-190-000-people-could-die-COVID-19-africa-if-not-controlled.
33. Ifeanyi Nsofor, and Adaeze Oreh, "Neglected Diseases Kill More People Than COVID-19—It's Time to Address Them," *Inter Press Service News Agency*, March 30, 2020, http://www.ipsnews.net/2020/03/neglected-diseases-kill-people-COVID-19-time-address/.
34. Kristofer Hamel, Baldwin Tong, and Martin Hofer, "Poverty in Africa Is Now Falling—But Not Fast Enough," *Brookings*, March 28, 2019, https://www.brookings.edu/blog/future-development/2019/03/28/poverty-in-africa-is-now-falling-but-not-fast-enough/.
35. "Policy Brief: Impact of COVID-19 in Africa," *United Nations*, May 20, 2020, https://unsdg.un.org/resources/policy-brief-impact-COVID-19-africa.
36. "Economic Impact of the COVID-19 on Africa," *United Nations Economic Commission for Africa*, May 31, 2020, https://www.uneca.org/sites/default/files/uploaded-documents/stories/eca_analysis_-_COVID-19_macroeconomiceffects.pdf. Accessed 3 June 2020.
37. "Policy Brief: Impact of COVID-19 in Africa," *United Nations*, May 20, 2020, https://unsdg.un.org/resources/policy-brief-impact-COVID-19-africa.
38. Yida Seydou Diall, "The effects of COVID-19 on the situation in Mali Political Unrest or Violence," *Accord*, September 30, 2020, https://www.accord.org.za/analysis/the-effects-of-COVID-19-on-the-situation-in-mali/.
39. Abdinor Hassan Dahir, "Africa and the Coronavirus Pandemic: Responses, Challenges and Consequences," *TRT World Research Centre,* April 3, 2020, https://researchcentre.trtworld.com/publications/info-packs/africa-and-the-coronavirus-pandemic-responses-challenges-and-consequences.
40. "Ethiopia's Tigray Crisis: PM Declares Assault on Regional Capital Mekelle," *BBC News*, November 27, 2020, https://www.bbc.com/news/world-africa-55083098.

41. Maru Mormina, and Ifeanyi M. Nsofor, "What Developing Countries Can Teach Rich Countries About How to Respond to a Pandemic," *The Conversation*, October 15, 2020, https://theconversation.com/what-developing-countries-can-teach-rich-countries-about-how-to-respond-to-a-pandemic-146784.
42. Muhammed O. Afolabi, et al., "Lessons from the Ebola Epidemics and Their Applications for COVID-19 Pandemic Response in Sub-Saharan Africa," *Developing world bioethics* (July 2020). doi.org/10.1111/dewb.12275.
43. Aloysius Uche Ordu, "The Coming of Age of the Africa Centers for Disease Control," *Brookings*, April 15, 2020, https://www.brookings.edu/blog/africa-in-focus/2020/04/15/the-coming-of-age-of-the-africa-centers-for-disease-control/.
44. Martin Farrer, "Coronavirus: Trump Says US Risk 'Very Low' as Australian PM Warns Pandemic Is 'Upon Us,'" *The Guardian*, February 27, 2020, https://www.theguardian.com/world/2020/feb/27/coronavirus-trump-says-risk-to-us-is-very-low-as-australia-enacts-emergency-plan.
45. Joe Penney, "African Nations Turn the Tables, Imposing Travel Restrictions Against US, Europe and China to Stave Off Coronavirus," *The Intercept*, March 15, 2020, https://theintercept.com/2020/03/15/african-nations-turn-the-tables-imposing-travel-restrictions-against-u-s-europe-and-china-to-stave-off-coronavirus/.
46. Freedom C. Onuoha, "Governments Response to COVID-19 and Citizens Security." Presented at the "6th Annual National People and Power Conference, organized by the Fled Leadership Institute, Abuja, NigeriaNigeria, November 5, 2020.
47. "Policy Brief: Impact of COVID-19 in Africa," *United Nations*, May 20, 2020, https://unsdg.un.org/resources/policy-brief-impact-COVID-19-africa.
48. "Ethiopia's Tigray Crisis: PM Declares Assault on Regional Capital Mekelle," *BBC News*, November 27, 2020, https://www.bbc.com/news/world-africa-55083098.
49. Héla Slim, "Electoral Process in Africa: The Impact of COVID-19 and Challenges for the EU," *European View* 19, no. 2 (November 2020): 212–221. https://doi.org/10.1177/1781685820971223.

50. Yida Seydou Diall, "The Effects of COVID-19 on the Situation in Mali Political Unrest or Violence," *Accord*, September 30, 2020, https://www.accord.org.za/analysis/the-effects-of-COVID-19-on-the-situation-in-mali/.
51. Isaac Mugabi, "COVID-19: Security Forces in Africa Brutalizing Civilians Under Lockdown," *Deutsche Welle*, April 20, 2020, https://www.dw.com/en/COVID-19.
52. URN, "Ugandan Security Have Killed 6 While Enforcing COVID Guidelines," *The Observer*, June 4, 2020, https://observer.ug/news/headlines/65127-ugandan-security-have-killed-6-while-enforcing-COVID-guidelines.
53. "African Lockdown Killings, Delayed Elections and a US Sexual Health Impasse". *The New Humanitarian*, June 5, 2020, https://www.thenewhumanitarian.org/news/2020/06/05/Africa-lockdown-killings.
54. Shalini Mittal, and Tushar Singh, "Gender Based Violence During COVID-19 Pandemic: A Mini Review," *Frontiers in Global Women Health* 4, (September 2020). https://doi.org/10.3389/fgwh.2020.00004.
55. Phumzile Mlambo-Ngcuka, "Violence Against Women and Girls: The Shadow Pandemic," *UN Women*, April 6, 2020, https://www.unwomen.org/en/newxs/stories/2020/4/statement-ed-phumzile-violence-against-women-during-pandemic.
56. Silja Fröhlich, "Violence Against Women: Africa's Shadow Pandemic," *Deutsche Welle*, May 10, 2020, https://www.dw.com/en/africa-pandemic-violence-rape-women/a-55174136.
57. Sunday Aborisade, "Nigeria Recorded 3, 600 Rape Cases During Lockdown—Minister," *Punch*, July 13, 2020, https://punchng.com/nigeria-recorded-3-600-rape-cases-during-lockdown-minister/.
58. Silja Fröhlich, "Violence Against Women: Africa's Shadow Pandemic," *Deutsche Welle*, May 10, 2020, https://www.dw.com/en/africa-pandemic-violence-rape-women/a-55174136.
59. Baldwin Tong, "COVID-19 Has Pushed Extreme Poverty Numbers in Africa to over Half a Billion," *OECD Development Matters*, October 12, 2020, https://oecd-development-matters.org/2020/10/12/COVID-19-has-pushed-extreme-poverty-numbers-in-africa-to-over-half-a-billion/.

60. "Africa Economic Outlook 2020 Supplement Amid COVID-19," *African Development Bank Group*, file:///C:/Users/onuoha/Downloads/afdb20-04_aeo_supplement_full_report_for_web_0705.pdf.
61. FAO, IFAD, UNICEF, WFP and WHO. 2019. The state of food security and nutrition in the world 2019. Rome, FAO.
62. Marisha Ramdeen, "Social and Political Protests, Exacerbated by the COVID-19 Pandemic, on the Increase in Africa," *Accord*, July 8, 2020, https://www.accord.org.za/analysis/social-and-political-protests-exacerbated-by-the-COVID-19-pandemic-on-the-increase-in-africa/.
63. "COVID-19 Alert: Disruptions Possible in Kindia, Guinea May 13 Due to Protests Against Movement Controls," *WorldAware*, May 13, 2020, https://www.worldaware.com/COVID-19-alert-disruptions-possible-kindia-guinea-may-13-due-protests-against-movement-controls.
64. AFP, "Lockdown: Senegal Arrests 74 People Over Violent Protests Against Coronavirus Curfew," *News24*, June 4, 2020, https://www.news24.com/news24/africa/news/lockdown-senegal-arrests-74-people-over-violent-protests-against-coronavirus-curfew-20200604.
65. Philip Kleinfeld, and Mohamed Salaha, "What's Behind the Mass Protests in Mali?," *The New Humanitarian*, July 10, 2020, https://www.thenewhumanitarian.org/news/2020/07/10/Mali-protests-Keita-Dicko.
66. Thomaz Favaro, "COVID-19—The Security Impacts in Africa," *Control Risks*, June 1, 2020, https://www.controlrisks.com/our-thinking/insights/COVID19-the-security-impacts-in-africa.
67. Maurice Stierl, "Migration: How Europe Is Using Coronavirus to Reinforce Its Hostile Environment in the Mediterranean," *The Conversation*, May 13, 2020, https://theconversation.com/migration-how-europe-is-using-coronavirus-to-reinforce-its-hostile-environment-in-the-mediterranean-137840.
68. "Migration Flows Across West and Central Africa Nearly Halved by COVID-19; Mobile Populations Economically Impacted," *International Organization for Migration*, June 16, 2020, https://www.iom.int/news/migration-flows-across-west.
69. Benjamine Bathke, "Europol: Migrant Smuggling Patterns Changing Due to Coronavirus," *Info Migrants*, May 18, 2020,

https://www.infomigrants.net/en/post/24819/europol-migrant-smuggling-patterns-changing-due-to-coronavirus.

70. Graham Keeley, "In COVID-19 Migration Surge, Africans Take a More Dangerous Route," *VOA News*, 2 September,2020, https://www.voanews.com/africa/COVID-19-migration-surge-africans-take-more-dangerous-route.
71. Ifesinachi Okafor-Yarwood, "COVID-19 in Africa: From Disruption to Opportunities for Sustainable Intra-African Maritime Security Cooperation," *Africa Leadership Centre* 2, no. 4 (May 2020): https://www.africanleadershipcentre.org/index.php/COVID-19-research/633-COVID-19-in-africa-from-disruption-to-opportunities-for-sustainable-intra-african-maritime-security-cooperation?fbclid=IwAR3EM3luf6Q4M6fIWiUbLcso_eH1wB0i7KGcpKrCxEzNaWXucfk7qBMT-TY.
72. "Pirates Are Kidnapping More Seafarers Off West Africa, IMB Reports," *International Chamber of Commerce*, October 14, 2020, https://iccwbo.org/media-wall/news-speeches/imb-piracy-report-2020/.
73. Freedom C. Onuoha, Chikodiri Nwangwu and Michael I. Ugwueze, "Counterinsurgency Operations of the Nigerian Military and Boko Haram Insurgency: Expounding the Viscid Manacle," *Security Journal* 33 (February 2020): 401–426, https://doi.org/10.1057/s41284-020-00234-6.
74. Freedom C. Onuoha, "Governments Response to COVID-19 and Citizens Security." Presented at the "6th Annual National People and Power Conference, organized by the Fled Leadership Institute, Abuja, NigeriaNigeria, November 5, 2020.
75. Yida Seydou Diall, "The Effects of COVID-19 on the Situation in Mali Political Unrest or Violence," *Accord*, September 30, 2020, https://www.accord.org.za/analysis/the-effects-of-COVID-19-on-the-situation-in-mali/.
76. "Policy Brief: Impact of COVID-19 in Africa," *United Nations*, May 20, 2020, https://unsdg.un.org/resources/policy-brief-impact-COVID-19-africa.
77. Edith M. Lederer, "UN Chief: COVID-19 Compounds Dire Situation in Mali, Sahel," *AP News*, June 5, 2020, https://apnews.com/article/221029e19c81e2a78e392e379e748164.
78. Fiifi Edu-Afful, "COVID-19 Exacerbates the Risk of Violent Extremism in the Sahel and West Africa," *Accord*, September

23, 2020, https://www.accord.org.za/analysis/COVID-19-exacerbates-the-risk-of-violent-extremism.
79. Cedric de Coning, "COVID-19 and Peacebuilding: Disruption, Adaptation and Transformation," *Accord*, July 8, 2020, https://www.accord.org.za/analysis/COVID-19-and-peacebuilding-disruption-adaptation-and-transformation/.
80. Daniel Forti, "How COVID-19 Has Impacted the UN peacekeeping Transition in Sudan," *Accord*, September 23, 2020, https://www.accord.org.za/analysis/how-COVID-19-has-impacted-the-un-peacekeeping-transition-in-sudan/
81. James Okuk, "The Impact of COVID-19 on the Delicate Peace Process in South Sudan," *Accord*, November 18, 2020, https://www.accord.org.za/analysis/the-impact-of-COVID-19-on-the-delicate-peace-process-in-south-sudan/.
82. Bulama Bukarti, "A Deadly Alliance: Coronavirus Makes Boko Haram More Dangerous Than Ever," *Telegraph*, June 7. https://www.telegraph.co.uk/global-health/science-and-disease/deadly-alliance-coronavirus-makes-boko-haram-dangerous-ever/.
83. Caleb Okereke, and Kelsey Nielsen, "The Problem with Predicting Coronavirus Apocalypse in Africa," *Aljazeera*, May 7, 2020, https://www.aljazeera.com/indepth/opinion/problem-predicting-coronavirus-apocalypse-africa-200505103847843.html.

Bibliography

"African Adaptations to the COVID-19 Response." *Africa Center for Strategic Studies*, April 15, 2020. https://africacenter.org/spotlight/african-adaptations-to-the-COVID-19-response/.

"Africans and Europeans Have Genetically Different Immune Systems... and Neanderthals Had Something to Do with It." *Institut Pasteu*, October 21, 2016. https://www.pasteur.fr/en/africans-and-europeans-have-genetically-different-immune-systems-and-neanderthals-had-something-do.

"COVID-19 Alert: Disruptions Possible in Kindia, Guinea May 13 Due to Protests Against Movement Controls." *WorldAware*, May 13, 2020. https://www.worldaware.com/COVID-19-alert-disruptions-possible-kindia-guinea-may-13-due-protests-against-movement-controls.

"Ethiopia's Tigray Crisis: PM Declares Assault on Regional Capital Mekelle." *BBC News*, November 27, 2020. https://www.bbc.com/news/world-africa-55083098.

"Exclusive: Melinda Gates on Fighting COVID-19, Searching for Vaccines." *YouTube*, April 10, 2020. https://www.youtube.com/watch?v=qSVse07y2O4.

"Freedom in The World 2015." *Freedom House*, February 2014. https://freedomhouse.org/sites/default/files/01152015_FIW_2015_final.pdf.

"Global Employment Trends for Youth 2020: Africa." *International Labour Organization*, March 9, 2020. https://www.ilo.org/wcmsp5/groups/public/---dgreports/---dcomm/documents/briefingnote/wcms_737670.pdf.

"Global: Amnesty Analysis reveals over 7,000 Health Workers Have Died from COVID-19." *Amnesty International*, September 3, 2020. https://www.amnesty.org/en/latest/news/2020/09/amnesty-analysis-7000-health-workers-have-died-from-COVID19/.

"Migration Flows Across West and Central Africa Nearly Halved by COVID-19; Mobile Populations Economically Impacted." *International Organization for Migration*, June 16, 2020. https://www.iom.int/news/migration-flows-across-west-and-central-africa-nearly.

"New WHO Estimates: Up to 190 000 People Could Die of COVID-19 in Africa if Not Controlled." *World Health Organization Regional Office for Africa*, May 7, 2020. https://www.afro.who.int/news/new-who-estimates-190-000-people-could-die-COVID-19-africa-if-not-controlled.

"Policy Brief: Impact of COVID-19 in Africa." *United Nations*, May 20, 2020. https://unsdg.un.org/resources/policy-brief-impact-COVID-19-africa.

"Regional Economic Outlook Sub Saharan Africa." *International Monetary Fund*, April 2018. https://www.imf.org/en/Publications/REO/SSA/Issues/2018/09/20/sreo1018.

"WHO Coronavirus Disease (COVID-19) Dashboard." *World Health Organization*, 2021. https://COVID19.who.int/.

"World Malaria Report 2019." *World Health Organization*, December 4, 2019. https://www.who.int/publications/i/item/9789241565721.

Aborisade, Sunday. "Nigeria Recorded 3, 600 Rape Cases During Lockdown—Minister." *Punch*, July 13,2020. https://punchng.com/nigeria-recorded-3-600-rape-cases-during-lockdown-minister/.

Afolabi, Muhammed O., Morenike Oluwatoyin Folayan, Nchangwi Syntia Munung, Aminu Yakubu, Gibril Ndow, Ayodele Jegede, Jennyfer Ambe, and Francis Kombe. "Lessons from the Ebola Epidemics and Their Applications for COVID-19 Pandemic Response in Sub-Saharan Africa." *Developing World Bioethics* 21, no. 1 (July 2020): 25–30. https://doi.org/10.1111/dewb.12275.

AFP. "Lockdown: Senegal Arrests 74 People over Violent Protests Against Coronavirus Curfew." *News24*, June 4, 2020. https://www.news24.com/news24/africa/news/lockdown-senegal-arrests-74-people-over-violent-protests-against-coronavirus-curfew-20200604.

Aidi, Hisham. "Public Trust, Capacity and COVID-19: Early Lessons from Africa." *Policy Center for the New South*, May 2020. https://www.policycenter.ma/sites/default/files/PB_20-45_Aidi.pdf.

Anjorin, AbdulAzeez A. "The Coronavirus Disease 2019 (COVID-19) Pandemic: A Review and an Update on Cases in Africa." *Asian Pacific Journal of Tropical Medicine* 13, no. 5 (April 2020): 199–203. doi:https://doi.org/10.4103/1995-7645.281612.

Bathke, Benjamine. "Europol: Migrant Smuggling Patterns Changing Due to Coronavirus." *Info Migrants*, May 18, 2020. https://www.infomigrants.net/en/post/24819/europol-migrant-smuggling-patterns-changing-due-to-coronavirus.

Bearak, Max. "Kenyan Factory Transforms into a Surgical Mask Assembly Line Overnight." *The Washington Post*, April 8. https://www.greenwichtime.com/news/article/Kenyan-factory-transforms-into-a-surgical-mask-15186523.php.

Beech, Hannah, Alissa J. Rubin, Anatoly Kurmanaev, and Ruth Maclean. "The COVID-19 Riddle: Why Does the Virus Wallop Some Places and Spare Others?." *New York Times*, May 3, 2020. https://www.nytimes.com/2020/05/03/world/asia/coronavirus-spread-where-why.html.

Bouet, Antoine, and David Laborde. "COVID-19 Border Policies Create Problems for African Trade and Economic Pain for Communities." *IFPRI WCAO*, May 14, 2020. https://wca.ifpri.info/2020/05/14/COVID-19-border-policies-create-problems-for-african-trade-and-economic-pain-for-communities/.

Bruton, Bronwyn. "What does the Coronavirus mean for Africa?." *Atlantic Council,* March 24, 2020. https://www.atlanticcouncil.org/blogs/africasource/what-does-the-coronavirus-mean-for-africa/.

Bukarti, Bulama. "A Deadly Alliance: Coronavirus Makes Boko Haram More Dangerous Than Ever." *Telegraph*, June 7. https://www.telegraph.co.uk/global-health/science-and-disease/deadly-alliance-coronavirus-makes-boko-haram-dangerous.

Chikwanah, Eveline. "Violence Against Women, Girls in Africa Spikes Amid COVID-19." *UM News*, September 10, 2020. https://www.umnews.org/en/news/gender-based-violence-in-africa-spikes-amid-COVID-19.

Cummings, Ryan. "The Calm Before a Spike in Coronavirus Cases in Africa." *IPI Global Observatory*, May 7, 2020. https://theglobalobservatory.org/2020/05/calm-before-spike-coronavirus-cases-africa/.

Dahir, Abdinor Hassan. "Africa and the Coronavirus Pandemic: Responses, Challenges and Consequences." *TRT World Research Centre*, April 3, 2020. https://researchcentre.trtworld.com/publications/info-packs/africa-and-the-coronavirus-pandemic-responses-challenges-and-consequences.

De Coning, Cedric. "COVID-19 and Peacebuilding: Disruption, Adaptation and Transformation." *Accord*, July 8, 2020. https://www.accord.org.za/analysis/COVID-19-and-peacebuilding-disruption-adaptation-and-transformation/.

Desjardins, Jeff. "Mapped: The Median Age of the Population on Every Continent." *World Economic Forum*, February 20, 2019. https://www.weforum.org/agenda/2019/02/mapped-the-median-age-of-the-population-on-every-continent/.

Diall, Yida Seydou. "The effects of COVID-19 on the situation in Mali Political Unrest or Violence." *Accord,* September 30, 2020. https://www.accord.org.za/analysis/the-effects-of-COVID-19-on-the-situation-in-mali/.

Ebiede, Tarila Marclint. "How to Ensure That Coronavirus Doesn't Stop Peace Efforts in Africa." *The Conversation*, April 26, 2020. https://theconversation.com/how-to-ensure-that-coronavirus-doesnt-stop-peace-efforts-in-africa-135859.

Edu-Afful, Fiifi. "COVID-19 Exacerbates the Risk of Violent Extremism in the Sahel and West Africa." *Accord*, September 23, 2020. https://www.accord.org.za/analysis/COVID-19-exacerbates-the-risk-of-violent-extremism-in-the-sahel-and-west-africa/elections-US-sexual-health-cheat-sheet.

Farrer, Martin. "Coronavirus: Trump Says US Risk 'Very Low' as Australian PM Warns Pandemic Is 'Upon Us.'" *The Guardian*, February 27, 2020. https://www.theguardian.com/world/2020/feb/27/coronavirus-trump-says-risk-to-us-is-very-low-as-australia-enacts-emergency-plan.

Favaro, Thomaz, "COVID-19—The Security Impacts in Africa." *Control Risks*, June 1, 2020. https://www.controlrisks.com/our-thinking/insights/COVID19-the-security-impacts-in-africa.

Folorunsho-Francis, Adebayo. "A We've Made Two Prototype Ventilators Locally, Says NDA." *Punch Healthwise*, April 20, 2020. https://healthwise.punchng.com/weve-made-two-prototype-ventilators-locally-says-nda/.forces-in-africa-brutalizing-civilians-under-lockdown/a-53192163.

Forti, Daniel. "How COVID-19 Has Impacted the UN Peacekeeping Transition in Sudan." *Accord*, September 23, 2020. https://www.accord.org.za/analysis/how-COVID-19-has-impacted-the-un-peacekeeping-transition-in-sudan/

Fröhlich, Silja. "Violence Against Women: Africa's Shadow Pandemic." *Deutsche Welle*, May 10, 2020. https://www.dw.com/en/africa-pandemic-violence-rape-women/a-55174136halved-COVID-19-mobile-populations.

Hamel, Kristofer, Baldwin Tong, and Martin Hofer. "Poverty in Africa Is Now Falling—But Not Fast Enough." *Brookings*, March 28, 2019. https://www.brookings.edu/blog/future-development/2019/03/28/poverty-in-africa-is-now-falling-but-not-fast-enough/.

Hewings-Martin, Yella. "Is There More Than One Strain of the New Coronavirus?." *Medical News Today*, May 22, 2020. https://www.medicalnewstoday.com/articles/is-there-more-than-one-strain-of-the-new-coronavirus.

Houreld, Katharine, David Lewis, Ryan McNeill, and Samuel Granados. "Understanding COVID-19: Virus Exposes Gaping Holes in Africa's Health

Systems." *Reuters*, May 7, 2020. https://graphics.reuters.com/HEALTH-CORONAVIRUS/AFRICA/yzdpxoqbdvx/.

Ifesinachi, K. "Neo-Liberal Foreign Economic Policy and Social Welfare in Nigeria." *University of Nigeria Journal of Political Economy* 2: 153–174.

Iweze, Daniel Olisa. "COVID-19 and Nigeria's Counterinsurgency Operations in the Northeast." *Kujenga Amani*, June 4, 2020. https://kujenga-amani.ssrc.org/2020/06/04/COVID-19-and-nigerias-counterinsurgency-operations-in-the-northeast/.

Keeley, Graham. "In COVID-19 Migration Surge, Africans Take a More Dangerous Route." *VOA News*, 2 September,2020. https://www.voanews.com/africa/COVID-19-migration-surge-africans-take-more-dangerous-route.

Kleinfeld, Philip, and Mohamed Salaha. "What's Behind the Mass Protests in Mali?." *The New Humanitarian*, July 10, 2020. https://www.thenewhumanitarian.org/news/2020/07/10/Mali-protests-Keita-Dicko.

Lederer, Edith M. "UN chief: COVID-19 Compounds Dire Situation in Mali, Sahel." *AP News*, June 5, 2020. https://apnews.com/article/221029e19c81e2a78e392e379e748164.

Marbot, Olivier. "Coronavirus: Unpacking the Theories Behind Africa's Low Infection Rate." *The Africa Report,* May 5, 2020. https://www.theafricareport.com/27470/coronavirus-unpacking-the-theories-behind-africas-low-infection-rate/.

Mazareanu, E. "Worldwide Air Passenger Traffic Share by Region 2019." *Statista*, November 19, 2020. https://www.statista.com/statistics/619777/air-passenger-traffic-by-region/.

Mishra, Mukesh Kumar. "The World After COVID-19 and Its Impact on Global Economy." *ZBW—Leibniz Information Centre for Economics*, 2020, https://www.econstor.eu/bitstream/10419/215931/1/MKM%20PAPER%20FOR%20COVID.pdf.

Mittal, Shalini, and Tushar Singh. "Gender Based Violence During COVID-19 Pandemic: A Mini Review." *Frontiers in Global Women Health* 4, (September 2020). https://doi.org/10.3389/fgwh.2020.00004.

Mlambo-Ngcuka, Phumzile. "Violence Against Women and Girls: The Shadow Pandemic." *UN Women*, April 6, 2020. https://www.unwomen.org/en/newxs/stories/2020/4/statement-ed-phumzile-violence-against-women-during-pandemic.

Mormina, Maru, and Ifeanyi M. Nsofor. "What Developing Countries Can Teach Rich Countries About How to Respond to a Pandemic." *The Conversation*, October 15, 2020. https://theconversation.com/what-developing-countries-can-teach-rich-countries-about-how-to-respond-to-a-pandemic-146784.

Muanya, Chukwuma. "Why Africa Is Least Affected by Deaths from COVID-19." *The Guardian*, May 19, 2020. https://guardian.ng/news/why-africa-is-least-affected-by-deaths-from-COVID-19/.

Mugabi, Isaac. "COVID-19: Security forces in Africa brutalizing civilians under lockdown." *New Humanitarian*, June 5, 2020. https://www.dw.com/en/covid-19-security-forces-in-africabrutalizing-civilians-under-lockdown/a-53192163.

Nsofor, Ifeanyi, and Adaeze Oreh. "Neglected Diseases Kill More People Than COVID-19—It's Time to Address Them." *Inter Press Service News Agency*, March 30, 2020. http://www.ipsnews.net/2020/03/neglected-diseases-kill-people-COVID-19-time-address/.

Odusola, Ayodele. "Investing in Africa Is Sound Business and a Sustainable Corporate Strategy." *United Nations Africa Renewal*, 2018. https://www.un.org/africarenewal/web-features/investing-africa-sound-business-and-sustainable-corporate-strategy.

Okafor-Yarwood, Ifesinachi. "COVID-19 in Africa: From Disruption to Opportunities for Sustainable Intra-African Maritime Security Cooperation." *Africa Leadership Centre* 2, no. 4 (May 2020). https://www.africanleadershipcentre.org/index.php/COVID-19-research/633-COVID-19-in-africa-from-disruption-to-opportunities-for-sustainable-intra-african-maritime-security-cooperation?fbclid=IwAR3EM3luf6Q4M6fIWiUbLcso_eH1wB0i7KGcpKrCxEzNaWXucfk7qBMT-TY.

Okereke, Caleb and Kelsey Nielsen. "The Problem with Predicting Coronavirus Apocalypse in Africa." *Aljazeera*, May 7, 2020. https://www.aljazeera.com/indepth/opinion/problem-predicting-coronavirus-apocalypse-africa-200505103847843.html.

Okuk, James. "The Impact of COVID-19 on the Delicate Peace Process in South Sudan." *Accord*, November 18, 2020. https://www.accord.org.za/analysis/the-impact-of-COVID-19-on-the-delicate-peace-process-in-south-sudan/.

Onuoha, Freedom C., Chikodiri Nwangwu, and Michael I. Ugwueze. "Counterinsurgency Operations of the Nigerian Military and Boko Haram Insurgency: Expounding the Viscid Manacle." *Security Journal* 33 (February 2020): 401–426. https://doi.org/10.1057/s41284-020-00234-6.

Onuoha, Freedom C., Gerald E. Ezirim, and Paul A. Onuh. "Extortionate Policing and the Futility of COVID-19 Pandemic Nationwide Lockdown in Nigeria: Insights from the South East Zone." *African Security Review* (September 2021). https://doi.org/10.1080/10246029.2021.1969961.

Onyekwena, Chukwuka and Mma Amara Ekeruche. "Is a Debt Crisis looming in Africa?" April 10, 2019. https://www.brookings.edu/blog/africa-in-focus/2019/04/10/is-a-debt-crisis-looming-in-africa/.

Ordu, Aloysius Uche. "The Coming of Age of the Africa Centers for Disease Control." *Brookings*, April 15, 2020. https://www.brookings.edu/blog/africa-in-focus/2020/04/15/the-coming-of-age-of-the-africa-centers-for-disease-control/.

Penney, Joe. "African Nations Turn the Tables, Imposing Travel Restrictions Against US, Europe, and China to Stave Off Coronavirus." *The Intercept*, March 15, 2020. https://theintercept.com/2020/03/15/african-nations-turn-the-tables-imposing-travel-restrictions-against-u-s-europe-and-china-to-stave-off-coronavirus/.

Quach, Hélène, Maxime Rotival, Julien Pothlichet, Yong-Hwee Eddie Loh, Michael Dannemann, Nora Zidane, Guillaume Laval, et al. "Genetic Adaptation and Neandertal Admixture Shaped the Immune System of Human Populations." *National Library of Medicine* 167, no. 3 (October 2016): 643–656. https://doi.org/10.1016/j.cell.2016.09.024.

Ramdeen, Marisha. "Social and Political Protests, Exacerbated by the COVID-19 Pandemic, on the Increase in Africa." *Accord*, July 8, 2020. https://www.accord.org.za/analysis/social-and-political-protests-exacerbated-by-the-COVID-19-pandemic-on-the-increase-in-africa/.

Sawlani, Samira. "COVID-19: Africa Told to Prepare for Worst: What's the Response?." *Aljazeera*, March 19, 2020. https://www.aljazeera.com/news/2020/03/COVID-19-africa-told-prepare-worst-response-200319085112877.html.

Slim, Héla. "Electoral Process in Africa: The Impact of COVID-19 and Challenges for the EU." *European View* 19, no. 2 (November 2020): 212–221. https://doi.org/10.1177/1781685820971223.

Stierl, Maurice. "Migration: How Europe Is Using Coronavirus to Reinforce Its Hostile Environment in the Mediterranean." *The Conversation*, May 13, 2020, https://theconversation.com/migration-how-europe-is-using-coronavirus-to-reinforce-its-hostile-environment-in-the-mediterranean-137840

Tih, Felix. "WHO Calls for Clinical Trial of Madagascar's Virus Cure." *Anadolu Agency*, May 7, 2020. https://www.aa.com.tr/en/africa/who-calls-for-clinical-trial-of-madagascars-virus-cure/1832600.

Tong, Baldwin. "COVID-19 Has Pushed Extreme Poverty Numbers in Africa to over Half a Billion." *OECD Development Matters*, October 12, 2020. https://oecd-development-matters.org/2020/10/12/COVID-19-has-pushed-extreme-poverty-numbers-in-africa-to-over-half-a-billion/.

URN. "Ugandan Security Have Killed 6 While Enforcing COVID Guidelines." *The Observer*, June 4,2020. https://observer.ug/news/headlines/65127-ugandan-security-have-killed-6-while-enforcing-COVID-guidelines.

Wilkinson, Nick. "Debt Relief for Pain Relief: Public Finances and COVID-19 in Low-Income Countries." *International Growth Centre*, April 3, 2020. https://www.theigc.org/blog/debt-relief-for-pain-relief-public-finances-and-COVID-19-in-low-income-countries/.

CHAPTER 6

Long COVID and the New Middle East

Mitchell Belfer

Introduction

The history of COVID-19 will likely be overshadowed by the residual impacts of the virus rather than the pandemic itself. This is because COVID-19 has not produced change per se, but rather reminds states, and publics, of the nature of international and regional political and economic life. In the Middle East, COVID-19 has exposed extreme variance between levels of national cohesion, political and economic stamina. It has also cemented some important security-related trends. Geopolitical brinkmanship involving regional and international actors continues uninterrupted, civil strife in Iraq, Libya, Syria and Yemen ebbs and flows while Lebanon teeters. Yet, at the same time, Israel has made peace with the United Arab Emirates (UAE), Bahrain and Morocco (and Sudan), the intra-Gulf Cooperation Council (GCC) crisis was resolved at the Al-Ula Summit and the arrival of the Biden team provided breathing space for Iran to re-engage the United States (US) and the Gulf countries. The years surrounding COVID-19 are proving to be exceptionally important

M. Belfer (✉)
Euro-Gulf Information Centre, Rome, Italy
e-mail: belfer@egic.info

C. Varin (ed.), *Global Security in Times of Covid-19*, New Security Challenges, https://doi.org/10.1007/978-3-030-82230-9_6

for the Middle East and the setting of the scene for the medium and long-term future of the region.

This chapter unpacks the security dynamics at play at the arrival of COVID-19 including a discussion of the main security challenges, regional rivalries, unfolding conflicts and crises. The chapter identifies and analyses two significant transitions that were accelerated by the pandemic: a transition in terms of the balance(s) of power (regional and international) and a transition in alliances and alliance clustering. Finally, this chapter seeks to anticipate what comes next. Of course, international politics is not an exact science, however the trends that have been accelerated by COVID-19 will produce likely outcomes and it is important to develop scenarios to better understand long-COVID in political and security terms. Before turning to the main argument of this chapter, this work takes a short detour to explain what and where the Middle East is. This is necessary since COVID-19 is not equally distributed and neither will its security impact be equally felt.

A Middle East of Parts

Scholars of the Middle East have had their hands full trying to agree on where the region starts and ends. This work identifies the Middle East as an umbrella term for a region composed of three subregions: North Africa, the Levant/East Mediterranean and the Arabian Peninsula/Gulf. This subdivision is important since each of these faced different circumstances going into, and will face different consequences as a result of, the pandemic. The subregions are broken-down as follows:

- *North Africa*: Algeria, Morocco, Libya and Tunisia but omits the Sahel states.[1]
- *The Levant/East Mediterranean*: Cyprus, Egypt, Israel, Jordan, Lebanon, Palestine, Syria and Turkey.
- *The Arabian Peninsula/Gulf*: Bahrain, Kuwait, Iran, Iraq, Oman, Qatar, Saudi Arabia, the UAE and Yemen.

This subdivision is set according to geopolitical conditions rather than strictly geographic determinism. For instance, the North African states remain an auxiliary of European political and economic life in ways that the Levantine and Arabian Peninsula states are not. The Middle East's only North Atlantic Treaty Organization (NATO) member, Turkey, is clustered together with the region's only European Union (EU) member, Cyprus, into the East Mediterranean where their strategic foci have been since the major gas finds in 2011. Turkey is, somewhat, focused on the Caucasus and Central Asia but to a far lesser extent. The rest of the subregional actors are defined entirely by their extended neighborhoods except for Iran, which is also immersed in the Caspian Sea/Central Asian and South Asia subcontinent's strategic life. Of course each state in the Middle East has international interests, however, their strategic views are very limited and regionally tied. Even the most populous state, Egypt, does not have a deep strategic awareness of non-peripheral regions and, despite being a key African state, identifies more as an Arab and Middle Eastern actor with its interests tied more to the Levant/East Mediterranean and the Arabian Peninsula.[2] COVID-19 has not changed much in terms of the Middle East states' pursuit of core security interests, but it has accelerated such pursuits as well as some of the roles played by exogenous actors such as the US, Russia, the EU27, the United Kingdom (UK) and China.

Fateful Years in the Middle East: 2020 and 2021

History will likely judge 2020 and 2021 as forging the international relations of the future. In the Middle East, the arrival of COVID-19 deeply impacted regional security conditions. Yet, even before the pandemic, the region was situated on the brink. On 3 January 2020, a US drone strike killed the Islamic Revolutionary Guard Corps (IRGC)-Al Quds Force Chief, Major General Qassem Soleimani, and Kataib Hezbollah Commander, Abu Mahdi al-Muhandis, in a targeted assassination. The operation reflected the growing frustration of the Trump Administration's inability to deter Iran, despite leaving the Joint Comprehensive Plan of Action (JCPoA, re: Iran nuclear deal) and applying a 'maximum pressure' strategy to force changes to Iran's regional policy.[3] In that context, the drone attack intended to do four things:

- Eliminate the most acute threat to US forces and diplomatic personnel in Iraq.
- Undermine Iran's operational hierarchy in Iraq.
- Punish Iran's security apparatus for the 2019 attacks on the Aramco sites in Saudi Arabia.

- Signal to Tehran the level of US resolve and its military-intelligence capabilities.

Iran's immediate response came with a missile barrage on US-staffed bases in Iraq. In the fog-o-war, an anti-aircraft missile downed Ukrainian International Airlines Flight 752, which had just taken off, killing all 176 people on board. US–Iran relations have come to dominate many international affairs debates as it seemed to have marked a new twist in their regional rivalry and led to renewed US efforts to confront Iran kinetically, economically and via concerted acts of sabotage and cyber-warfare. The US–Iran rivalry has even persisted through the transition from the Trump to the Biden Administrations and despite the progress made in the JCPoA II talks, both Washington and Tehran remain deeply suspicious of each other. This suspicion has been exacerbated by the June 2021 election of Ibrahim Raisi to President of Iran as he is widely seen as a champion of Iran's revolutionary politics and has adopted a hardline in relations with the West. Nonetheless, the pandemic has exposed massive differences between the subregions of the Middle East and is set to impact some wider strategic questions as well.

The outbreak of COVID-19 may eventually be heralded as providing important breathing space in the Middle East. While accusations of 'healthcare nationalism' may be used to denounce those European states that enacted protective measures at the onset of the pandemic, in some ways COVID-19 could not have come at a better time. Nationalist narratives were developed in the Middle East to deal with the pandemic. Some of the manifestations of COVID-19 nationalism have helped enhance internal political cohesion and strengthen subregional stability while others have done the opposite. In the Arabian Peninsula/Gulf subregion, all six GCC members were quick to enact far-reaching early warning systems, testing, specialized health units, tracing applications, border closures and, eventually, comprehensive vaccine roll-out programmes. Bahrain and the UAE emerged as world leaders for both their testing and vaccination regimes. This was made possible by the type of nationalism honed during the pandemic throughout the GCC—non-aggressive, community focused and determined. However, this was not the norm and while some states dealt with COVID-19 in a haphazard way, others have been accused of simply ignoring it. After all, it is difficult to deal with a health emergency when civil war is gripping the country as in Yemen. A quick glance at the at the COVID data from 1 January 2020 until 18

Table 6.1 Arab Peninsula/Gulf COVID data

Country	*Infections*	*Fatalities*
Iran	2,765,485	77,222
Iraq	1,142,925	15,997
Saudi Arabia	433,980	7,174
Oman	206,297	2,206
Kuwait	292,490	1,696
UAE	547,411	1,633
Yemen	6,572	1,295
Bahrain	202,556	752
Qatar	213, 485	532

Source This data is derived from the World Health Organization and is available at: https://covid19.who.int/table

May 2021 shows the huge disparity of infections and deaths within the subregions (see Table 6.1).

In the Arabian Peninsula/Gulf, while the GCC states have considerably smaller populations than Iran, even if viewed on a per capita basis, the outbreak of COVID-19 was more acutely felt in Iran than among the GCC states. It is also worth noting that Iran has refused to import vaccinations from the US and the UK, which has meant that it relies entirely on the Russian Sputnik V and the Chinese Sinovac and does not have widespread access to Pfizer-BioNTech or Moderna—the more effective vaccines.[4] Also, Iraq (39 million) and Saudi Arabia (34 million) are proximate in population size, and yet the former has seen more than double the cases and fatalities than the later. The data on Yemen is incomplete given the unfolding civil war and the numbers shown below are inaccurate. As Table 6.1 indicates, the GCC states' capability to deal with the pandemic surpassed the others in the subregion.

Similar situations are visible in the other subregions as well, with a few states outpacing the others in terms of testing and vaccinations while keeping their case numbers relatively low.

In the Levant, the numbers are largely inaccurate as they rely on governmental reporting to the World Health Organization (WHO). Only Cyprus, Egypt, Israel, Jordan and Turkey have managed to undertake adequate accounting of COVID-19 while Lebanon, Palestine and Syria are either unable, or unwilling, to treat the pandemic seriously. This shows an important discrepancy among the Levantine countries—those states that generally have accountability mechanisms are faring better than the

Table 6.2 Levant COVID data

Country	*Infections*	*Dead*
Turkey	5,151,038	45,419
Israel	839,162	6,395
Lebanon	537,437	7,658
Jordan	728,549	9,328
Palestine	333,598	3,718
Egypt	250,391	14,559
Cyprus	71,533	348
Syria	23,939	1,720

Source Emadeddin Badi, "Coronavirus in Libya: The Contagion of Instability," ***Italian Institute for International Political Studies (ISPI)***, May 7, 2020, https://www.ispionline.it/it/pubblicazione/coronavirus-libya-contagion-instability-25963

others. In the case of Israel and, especially, Cyprus, the number of dead versus the number of infections speaks to the quality of their healthcare systems and rapid responses to the pandemic.

In North Africa, both Morocco and Tunisia were quick to adopt policies to restrict the spread of COVID-19 and the infections: death ratio is in line with other similar sized states, though when compared to the GCC they fare poorly. In Libya, COVID-19 has been 'securitized' and is being deployed as a legitimacy-generating mechanism for the various factions operating there.[5] This may explain the low figures as each faction—armed with EU and UNDP testing kits and vaccines (since April 2021)—aims to illustrate its authority in the areas it operates from. Likewise, Algeria has fared better than others due to the rapid support provided by external actors, notably the EU, which reinforced its healthcare system.

This brief review of the COVID-19 situation is an indication of the balance of responsibility in the wider region. It shows which states have prioritized social sustainability and which prioritize other policy areas. In some ways, COVID-19 is exposing the internal (regional) balance of power: North Africa gravitates to Europe and relies on European economic ties, the Levant is fractured but Turkey, Israel and Egypt remain stable poles. Cyprus is special owing to its EU membership. In the Arabian Peninsula/Gulf the states of the GCC expend their vast resources for their populations while the others are either going through messy political transitions (re: Lebanon), are in a state of war (re: Yemen and

Table 6.3 North Africa COVID data

Country	*Infections*	*Dead*
Morocco	516,091	9,109
Tunisia	331,674	12,089
Libya	182,649	3,102
Algeria	125,896	3,395

Source Emadeddin Badi, "Coronavirus in Libya: The Contagion of Instability," *Italian Institute for International Political Studies (ISPI)*, May 7, 2020, https://www.ispionline.it/it/pubblicazione/coronavirus-libya-contagion-instability-25963

Iraq) or are motivated by other ideological factors (re: Iran) (Table 6.2 and 6.3).

Just as COVID-19 exposed variance between states in the region, it has also adjusted the strategic environment in terms of the balance of power and alliances.

Balance of Power

COVID-19 did not change the balance of power but it has impacted regional stability. This section reviews the four main exogenous powers and assesses how COVID-19 altered their behaviors in the Middle East.

United States of America

The US extended the gap between itself and potential rivals. This is due to a number of policy advancements made during 2020/2021, despite the COVID-19 crisis and the transfer of power from the Trump to the Biden Administration. Two key policy areas stand out: the Abraham Accords and further restricting Iran's strategic movements. In relation to the Abraham Accords, the US developed a stabilization approach that further integrated the wider Middle East via the normalization process with Israel (on the one side) and the UAE, Bahrain, Morocco and Sudan (on the other) and is generally helping resolve other regional conflicts. For instance, the Accords resolved, de facto, the territorial conflict in Western Sahara by recognizing Moroccan sovereignty over the territory, they reintegrated Sudan into the international community by removing it from the US terrorist designation and sanctions lists and, through these moves, heightened deterrence capabilities across the region. Unlike the Camp David

Accords (with Egypt, 1979) and the Wada Araba Treaty (with Jordan, 1994), the Abraham Accords also included important society-to-society contact points so that normalization was not relegated to high-level politics alone. Israel is now working closely with the UAE and Bahrain towards economic and security-related objectives. Saudi Arabia does not oppose the Abraham Accords (although it will likely not join for some time) and now has reliable partners to convey messages to Israel. Oman and Qatar are both eyeing the Accords and, probably, will seek to join in the coming years. Only Kuwait fully rejects the idea of normalizing relations with Israel before the Israel–Palestine conflict is resolved.

The Abraham Accords also enhanced US efforts against its two main regional adversaries: the nexus of radical Sunni Islamist groups (re: Al Qaeda, ISIS) and the Islamic Republic of Iran with its many proxies (re: Hezbollah, Kata'ib Hezbollah [Iraq], Ansar Allah aka Houthi [Yemen], Saraya al-Ashtar [Bahrain]). Alienating Iran is a key part of the US's Iran Dossier, which includes four dimensions: preventing Iran's nuclear breakout (re: JCPoA), limiting its ballistic missile capabilities, rolling back its support for proxy insurgents and interdicting acts of international terrorism. By forming a network of states that share similar threat perceptions, the US built a strategic bulwark to assist its main missions and free-up resources to develop other aspects of its foreign policy and pushed further away from its competitors—regional and international. The COVID-19 years further entrenched the US position in the Middle East and therefore reinforced the balance of power *status quo*, which favors Washington.

Russia

In contrast, Russia slowed its regional engagement and is repositioning. There had been consensus that Russia's involvement in Syria marked the beginning of its renewed interest in returning to a Cold War-time balance of power with the US in the Middle East. This thinking did not match Russian behavior and instead of seeking to edge into the US' sphere of influence, Russia learned the lesson of overextension and carved out a space in Syria, from which the US has traditionally been absent, while engaging with the others strictly on an economic and soft power level. Of course, it did not shy away from trying to twist some of the US' allies out of Washington's sphere of influence—but it never managed to achieve this goal. The most important case in point was the Russian sale of its most advanced anti-aircraft missiles, the S-400s, to Turkey. Many speculated that Ankara would abandon NATO or that the bloc would suspend it for its military purchases from Russia. However, Turkey and Russia were engaged in proxy conflict in Syria which had, twice, nearly morphed into a direct confrontation. As part of its de-escalation strategy, Turkey purchased the S-400s as a face-saving, confidence-building mechanism.[6] As for other arms sales that Russia sought to finalize during the COVID-19 crisis, such as with Saudi Arabia and the UAE, they should be viewed as fulfilling commercial, rather than political, objectives. The only real exception to this is with regards to Russia's energy diplomacy and participation in the OPEC+ configuration; Moscow has expended tremendous political energy in trying to stabilize the oil markets on which it heavily relies. The March 2021 regional tour of Russian Foreign Minister, Sergei Lavrov, followed by the visit of Israeli Foreign Minister, Gabi Ashkenazi, to Moscow seems to have cemented Russia's role in the Middle East as a secondary power, able to affect a limited number of theaters and outcomes but by no means seeking to establish an alternative strategic pole (to the US). COVID-19 has encouraged Russia to limit its engagements in the region but this has not significantly impacted the balance of power.

The EU27 and UK

The EU27 countries and the UK have spent the COVID-19 years largely dealing with internal issues such as Brexit, growing totalitarian practices in parts of Central/East Europe, internal economic strains and coordinating healthcare strategies. To be sure, the EU27 and UK tend to deploy the language of value-driven foreign affairs, however their aspirations do not match their capabilities, which has led to an underperforming Europe, especially in relation to security affairs in the Middle East. The concept of a Europe with strategic autonomy [from the US and NATO] is, again, being popularized but it remains vague.[7] For instance, the EU was entirely absent from the Abraham Accords and its members have undertaken very few steps to help encourage further Arab–Israeli rapprochement. Even in Western Sahara, European stakeholders remained on the sidelines. In Libya, the EU helped provide legitimacy for national elections but has done relatively little in terms of capacity building. Regarding tensions over gas off the territorial waters of Cyprus, the EU has made a few statements but offered little else. Only in relation to Iran has the EU developed a clear plan though it remains based on unequivocal support for the JCPoA. For the most part, the EU's confused foreign policy is reducible to the intentions-capability gap and while most of the middle and larger powers in the Union seek to affect global affairs, they have not invested enough into modernizing their militaries or mobilizing their soft-power capabilities. The result is an EU of versions with only France—and non-EU member, UK—capable of affecting regional politics but unable to due to political and social constraints. COVID-19, and the many intra-European squabbles it generated, have clearly illustrated that the EU (and the UK) are underperforming and not serious about being a significant power in the Middle East. Even its role in the COVAX programme has not changed that. COVID-19 has not (yet) altered the EU+UK roles in the balance of power.

China

During this balance of power, China has not sought any real role in the Middle East. However, with its economic prowess, Beijing's actions matter and COVID-19 is increasing its importance for regional actors. Despite its restive western districts where ethnic Uyghurs—Muslim by religion—have been brutally repressed, the attractiveness of the Chinese marketplace and China's investments in Middle Eastern states remains unchanged. China seeks to secure resources for its ever-expanding middle class and, as a result, does not weigh into other discourses that ideologically divide the region. China is interested in Chinese growth and development. As a result, Beijing enjoys healthy relationships with nearly all the states in the region. For example, Israeli start-ups have assisted China in dealing with environmental challenges just as Chinese investments have pushed Israeli technology and infrastructure to new heights.[8] And, China is deeply engaged to Iran and has finalized their 25-year *Strategic Cooperation Agreement* that provides Beijing with access to Iran's resources and gives Tehran access to China's marketplace. Similarly, with the Arab states and Turkey—China is ever-present. However, China is not a security actor and neither has COVID-19 facilitated that role. This may not last long. COVID-19 exposed a growing international distrust of China and produced a call for deglobalization: to decouple international trade and production from China. The arrival of the Biden team (2021), coupled with heightened tensions between China and the EU/UK is increasing uncertainty. The states of the Middle East may soon be limited in their choice of strategic partners. In this eventuality, it is likely that China will affect the balance of power and regional polarity with much of the GCC, Levant and North Africa opting to deepen their relationship with the US, even at the expense of relations to China, while Iran, Syria, Lebanon and Palestine will probably do the opposite. China may already anticipate what comes next. It has embarked on a COVID-19 charm offensive—with mask and vaccine diplomacy being prioritized—in part to brush over its role in sparking the pandemic in the first place and, possibly, to cushion itself from growing pressure to decouple European and US economic activities from China—it may be trying to woo the states of the Middle East in anticipation of capital retreat by the West. In this way, COVID-19 may be dragging China into the balance of power against its better judgment.

The Impact on Alliances

The Middle East is not known for its stabilizing, multilateral institutions. With the exception of the GCC—which is also periodically paralyzed by internal crises (re: 2013–2014 and 2017–2020)—all other regional institutions have failed to fulfil their mandates. This is largely due to the self-interests being pursued and hence looking at alliances[9] and alliance clusters[10] may better illustrate the strategic situation on the ground and help in evaluating the impact of COVID-19. The epidemic impacted the process of alliance formation and alliance clustering throughout the Middle East. In the East Mediterranean–Arabian Peninsula this process has been most obvious and has generated some very interesting outcomes.

As COVID-19 broke, several alliances were in the process of tightening, notably: the Cyprus–Greece–Israel, the Bahrain–Egypt–Saudi Arabia–UAE and the Turkey–Qatar alliances. These alliances were based on providing material security (re: economic and military) for their members and a degree of ideological cushioning. For instance, Cyprus–Greece–Israel largely share threat perceptions in regard to Turkey and seek to contain it. Of course, each member of the alliance considers different aspects of Turkish foreign policy challenging. For Cyprus, Turkey continues to occupy the northern parts of the country and has threatened to expand its 'line of control' in and around its territorial waters (re: gas) and is therefore an existential threat.[11] For Greece, Ankara's use of migrant flows and the mobilization of military forces to destabilize the frontier is a key security threat. And, for Israel, Turkey's support to Hamas and other Muslim Brotherhood affiliated groups has led Tel Aviv to regard Ankara as a security challenge—not nearly as pronounced as for Greece and Cyprus just as Iran is not regarded as a core challenge in Nicosia or Athens.[12] In this case though, Turkey was the glue. The Bahrain–Egypt–Saudi Arabia–UAE alliance, the so-called Quartet, began to liaise long-before the 2017 Qatar crisis, however it was that crisis that brought Egypt into the fold and structured aspects of their security policies to reflect their alliance. This morphed into an important bloc that traverses the East Mediterranean, Red Sea and Arabian Gulf and extends over the Arabian Peninsula. The two pillars of this relationship are: (1) containing radical Islamist organizations (notably those connected to the Muslim Brotherhood) and (2) preventing the emergence of a non-Arab regional hegemon (re: Iran, Turkey). The Turkey–Qatar alliance is, in part, a reflection of the far-reaching geostrategic importance of Turkey and the combination of the extreme wealth and global ambitions of Qatar. Ankara, long interested in entering the Arabian Peninsula/Gulf, constructed a large military facility just south of Doha—sending clear signals to both Iran and Saudi Arabia (and the rest of the GCC). This facility was especially important for Qatar during the political and economic embargo enforced by the Quartet as it offered Doha an important strategic lifeline and enhanced its deterrence capabilities while Ankara became a Gulf actor. These alliances preclude economic partnerships and other forms of engagement that have been affected by COVID-19. For instance, since 2017, Qatar and Iran began a short-lived affair based mostly on economic activities and investments but also, periodically, spilling over into the political realm. This was particularly evident in the aftermath of the US targeted assassination of Qassem Soleimani.

Interestingly, COVID-19 opened a host of opportunities for alliances to change. A clustering took place that strategically moored the Cyprus–Greece–Israel alliance to the Quartet. The Abraham Accords may have officially rubber-stamped the Bahrain–Israel and UAE–Israel relationship, but tacit cooperation was already evidenced and it included Saudi Arabia. Together, these seven states have begun to share intelligence, jointly train and provide each other with early warnings.[13] The cluster aims to restrict both Iran and Turkey, increase deterrence capabilities and generally stabilize the region. COVID-19 helped this process. It also helped temper the Qatar–Turkey alliance because it slowed down the pace of engagement and reminded Qatar—and the rest of the GCC—that it remains an essential part of the Peninsula; that it's social, political and military health more obviously relies on the region than beyond it. This prodded the reconciliation efforts between Doha and Riyadh, which led to a general scaling-back of the embargo imposed on Qatar by the other Quartet states. The Al 'Ula GCC Summit (5 January 2021) formally ended the GCC crisis and, in some ways, brought Qatar into the East Mediterranean–Peninsula cluster at the expense of an alliance with Turkey, which is increasingly geopolitically isolated.

In short, COVID-19 has helped stabilize the Middle East through treaty (re: the Abraham Accords), practice (re: Al 'Ula Summit) and the process of clustering. These changed the regional balance of power. The GCC-Iran balance now favors the GCC and reconciliation with Qatar underscores this dynamic well. This has been enhanced by the Abraham Accords. This process has not impeded Iran's ability to target the GCC or Israel. The latest round of the Israel–Hamas conflict, the increase of Houthis violence against Saudi Arabia and attacks on Israeli shipping in the Arabian Sea speak to Iran's breakout policy. This dynamic will become more interesting if, as anticipated, Qatar joins the Abraham Accords, and turns its back on Tehran for an enhanced relationship with Tel Aviv. In this way, Qatar is a lynchpin and can change the course of regional affairs. Its armed forces are irrelevant in this case. It is the legitimacy of stabilization it would produce by shifting away from Turkish and Iranian adventurism and leaning into the GCC and the Cyprus–Greece–Israel cluster that would raise its influence in regional and international affairs. However, with a heavily invested and increasingly agitated Ankara, together with an impatient and increasingly impoverished Iran, Qatar's options may be severely limited.

What Next in the New Middle East

With continued uncertainty, as it became increasingly clear that COVID-19 is here to stay, countries in the Middle East have sought ways to limit the threat in the long-run. Vaccination machinery is in motion and the logistics are slowly being worked out. However, with COVID-19 respite will also come the return to more 'normal' international relations but in a changed geopolitical environment. Healthcare nationalism has generated immense mobilization among the Arab Peninsula/Gulf, which has enabled enhanced social cohesion. The spirit of national unity helped unstick one of the most pervasive regional conflicts—between Israel–Palestine and even the recent Hamas–Israel conflict will not turn back the clock. By normalizing relations with Tel Aviv, Bahrain, Morocco, Sudan and the UAE fast forwarded to a new Middle East, where local actors have more agency than ever before and super powers need partners to participate. It was likely the UAE–Qatar rivalry brought Abu Dhabi to formalize relations with Tel Aviv. Ironically, doing so likely brought Qatar to return to the GCC fold and limit its burgeoning relationship with Turkey and Iran.

COVID-19 began and will end with heightened uncertainty in Iran. The ink on the China–Iran *Strategic Cooperation Agreement* may have dried, but the double-edged sword of internal combustion and failed brinkmanship (with the US, the GCC and Israel) is driving Iran to recalibrate its own strategic awareness. COVID-19 deeply wounded Iran and its leadership is cagier than ever—a point reinforced by the failure to (so far) convince the Biden Administration to rejoin the JCPoA. Predictably, Iran has reacted by flouting its international obligations and recommenced its uranium enrichment programme at a heightened pace. The EU, Russia and the UK have all expressed their concern at Iran's growing intransigence while the regional powers cluster together as a deterrent.

Unfortunately, COVID-19 did not dent the civil wars raging on in Yemen or Syria and the ten-year anniversary of the later conflict should cause some reflection in the international community—with at least 500,000 killed and millions displaced, Syria remains a dark chapter. In Yemen, Saudi Arabia and its coalition allies have tried to use the COVID-19 pandemic to relaunch ceasefire efforts; all of which have been rejected by Ansar Allah and their backers in Iran. Instead, such overtures have been met with increased attacks on Saudi Arabia and an offensive in the Mahrib area of Yemen. Despite the heavy toll in civilian lives, there is a reluctance from the international community to properly commit to its resolution and the conflict shows no signs of abating. In Libya, COVID-19, the reduction of French and Italian engagements and a series of military setbacks by General Khalifa Haftar, led to new elections, and they have produced a new government.

All in all, there is scope for guarded optimism. COVID-19 has taught the international community to prepare for the worst but hope for the best. This is applicable on the individual and the strategic levels alike. With the number of hotspots dwindling downwards, perhaps the COVID-19 mid-term surprise will be a more stabilized Middle East, more lives saved, wealth generated, trust restored and peace facilitated. Without a crystal ball, it is hard to tell, but it is worth imagining.

Notes

1. This work accepts the UN definition of the Sahel as containing: Burkina Faso, Cameroon, Chad, The Gambia, Guinea Mauritania, Mali, Niger, Nigeria and Senegal. See: UN, "The Sahel: Land of Opportunities," available at: https://www.un.org/africarenewal/sahel.
2. Tamim K. Kashgari, "The African Dimension of Egyptian Foreign Policy," *Inquiries Journal* 3, no. 9 (2011): 1–21.
3. Hamidreza Azizi, Vali Golmohammadi and Amir Hossein Vazirian, 'Trump's "'Maximum Pressure' and Anti-Containment in Iran's Regional Policy," *Digest of Middle East Studies* 29, no. 2 (October 27, 2020): 150–166, https://doi.org/10.1111/dome.12219.
4. Yasna Haghdoost, "Iran Bans U.S., U.K. Covid-19 Vaccines in Feud With West," *Bloomberg*, January 8, 2021, https://www.bloomberg.com/news/articles/2021-01-08/khamenei-bans-u-s-u-k-covid-19-vaccines-amid-feud-with-west.
5. Emadeddin Badi, "'Coronavirus in Libya: The Contagion of Instability," *Italian Institute for International Political Studies (ISPI)*, May 7, 2020, https://www.ispionline.it/it/pubblicazione/coronavirus-libya-contagion-instability-25963.
6. Reuters Staff, "Turkey Says It Bought Russian S-400 s to Use Them, Not Put Them Aside," *Reuters*, November 16, 2019, https://www.reuters.com/article/us-usa-turkey-russia-idUSKBN1XQ07Z.
7. The term 'strategic autonomy' as it refers to the EU and EU member states dates back to the Balkan conflicts in the early 1990s when the US and NATO were seen as war-fighting agents and the EU as a civilian power. Since then, each time there is a strategic disconnect between the various part of the transatlantic relationship the concept is revived (re: in 2003 over Iraq and throughout the Trump Administration). Daniel Fiott, "Strategic Autonomy: Towards "European Sovereignty" in Defence?" (European Union Institute for Security Studies, November 2018), https://www.iss.europa.eu/sites/default/files/EUISSFiles/Brief%2012__Strategic%20Autonomy.pdf.

8. Shira Efron, Karen Schwindt and Emily Haskel, "Chinese Investment in Israeli Technology and Infrastructure: Security Implications for Israel and the United States" (RAND Corporation, 2020), https://www.rand.org/content/dam/rand/pubs/research_reports/RR3100/RR3176/RAND_RR3176.pdf.
9. Alliance here describes a bilateral or multilateral relationship in security affairs (formal or informal) that entails policy and asset coordination.
10. Alliance clustering is the tactical merger of two or more existing alliances—a form of polarity. Alliance clustering does not entail frequent alliance-to-alliance communications or coordination but does require political expressions of cooperation and/or financial support.
11. Nikola Zukalová, "Gas Leak: The Story of Turkey's Theft of Cyprus' Gas," *Euro-Gulf Information Centre*, July 15, 2019, https://www.egic.info/turkey-gas-theft-cyprus-article; Melissa Rossi, "East Mediterranean Tensions Continue to Rise: Turkey Sends Drillship Yavuz Back into Cyprus' Waters," *Euro-Gulf Information Centre*, January 22, 2020, https://www.egic.info/east-mediterranean-tensions-continu.
12. Steven Merley, "Turkey, the Global Muslim Brotherhood, and the Gaza Flotilla," *Jerusalem Center for Public Affairs*, 2011; Gallia Lindenstrauss and Sufyan Kadir Kivam, "Turkish–Hamas Relations: Between Strategic Calculations and Ideological Affinity," *Institute for National Security Studies*, Strategic Assessment 17, no 2 (July 2014); Nazir Magally, "Turkey's Support to Hamas Hinders Improvement of Relations with Israel," *Asharq Al-awsat*, 28 December 2020, https://english.aawsat.com/home/article/2707636/turkey's-support-hamas-hinders-improvement-relations-israel.
13. "Mossad Chief Visits Bahrain," *Bahrain News Agency*, October 1, 2020, https://www.bna.bh/en/MossadchiefvisitsBahrain.aspx?cms=q8FmFJgiscL2fwIzON1%2BDotd8LRx70R338NyFrUL%2BLI%3D; Seth Frantzman, "Joint Egyptian Military Drills with Jordan, UAE, Bahrain Are Regional Gamechanger," *The Jerusalem Post*, November 19, 2020, https://www.jpost.com/middle-east/joint-egyptian-military-drills-with-jordan-uae-bahrain-are-regional-gamechanger-649582; Bradley Bowman and Ryan Brobst, "The Iniochos Military Exercise in Greece Is Bad News for Iran,"

Defense News, April 30, 2021, https://www.defensenews.com/opinion/commentary/2021/04/30/the-iniochos-military-exercise-in-greece-is-bad-news-for-iran/.

Bibliography

"Mossad Chief Visits Bahrain." *Bahrain News Agency*, October 1, 2020. https://www.bna.bh/en/MossadchiefvisitsBahrain.aspx?cms=q8FmFJgiscL2fwIzON1%2BDotd8LRx70R338NyFrUL%2BLI%3D.

"Turkey Says It Bought Russian S-400s to Use Them, Not Put Them Aside." *Reuters*, November 16, 2019. https://www.reuters.com/article/us-usa-turkey-russia-idUSKBN1XQ07Z.

"WHO Coronavirus (COVID-19) Dashboard." *World Health Organisation*, 2020. https://covid19.who.int/.

Azizi, Hamidreza, Vali Golmohammadi, and Amir Hossein Vazirian. "Trump's 'Maximum Pressure' and Anti-Containment in Iran's Regional Policy." *Digest of Middle East Studies* 29, no. 2 (October, 2020): 150–166.

Badi, Emadeddin. "Coronavirus in Libya: The Contagion of Instability." *Italian Institute for International Political Studies (ISPI)*, May 7, 2020. https://www.ispionline.it/it/pubblicazione/coronavirus-libya-contagion-instability-25963.

Bowman, Bradley, and Ryan Brobst. "The Iniochos Military Exercise in Greece Is Bad News for Iran." *Defense News*, April 30, 2021. https://www.defensenews.com/opinion/commentary/2021/04/30/the-iniochos-military-exercise-in-greece-is-bad-news-for-iran/.

Efron, Shira, Karen Schwindt, and Emily Haskel. "Chinese Investment in Israeli Technology and Infrastructure: Security Implications for Israel and the United States." *RAND Corporation*, 2020. https://www.rand.org/content/dam/rand/pubs/research_reports/RR3100/RR3176/RAND_RR3176.pdf.

Fiott, Daniel. "Strategic Autonomy: Towards 'European Sovereignt'y in Defence?" *European Union Institute for Security Studies (EUISS)*, November 2018. https://www.iss.europa.eu/sites/default/files/EUISSFiles/Brief%2012__Strategic%20Autonomy.pdf.

Frantzman, Seth. "Joint Egyptian Military Drills with Jordan, UAE, Bahrain Are Regional Gamechanger." *The Jerusalem Post*, November 19, 2020. https://www.jpost.com/middle-east/joint-egyptian-military-drills-with-jordan-uae-bahrain-are-regional-gamechanger-649582.

Guerin, Orla. "ISIS in Iraq: Militants Getting Stronger Again." *BBC News*, December 23, 2019. https://www.bbc.com/news/world-middle-east-50850325.

Haghdoost, Yasna. "Iran Bans U.S., U.K. Covid-19 Vaccines in Feud With West." *Bloomberg*, January 8, 2021. https://www.bloomberg.com/news/articles/2021-01-08/khamenei-bans-u-s-u-k-covid-19-vaccines-amid-feud-with-west.

Kashgari, Tamim K. "The African Dimension of Egyptian Foreign Policy." *Inquiries Journal* 3, no. 9 (2011): 1–21.

Rossi, Melissa. "East Mediterranean Tensions Continue to Rise: Turkey Sends Drillship Yavuz Back into Cyprus' Waters." Euro-Gulf Information Centre, January 22, 2020. https://www.egic.info/east-mediterranean-tensions-continu.

Zukalová, Nikola. "Gas Leak: The Story of Turkey's Theft of Cyprus' Gas." Euro-Gulf Information Centre, July 15, 2019. https://www.egic.info/turkey-gas-theft-cyprus-article.

CHAPTER 7

The Securitization of the Coronavirus in Asian Countries: A Paradox of National Security and Human Security During the COVID-19 Crisis

Sipim Sornbanlang

Introduction

Starting with COVID-19 case zero in Wuhan, China, before this novel coronavirus even began to travel throughout the world, many scientists and public health experts realized that this new communicable disease had the potential to threaten every country within a short period of time. As of the beginning of the first week of March 2021, there were 114,140,104 COVID-19 cases as well as 2,535,520 deaths reported worldwide.[1] Initially, the number of reported COVID-19 cases and deaths in Asia had been considerably lower than in almost any other

S. Sornbanlang (✉)
Department of Political Science, Faculty of Social Sciences, Srinakharinwirot University, Bangkok, Thailand
e-mail: sipim@g.swu.ac.th

C. Varin (ed.), *Global Security in Times of Covid-19*, New Security Challenges, https://doi.org/10.1007/978-3-030-82230-9_7

part of the world. In addition to causing high morbidity and mortality rates, as well as dramatically overloading national and local health care delivery systems and thus preventing them from operating normally or at an optimal level, the COVID-19 pandemic has created a great deal of fear among people throughout the world as there is presently no definitive cure for this illness.[2] Several vaccines, produced in the USA, England, China, and Russia, were introduced as of the latter part of December 2020. However, there are a great many practical logistical issues and problems that may affect the production, distribution, and storage of adequate amounts of vaccine to ensure that most people, in Asian countries, and many other parts of the world, can be shortly protected against this deadly virus.[3] In the second quarter of 2021, however, increased production of vaccines offered a more optimistic picture, but for many people living in rural areas, as well as most parts of Asia, vaccines would not be available for many months.

Although a great deal is now known about the COVID-19 virus with respect to (a) its mode of transmission, (b) more effective ways to treat certain severe signs and symptoms, and (c) practical public health measures to reduce transmission in a given population, it seems that scientists and medical personnel are nevertheless continuing to learn many new things about this new and at times very strange virus.[4] The novel virus has thus been labeled as a "threat" to every country around the world once it was proclaimed to constitute a "global pandemic."[5] This meant that COVID-19 was potentially capable of harming anyone living in any part of the world.

Within a year of the outbreak however, many pharmaceutical companies were claiming that their vaccine was more than 90% effective; and the UK, US, Russia, and China, have approved the newly developed vaccines for immediate use among their population as well as exporting their version of the vaccine to their allies and/or other countries. As expected, there have been several reported cases of vaccine recipients experiencing adverse reactions or side effects; but this phenomenon usually occurs with most vaccines as there is always a tiny percentage of individuals, who for a variety of reasons, react adversely to vaccines.[6]

Another potential problem is the virus' ability to constantly mutate. In 2021, several new variants of the COVID-19 virus were identified such as the variants from India, the UK, Brazil, and South Africa. There is real concern that the new vaccines developed by, for example,

Pfizer/BioNTech, Moderna, AstraZenaca, and Sinovac, may not be effective against these new strains of COVID-19 and others that may develop in the future.[7] Another important issue, which scientists presently cannot answer, is the length of time that these new vaccines will be able to provide protection against the COVID-19 virus. Will the vaccines, for example, be effective for only a few years or many years, or perhaps for one's entire lifetime?

Nearly every country in Asia found itself initially unprepared to tackle the threat posed by the arrival of the COVID-19 virus.[8] Although the response to this crisis has varied considerably between different countries, most have viewed the COVID-19 pandemic as an existential threat. Asian countries more or less felt that the new virus could affect not only the wellbeing of its citizens but also national security. Hence, in order to protect both human security and national security, countries have responded by implementing a wide range of measures, never before enacted, to deal with a global pandemic. Most Asian countries have put much of their society and economy into "lockdown" to prevent the continued spread of the disease and to accordingly prevent illness and death.[9] As a result, much of Asia seems to be frozen in time, often appearing to be on a prolonged vacation. Under these national "lockdown" policies, people are no longer able to move about domestically and internationally and the global economy in many ways screeched to a halt. A term "borderless" often associated with the term "globalization" has suddenly become suspect as most countries have closed all of their borders, and people are no longer moving freely from place to place. Many people have also begun to question whether "globalization," which has been the most dominant driving political, economic, and social force since the end of the Cold War in the early 1990s, and which projected a sense of freedom to transport goods and services as well as people around the world, needs to be reconsidered in a new light.[10] In other words, the COVID-19 crisis, or the chance of another such pandemic, has created greater fear among human beings beyond what had prevailed earlier, and has forced statesmen in Asian countries and their citizens to rethink their interaction with others in order to ensure that their existence is not threatened both now as well as in the future.[11]

While lockdowns have also paralyzed globalized international affairs that had been steadily increasing since the end of Cold War, globalization itself undoubtedly ensured that the novel coronavirus could spread to almost every corner of the world in an extremely short period of time as infected people (usually not exhibiting overt signs or symptoms) traveled from one country to another.[12] The outbreak that started in Wuhan China had in a matter of weeks physically traveled to Europe, other parts of Asia, and the USA, before eventually finding its way to Africa and South America. In fact, globalization and the refusal of many countries to prepare for a communicable disease pandemic illustrated the constant tension that exists between public health experts who are concerned with human security and governments that emphasize national security concerns, especially those dealing with economic security. This is the reason why countries in Asia like Japan and South Korea have been reluctant to implement adequate preventive measures even though they had already received adequate warnings about the harmful effects of this new virus; resulting in massive outbreaks that occurred beyond China's borders all around the world. Political leaders in Asian countries have reacted to the COVID-19 pandemic by prioritizing the survival and livelihood of their citizens by securitizing the most dangerous health threat of this era, through announcing a state of emergency, which unfortunately also affects the human security of their citizens, especially in the realm of social, economic and political rights.

Securitizing COVID-19: The Success of the Asian Countries' Responses

Asian countries are justified in claiming success in their management of the COVID-19 pandemic; their COVID-19 securitization strategies have clearly resulted in very low numbers of reported cases, hospitalizations, and deaths. This was especially the case in China, Taiwan, Hong Kong, Laos, Singapore, and Thailand. The success of Asian countries is not exaggerated, if one merely looks at the numbers of COVID-19 cases, hospitalizations, and deaths, as this development probably came about due to the implementation of early securitization measures as compared to the initially less robust and slow response to the COVID-19 pandemic that emerged in the West.

The COVID-19 crisis, after it originally unfolded in Wuhan, encouraged other Asian countries beyond China to securitize the novel virus respectively.[13] In fact, Asian countries reacted to the pandemic earlier than other parts of the world by securitizing the novel virus with many effective measures; these included the announcement of emergency decrees, lockdowns, state-sponsored quarantines, closure of crowded public/private venues, etc. Taiwan, Hong Kong, and Thailand responded extremely rapidly to the COVID-19 crisis by closing their respective borders and implementing very strict security measures, while Japan and South Korea at first chose a more nuanced and guarded approach before finding that they too needed to announce stricter emergency measures.

It should be noted that apart from domestic regulations, Asian authorities were at the time also following international COVID-19 guidelines, such as those related to physical distancing, public gatherings, state quarantine, etc.[14] In Thailand, for example, senior government officials, from the national level down to districts and sub-districts made daily public announcements illustrating the need for citizens to follow the emergency decrees in order to deal with the crisis. They emphasized how easily the virus could be transmitted and accordingly reminded citizens to keep social distancing, frequently wash hands and/or use hand-sanitizers, and to wear face masks to reduce transmission. Of course, by emphasizing new lifestyles, or behaviors, many essential items (such as face masks and hand sanitizers) shortly became unavailable as the normal supply chain was not prepared to deal with this dramatic increase in demand.[15] Thus, in many urban areas, panic ensued as local residents rushed around town trying to purchase supplies or to make sure there were stocks of essential items (such as food and water in addition to face masks, hand sanitizers, soap, etc.) at home, if the situation truly turned into a "life and death" crisis.

Generally, China's lockdown measures are perceived as an example of good management for other Asian countries to emulate, in order to impede the outbreak of the pandemic as the number of reported cases, hospitalizations, and deaths in China dramatically declined in a very short period of time after parts of the country were placed under strict lockdown. China also closed its borders, except for special restricted "repatriation flights" that were available only to Chinese citizens. The lockdowns curtailed virtually all outdoor activity. Guards, which are normally posted at the entrances to housing complexes, became very vigilant in stopping anyone not registered as a resident from entering and even searched vehicles to make sure that nobody was being smuggled in. If somebody was discovered trying to smuggle out of Wuhan, as in the case of one Wuhan resident who somehow managed to leave the city to move in with relatives, the regular police were immediately summoned, and the person could be detained as soon as they arrived at their new destination. Households were issued with no more than two special identity cards and only one person per household could be out at any time (logged in and out by guards) to buy groceries or medicine. These measures sound quite harsh and at times they were, but at the same time some authorities tried to ameliorate the restrictions. In Wuhan, as drones were being used to ensure that outdoor activities were not taking place, police officers speaking through loudspeakers attached to the drones, spoke in a mild tone to clearly confused elderly residents telling them they must wear face masks and must return home right away. Some officers very politely referred to the older people they addressed as "Uncle and Auntie," in an attempt to take the sting out of what were clearly commands.[16]

Other countries in the region such as South Korea, Taiwan, and Singapore also implemented lockdowns, but their measures were not as strict and did not generally disrupt the lives of most citizens and/or interfere with daily economic activity. In Taiwan, citizens were able to take care of themselves and other family members without having to undergo some of the more stringent lockdown measures. The management of the COVID-19 crisis in Japan was also interesting to observe as its leaders promulgated "pandemic guidelines" for citizens to follow but they did not choose to impose a lockdown until the early part of 2021. They nevertheless were able to successfully control the number of infections quite well during its first wave.[17]

Although the Thai government generally followed many of the international guidelines, a major difference was that it did not, as was the case in Korea or Taiwan, pursue active case findings until the latter half of December 2020 when a second surge or COVID-19 outbreak occurred. Active case findings only began in Thailand after a large number of migrant workers from Myanmar, working in Samut Sakorn province, were found to be COVID-19 positive. By the beginning of the first week of March 2021, the number of reported COVID-19 cases in Thailand had jumped to 26,031. However, of this number, 25,324 patients had recovered while 624 were receiving treatment and/or were in isolation. There had been only 83 deaths in Thailand a year after the outbreak started, and in March 2021, the number of daily reported new cases was under 100.

To cope with a potential serious situation, some Asian governments may have overreacted, earlier than circumstances warranted, by issuing public warnings that emphasized the need to take specific actions to reduce transmission. Daily press briefings by Thailand's CCSA made people aware of the dangers of this new virus by reporting the number of cases, hospitalizations, and deaths every day, throughout the day, on TV, radio, and via social media. People automatically became highly motivated to adopt behaviors that could prevent them from becoming infected with COVID-19. Under the state of emergency regulations, all people were required to wear face masks whenever they entered public areas. This regulation inadvertently created supply chain shortages. As prices skyrocketed, fake products began to appear, and enterprising criminal gangs even began collecting used masks from landfills; washing and then reselling them as new items until the police finally intervened.[18]

The response of Asian governments to the COVID-19 crisis has varied considerably, ranging from the extremely restrictive measures, which took the form of "National Emergency Decrees" to milder measures that included selective lockdowns and the closure of crowded venues; as well as maintaining social distancing and putting facemask on at all times while in public. Thailand, which was the second country outside of China to report a COVID-19 case, was among the first countries to announce a National Emergency Decree on 26 March 2020. Although Taiwan, Hong Kong, Japan, and South Korea have applied milder restrictive measures, their respective COVID-19 case rates have remained very low. Moreover, Hong Kong's and Taiwan's response to the COVID-19 pandemic occurred very early in this new global health crisis as Hong Kong shares a border with mainland China while many Taiwanese businessmen frequently travel back and forth to the mainland. As such, once COVID-19 "case zero" was confirmed in Wuhan, both Taiwan and Hong Kong undertook immediate action to prevent widespread transmission of this new virus into their own countries.

In summary, the early response of many East Asian countries to confront the new virus through their securitization of COVID-19 appears to be a key factor in Asia's success in effectively managing the pandemic, as these countries encountered only a fraction of the number of reported cases, hospitalizations, and deaths when compared to what happened in the West and other parts of the world.[19] Asian governments, as securitizing actors, have produced directive and declarative speech acts claiming in many ways to demonstrate that the new virus is extremely dangerous. This has resulted in their citizens acquiring the same perception as their government; namely that the COVID-19 virus is an existential threat to state security. Directive and declarative speech acts have been repeated over and over by government' representatives (i.e. the Prime Minister, the Minister of Public Health, the Director of COVID-19 Management Center, etc.) via every media channel, that includes social media, television, radio, posters, etc. These actions have also resulted in the promulgation of national emergency measures that have been arbitrary in nature and which threaten the human security of Asian citizens. Initially, certain Asian governments began the process of securitization as a reaction to the Coronavirus by repeatedly providing the public with information about the dangers of COVID-19. This allowed the government to become legitimated in operating new policies in response to the pandemic as the latter was viewed as a national threat. In fact, every country has securitized this threat and put their own efforts into combating the pandemic with various measures, which include, (a) the screening of travelers, (b) the announcement of a state of emergency (c) the establishment of COVID-19 management centers and (d) the development of a digital platform to support government during the crisis. Some of these measures have been more intrusive than others.

The Screening of Travelers

Reports coming out of China confirming the existence of a new infectious respiratory disease quickly caused concern in several nearby Asian countries. This development prompted them to take measures to securitize the pandemic as a threat to their national security. The easiest and most logical policy was to start screening travelers entering their country; especially visitors coming from China. Thus, certain countries that served as favorite destinations for Chinese tourists (such as Hong Kong, Taiwan, and Thailand,) immediately began to restrict and screen travelers as they entered their countries.

The Establishment of COVID-19 Management Centre

The stated objectives of these management centers were to effectively manage the flow of information as well as report the on-going situation about the COVID-19 crisis, so that the public would know what is currently occurring with respect to the number of COVID-19 cases, hospitalizations, and deaths nationally, as well as any other important information concerning this new viral infection. By providing routine reports and updating citizens about the measures being implemented to control transmission of the COVID-19 virus, the centers hoped to educate the public so that they would have an accurate understanding and awareness of the COVID-19 situation. Most important, apart from establishing a communication link between government and citizens, the management centers also served to facilitate and coordinate central governments and local agencies to control and manage the spread of the virus in each nation. These management centers are referred to differently in each country. For example, in China it is called the Chinese Center for Disease Control and Prevention (CCDC), while in Thailand it is referred to as the Center of COVID-19 Situational Administration (CCSA), and in Taiwan it is the Central Epidemic Command Center (CECC).

The Announcement of States of Emergency

A state of emergency was primarily announced when governments decided that the present situation could potentially get much worse. Although many Asian countries chose to establish a shield against the virus by declaring lockdowns that usually took the form of border closures to prevent external visitors from entering, other countries also announced a state of emergency or even established strict curfews that kept their citizens at home for part or all of the day. Critics have, however, questioned whether the curfews, enacted under the national emergency decrees or strict social distancing measures, were in fact aimed at preventing the domestic transmission of the COVID-19 virus or whether, as in the case of Hong Kong and Thailand, they were put into place as a strategy to prevent domestic political protests against the current governments.[20]

The Development of a Digital Platform

Certain Asian countries, such as Taiwan, South Korea, Singapore, and Thailand, have developed a digital platform, for mobile phones, aimed at helping the government manage their COVID-19 situation. There are two major functions of mobile applications that relate to COVID-19; namely (a) a mobile app that provides information and tracking symptoms[21] and (b) a mobile app that traces users who have interacted with others supposed to be infected with the virus so that the former can learn if they need to undergo quarantine and/or whether or not to closely observe any signs and symptoms that arise. However, the creation of this mobile app can be used to invade the privacy of the users.

Asian countries responded to the novel virus by securitizing the pandemic as a national security issue and applying different measures accordingly. Unfortunately, the securitization, as expressed in the above-mentioned measures, has adversely affected the human security of people living in certain Asian countries, which is obviously in opposition to the notion of improving national security.

Impacts of Securitization on Human Security

The rapid spread of the virus in Europe and the US could certainly give cause for concern for governmental authorities in Asia trying to prevent a similar situation from developing in their own countries. As time went by, there did not appear to be much local transmission of COVID-19 infection in many Asian countries when compared to the very high infection rates witnessed in Western countries; especially those in Europe and the USA. The total number of reported cases when comparing Asia to the West was strikingly different as of March 2021. Thus while the total number of reported cases in certain European countries (e.g. UK, Germany, Italy, and France) were above 3,000,000, while that of the US exceeded 28,000,000, the total number of reported cases in different parts of Asia was very low: Taiwan with less than 1000 cases, Vietnam with 2500 reported cases, Hong Kong with 11,000, and Thailand with approximately 26,000 cases.[22] While other countries were enjoying the new year celebrations, Taiwan had taken action very rapidly since the end of December 2019, launching mobile applications, preparing for a facemask shortage, and starting the screening and monitoring of travelers entering into the country. South Korea and Singapore also developed mobile applications in tracking and tracing their people who were potentially exposed to the COVID-19 virus. In fact, the mobile application played an important role not only in providing information on COVID-19 to citizens, but also effectively helped to physically monitor their citizens or even visitors who entered into the countries. Without massive nationwide lockdowns, or simply by applying select semi-lockdown measures, these countries managed to contain the transmission of the novel virus through a combination of measures, including aggressive testing, tracing via mobile application, or even tracking locations of citizens from credit card usages after obtaining the consent of their citizens.[23] In summary, they were able to avoid a serious COVID-19 crisis from engulfing their society with less disruption to daily life or the national economic wellbeing of the country.

Some countries, worried about their respective public health care delivery system's ability to cope with the pandemic—especially if the virus rapidly spread throughout the countries where the number of doctors, hospital beds, and medical equipment are insufficient to address a nation-wide health crisis of this nature—felt the need to enact stringent laws to deal with this unusual situation.[24] Nevertheless, the success of Asian countries in their securitization of COVID-19 has also resulted in the promulgation of a number of different draconian measures that has paradoxically negatively impacted upon people's freedoms. Some countries' responses to managing the pandemic have adversely impacted human security by impinging on human rights, including civil and political rights as well as social, economic, and cultural rights.

Human security includes "freedom from fear" and "freedom from want."[25] The emphasis on human security was introduced in the global Human Development Report (HDR) in 1944, which has become an important topic of many discussions at the United Nations ever since. The HDR has described human security as seven dimensions including: (1) economic (2) health (3) personal (4) political (5) food (6) environmental and (7) community.[26] Human security is also rooted in the four fundamental freedoms, originally proposed by US President Franklin D. Roosevelt in 1941, including (a) freedom of speech (b) freedom of worship (c) freedom from fear and (d) freedom from want. The four freedoms became not only a "founding stone" of the United Nations in 1945 but also for the drafting of the Universal Declaration of Human Rights (UDHR) in 1948, which focuses on the two scopes of freedom, the freedom from fear and the freedom from want.[27] According to the UDHR, the concept of human security derives from the two covenants on the principles of human rights (The International Covenants on Economic, Social, and Cultural Rights or ICESCR and the International Covenants on Civil and Political Rights or ICCPR). While freedom from fear mainly relates to civil and political rights, freedom from want relates to the social, economic, and cultural rights.[28] Therefore, when COVID-19 hit the Asian region and the governments securitized the pandemic with different measures in order to protect the security and wellbeing of their own citizens—whether in the establishment of COVID-19 centers, screening travelers, restriction of assembly, and development of digital platform—the securitization also had a negative impact on the human security of people living in Asia.

Impact on the Political and Personal Dimension

The securitization of COVID-19 in Asian countries has affected human security problems in the political and personal dimensions, especially with regards to civil rights and political rights under the International Covenant on Civil and Political Rights, which includes rights to liberty and freedom of thought, expression, political participation, peaceful assembly, and right to associate with other.[29]

When investigating the impact of securitization on human security, it becomes apparent that Hong Kong and Thailand have securitized COVID-19 as a tool to prevent the growing political opposition movements from expanding and gaining popularity in their countries.

The early response of closing borders and even the initial lockdown measures made perfect sense, given what was observed in China and the way the Chinese authorities dealt with their problem as reflected in their ability to control the transmission of this new infectious disease, preventing it dramatically and successfully from traveling to and infecting other parts of the country. In China, the government, though criticized for responding too slowly, had implemented a strict lockdown that lasted for 76 days with a 24 h curfew in Wuhan and every city in Hubei province quarantining more than 50 million people. During the strict lockdown, people could not leave their residence except for the purpose of buying necessary supplies with the government's permission and public transportation was completely closed. Moreover, the government also equipped drones everywhere to detect and give warnings to people not wearing masks in public areas. In addition to the strict measures, the Chinese government also set up an effective national system to combat the novel virus, and finally successfully decreased the number of infections to zero in April 2020.[30]

While many countries have admired the way that China has dealt with COVID-19, rapidly and effectively, some have also criticized the strict measures that violate the personal and political human security of Chinese people. In fact, China has been widely attacked for its political regime and authoritarianism for many decades. Chinese people were not allowed to give negative opinions on the government's administration. Moreover, people can use the internet only in a restricted manner with the so-called "Great Firewall of China" monitoring all online activities of citizens. During the COVID-19 crisis, the government not only delayed the state media from publishing news about the novel virus, but also censored related media that was revealing another side of truth to the rest of the world. Articles and video clips showing what really was happening in China published by local news reporters, journalists, bloggers, and youtubers, have been censored and later these people were arrested.[31]

In protecting the nation from COVID-19, the Chinese government has also deployed advanced technological measures in addition to lockdown and media censorship: mobile applications, street cameras, and drone systems. These technological measures have disrupted the privacy of citizens. The government has used facial recognition to record, track, give warnings, and categorize the health status of individuals, whether they need to quarantine or not. People who are not wearing masks in public areas risk getting tickets or letters of warning from their government.

Contrary to China, the government in Hong Kong has responded to COVID-19 differently with more relaxed measures, although still effectively operating in China's shadow. In the case of Hong Kong, the government did not choose to implement a strict lockdown but decided to restrict assembly and control its borders more decisively together with the use of mobile applications and digital wristbands, which could track people undergoing self-quarantine in their residences. The success of Hong Kong in beating the novel virus was evident by May 2020 as new infections had largely been stamped out and no new infected cases had been reported.[32] In fact, many observed that Hong Kong's residents played a crucial role in combating COVID-19, as they had earlier experience from the SARS outbreak and were very alert to the threat of infection. However, it could be said that the way China/Hong Kong securitized the pandemic has also violated the political and personal security of individuals living on the island.

In the case of Hong Kong, the securitization of COVID-19 by the government affected the political participation of the youth in the country. The pro-democracy political movement led mostly by young generations opposing the government efforts to break down the separation agreement between Hong Kong and China were clearly affected by restrictions on the right to assemble. The political demonstrations in Hong Kong that began in the summer of 2019 were put on hold when the first case of COVID in Hong Kong was confirmed on 22 January 2020; the government subsequently implemented a semi-lockdown without the announcement of an emergency decree but with the closure of many public areas, while public transport remained open.

During the pandemic crisis between 2020 and 2021, even though pro-democracy activists in Hong Kong had changed their political movement strategy to be online, many of them were still arrested. Therefore, according to the young protesters, it seemed the government measures had been used as a "golden opportunity" to crackdown on the political movement and keep them from gathering, since those who participated in prohibited groups faced arrests and/or fines up to the amount of $5,000.[33]

A similar situation can be observed in Thailand. The various lockdown measures prevented people from congregating, even in small numbers. Closing schools and universities also disrupted the new political movement as these sites served as public forums to allow different stakeholders to express their views as well as register their dissatisfaction with the current government and its policies. In recent years, Thailand had been trying to reorient itself onto a more conventional political path, ever since the military's coup d'état in May 2014. The latest national elections, that supposedly would return the country to democracy, only took place in the latter part of 2018 and this effort did not satisfy many citizens as the new prime minister, and leader of the new government was the same person who had led the military coup in 2014. In general, the Thai government has consistently enforced censorship in the media if there is any content related to the monarchy, military rule, or issues considered to be sensitive to national security.[34] Moreover, the government usually sends officers to observe academic seminars and public forums; especially those dealing with human rights and democracy.[35]

The arrival of the COVID-19 virus, in early 2020, coincided with a burgeoning political movement demanding more democratic governance. Hence there is the possibility that some measures ostensibly implemented as public health measures were also used to suppress dissent and public demonstrations. For several months, during mid/late 2020, huge daily rallies composed primarily of students but also other members of Thai society, marched throughout sections of the nation's capital as well as in nearly every other province in the country demanding change. This was the first time that students were able to organize such a widespread political movement to discuss important issues affecting the country as well as their hopes for the future. What started off as a relatively small group of protestors had in a very short period of time burgeoned into a nation-wide call for important changes in the constitution, as well as for modifications in sacred institutions such as the Thai monarchy. It is difficult to determine how this movement would have evolved had it not been for the implementation of renewed state of emergency measures, which made it extremely difficult for the students to continue their fight to promote greater democracy and social justice.

In the case of Thailand, a large segment of this movement represented the views of the younger generation. When the government initially announced the national emergency decrees, most people were extremely worried about this unknown new virus and deeply concerned about their safety and health. As such, they strictly followed the daily health-related instructions announced by government spokespersons. What had begun to be a surging political movement that had emerged before the COVID-19 crisis had simply been put on the backburner as it was not possible to convene meetings or organize public events. Instead, the movement went online while the emergency decrees forced people to remain indoors and focus on dealing with the essentials of daily life from their homes. Some of the lockdown decrees were probably not necessary, from a public health point of view, as there never had been a problem with Thais wearing face masks, and alcohol-based hand sanitizers could be found at nearly every public and private venue. Thais, like their counterparts in other countries that adopted successful COVID-19 prevention strategies, were in general practicing social distancing.

Once the government began to loosen the state of emergency measures, the students led flash mobs once again on a regular basis. This may be a result of schools and universities reopening, which allowed students to leave their homes to study and to mingle with their friends. Schools and campuses became important student assembly points as they began to engage in a much broader range of discussions than merely criticizing the government. As a matter of fact, student-led demonstrations re-emerged as an important political movement and soon gained wide public support.[36] Some observers even commented that without the onset of the second wave of COVID-19 crisis, Thailand might have already changed its government since the political clout of the younger generation was gathering steam all over the country and it looked as if their movement might have some success in promoting political change. Nevertheless, it should be noted that the local elections conducted in November 2020 resulted in none of the Future Forward Party members being elected to provincial level administrative offices. An important question is whether the government was justified in enacting the national emergency decrees to prevent the COVID-19 situation from turning into a true catastrophe in Thailand. Many countries, and outside observers, have praised Thailand's efforts to enact emergency decrees, which in effect put huge segments of its society in lockdown to prevent COVID-19 from raging throughout the country. However, one could query whether some of the measures were enacted more for political than public health reasons.

Impact on the Economic Dimension

The COVID-19 pandemic has created extreme economic problems for nearly every country in the world, including Asian countries. Whether this situation will eventually lead to a global recession or depression is still too early to assess as the pandemic may enter a new wave later. The restriction of assembly and national emergency decrees have nevertheless adversely affected the economic rights of people living in the region, as the lockdown policy prevented many people from leaving their homes and going to work. In the former, all department stores, shopping malls, restaurants, spas, hotels, guest houses, coffee shops, beauty salons/barber shops, and many offices and factories were closed almost immediately after each Asian government gradually announced its lockdown policy starting with China.

These emergency decrees, or lockdown measures in Asian countries have accordingly caused grave hardship on citizens with a large number of businesses declaring bankruptcy or simply closing their doors with little if any hope of reopening in the future. At least 240,000 businesses in China[37] and nearly 8700 in Hong Kong are filing for bankruptcy.[38] The lockdowns especially hurt the hospitality and real estate industries. In the case of tourist destinations like Japan, Hong Kong, and Thailand, which have for many decades been tourist hubs for Asia, Europe and Australia, within a matter of weeks, a vibrant industry catering to millions of foreign and domestic tourists found itself with no customers as hotels, guest houses, restaurants, spas, resorts, and curio shops were closed for business. Nobody had expected such grave actions from the government, and accordingly millions of people all of a sudden found themselves jobless and without any prospects of earning an income. Many companies similarly did not have any cash flow during the lockdown and accordingly found themselves laying off their employees. A large number of people in Asian countries were suddenly unemployed, as some governments had not effectively thought through how they would provide COVID-19 financial assistance to their people adversely affected by the lockdown measures.

According to the International Labor Organization, at least 11 million people across the region were affected by the COVID-19 crisis and fell into poverty in 2020.[39] Almost 260,000 people were unemployed in Hong Kong between August and October 2020,[40] and at least one million workers in Thailand's hospitality sector have been laid off.[41] While COVID-19 affects the unemployment rate and the closure of many companies in Asian countries, it should be noted that some countries in Asia have very little in the way of an economic safety net such as, for example, unemployment insurance. This dire situation forced many individuals and families to flee back from the cities and tourist venues to their homes in the countryside. However, this development was obviously not the best way to contain a highly infectious new communicable disease from spreading across the country. Other less fortunate people had nowhere to go and no idea how they would survive. This situation also affected o the increase in suicide rates in some Asian countries such as India, Japan, Thailand, and the Philippines.[42]

To counter the economic impact of COVID-19, governments in Asian countries have also launched various economic relief measures and stimulus packages to support businesses and individuals in their countries: some have used cash payments while others rolled out grant support measures, and some countries have done both.[43] Nevertheless, as the COVID-19 pandemic created the worst economic and human crisis in global history, the impact of COVID-19 and the way each government in Asia securitized the pandemic has also increased economic inequality, particularly among the vulnerable group of workers in informal sectors who have inadequate employment protection and access to social protection,[44] i.e. daily-wage workers, the poor, elderlies, disabled people, minorities, migrant workers, etc.

These vulnerable people in every country in Asia have been dramatically affected by the governments' securitization of COVID-19. The lockdown measures tend to lower income which push people further into poverty. Among these, the most vulnerable to the impact of COVID-19 are migrant workers, who, with limited access to public services and social protection, are not only treated discriminately but also facing more opportunities to be laid off. In addition, minorities and migrant workers are perceived by local people as "the others" in the society.[45] These "other people" such as Uyghurs in China and Myanmar laborers in Thailand, could be an explicit example showing the more difficulties of minorities and migrant workers' livelihood in relation to the human security impact from COVID-19.

During the COVID-19 crisis, some governments in Asia did not provide assistance to the large number of migrant workers that perform essential jobs in their countries. In the case of China, Uyghurs, in the Xinjiang Uyghur Autonomous Region (XUAR), are among the hardest hit by the COVID-19 outbreak, with camps operated by the Chinese government forcing them to live in deplorable conditions without access to basic social assistance.[46] In the case of Thailand, there are about three or more million migrants working in the country, however, these individuals (most of who originate from neighboring countries especially from Myanmar) similarly found themselves unemployed and without any means of support during the pandemic crisis. Due to the travel restrictions, these people could not return to their homes in Myanmar, Laos, or Cambodia, nor were they entitled to financial assistance provided to Thai citizens. Some were confined to their premises (dormitories, farms, apartments, etc.) often in very crowded conditions. This was just the situation one wished to avoid in order to prevent further COVID-19 transmission, as we saw emerge in late December 2020 in Samut Sakorn province. Moreover, because of the political conflict in Myanmar, it is likely that more people from Myanmar will become migrant workers in Thailand, despite the difficulties they face including a low standard of living and endemic discrimination.

The impact of the disease on human security in India has been particularly devastating. When India was hit by COVID-19 in the first wave, although the Indian government provided immediate economic relief measures by transferring cash to vulnerable people, it was not sufficient to cover the needs of millions already living in poverty and working in the informal sector. The unemployment rate increased while working hours decreased, resulting in lower wages and household incomes. Around 75 million people in India fell into poverty in the year 2020 because of the strict lockdown during the pandemic crisis.[47]

In the case of Thailand, the government had created a digital platform called "Rao Mai Ting Kan." which aimed at providing financial assistance to 4 groups of self-employed citizens including taxi drivers, motorbike riders, tourist guides, and lottery vendors. Unfortunately, the registration process for the "Rao Mai Ting Kan" initiative caused a great deal of confusion as many people adversely affected by the COVID-19 crisis did not receive any assistance while others that had not suffered any economic hardship were able to do so.[48] In fact, the Thai government has spent an enormous amount of money trying to deal with the economic outcome of its emergency measures, but these funds have actually not stimulated the economy and instead became merely "populist policies" aimed at dampening potential dissent from ordinary citizens instead of improving the economic situation for most Thais.[49]

Conclusion

As a case study of the impact of securitizing of COVID on human security, China, Hong Kong, Taiwan, and Thailand could become representatives of Asian countries that took a quick and strict response to the novel coronavirus, partly because these countries are the popular destinations of Chinese tourists while Thailand is the first place outside China where an infectious case was reported in the middle of January 2020. However, the ways in which countries in this region combat the novel virus threat in order to protect their national security have unfortunately had a negative impact on their citizens' rights and livelihood. Asian countries' pandemic management can claim their success only if their governments defend their citizens' freedoms under the human security's principle; the freedom from fear and the freedom from want.

In conclusion, while protecting national security from the Coronavirus, many countries in Asia decided to securitize the pandemic much earlier than other governments in other parts of the world. Up until now, these actions have generally been lauded by outsiders as being highly effective and successful in controlling the spread of the COVID-19 virus, which has ensured that the pandemic was relatively mild in Asia. Nonetheless, Asia's apparent success story may contain several "darker" lesions when it comes to dealing with human security challenges that arose through the securitization of the COVID-19 crisis and the infringements and impact on the socio-economic, political, and civil rights of the citizens.

Notes

1. "WHO Coronavirus (COVID-19) Dashboard," *World Health Organization*, March 17, 2021, https://COVID19.who.int.
2. Marc Siegel, *COVID: The Politics of Fear and the Power of Science* (Tennessee: Turner, 2021).

3. James Gallagher, "Coronavirus Cure: What Progress are We Making on Treatments?," *BBC,* January 13, 2021, https://www.bbc.com/news/health-52354520.
4. "KHN Morning Briefing," *KHN,* March 26, 2020, https://khn.org/morning-breakout/scientists-are-learning-hard-and-valuable-lessons-about-COVID-19-but-many-questions-are-still-unanswered/.
5. Francois Very, and Hussein Solomon, "COVID-19 as a Security Threat: Some Initial Perspectives," *Security Institute for Governance and Leadership in Africa* (July 2020) https://www.ufs.ac.za/docs/default-source/coronavirus-COVID-19-sars-cov-2/brief-7-COVID19.pdf?sfvrsn=a0979721_2.
6. Karen Weintraub, "'Very Inconsistent': 2 Allergic Reactions in the UK to COVID-19 Vaccine Puzzle Researchers," *USA Today News,* September 12, 2020, https://eu.usatoday.com/story/news/health/2020/12/09/COVID-pfizer-vaccine-allergic-reaction-uk/6505867002/.
7. Noah Higgins-Dunn, "Dr. Fauci Says New Data Shows COVID Vaccines Appear to be Less Effective Against Some New Strains," *CNBC,* January 22, 2021, https://www.cnbc.com/2021/01/21/dr-fauci-says-COVID-vaccines-appear-to-be-less-effective-against-some-new-strains.html.
8. Michael Le Page, "Coronavirus: How Well Prepared are Countries for a COVID-19 Pandemic?," *New Scientist,* February 12, 2020, https://www.newscientist.com/article/mg24532693-500-coronavirus-how-well-prepared-are-countries-for-a-COVID-19-pandemic/#ixzz6V71dC1S7.
9. Daniel Dunford et al., "Coronavirus: The World in Lockdown in Maps and Charts," *BBC,* April 7, 2020, https://www.bbc.com/news/world-52103747.
10. Seleman Yusuph Kitenge, "Globalization and the COVID-19 Pandemic: How Is Africa's Economy Impacted?," *Policy Center for the New South Publications* (April 2020) https://www.policycenter.ma/sites/default/files/PB_20-37_Seleman.pdf. p. 2.
11. John Micklethwait, and Adrian Woolridge, *The Wake-Up Call: Why the Pandemic Has Exposed the Weakness of the West and How to Fix It* (New York: Harper Collins, 2020), 2.

12. Lisa Saa, and Kenneth Iwuji, "Coronavirus Disease 2019: A Threat to Global Health," *Southwest Respiratory and Critical Care Chronicles* (May 2020) https://doi.org/10.12746/swrccc.v8i34.673.
13. William Yang, Marwaan Macan-Markar, Akane Okutsu, and Cliff Venzon, "Coronavirus: Economic Contagion Is Already Rippling Through Asia," *Nikkei Asia,* January 29, 2020, https://asia.nikkei.com/Spotlight/The-Big-Story/Coronavirus-Economic-contagion-is-already-rippling-through-Asia.
14. "Coronavirus Disease (COVID-19): Small Public Gatherings," *World Health Organization,* August 6, 2020, https://www.who.int/emergencies/diseases/novel-coronavirus-2019/question-and-answers-hub/q-a-detail/coronavirus-disease-COVID-19-small-public-gatherings.
15. Phusadee Arunmas, Dumrongkiat Mala, and Penchan Charoensuthipan, "Mask Shortage 'Baffling,'" *Bangkok Post,* March 15, 2020, https://www.bangkokpost.com/thailand/special-reports/1878975.
16. "Expat Working in China," interview by S. Sipim, November 15, 2020.
17. Rupert Wingfield-Hayes, "COVID-19: No Lockdown. Plus There Is a Very Old Age Population But Why Does Japan Have a Low Mortality?," *BBC,* July 7, 2020, https://www.bbc.com/thai/international-53307060.
18. "Raid on Junk Shop Suspected of Recycling Used Face Masks," *Thai PBS World,* March 2, 2020, https://www.thaipbsworld.com/raid-on-junk-shop-suspected-of-recycling-used-face-masks/.
19. John Micklethwait, and Adrian Woolridge, *The Wake-Up Call: Why the Pandemic Has Exposed the Weakness of the West and How to Fix It* (New York: Harper Collins, 2020), 145.
20. "World Report 2019: Thailand," *Human Rights Watch,* https://www.hrw.org/world-report/2019/country-chapters/Thailand.; Meenakshi Ganguly, "Sri Lanka Uses Pandemic to Curtail Free Expression," *Human Rights Watch,* April 3, 2020, https://www.hrw.org/news/2020/04/03/sri-lanka-uses-pandemic-curtail-free-expression.
21. "Coronavirus Apps and Dashboard," *WebMD,* 2020, https://www.webmd.com/lung/coronavirus-apps#1.
22. "COVID-19 Coronavirus Pandemic," *Worldometers,* March 19, 2021, https://www.worldometers.info/coronavirus/.

23. Jun Jie Woo, *Capacity Building and Pandemic: Singapore's Response to COVID-19* (Singapore: Palgrave Macmillan, 2020), 70–82.
24. "COVID-19: How You Can Conveniently Help?," *Bangkok Post,* March 26, 2020, https://www.bangkokpost.com/life/social-and-lifestyle/1886775/COVID-19-how-you-can-conveniently-help.
25. David Anderson-Rodgers, and Kerry Crawford, *Human Security: Theory and Action* (London, UK: Rowman & Littlefield, 2018), Kindle Edition.
26. "Human Development Report," *UNDP*, http://hdr.undp.org/sites/default/files/human_security_guidance_note_r-nhdrs.pdf, 2013.
27. *OHCHR*, https://2covenants.ohchr.org/Fundamental-Freedoms.html.
28. David Anderson-Rodgers, and Kerry Crawford, *Human Security: Theory and Action* (London, UK: Rowman & Littlefield, 2018), Kindle Edition. and "Universal Declaration of Human Rights," *United Nations*, https://www.un.org/en/about-us/universal-declaration-of-human-rights.
29. "ICJ Legal Briefing the Implementation of Thailand's Emergency Decree in Response to Protest in 2020," *International Commission of Jurists*, https://www.icj.org/wp-content/uploads/2020/10/Thailand-Protests-Legal-Briefing-2020-ENG.pdf. p. 2.
30. "Coronavirus: China Reports No COVID-19 Deaths for First Time," *BBC*, https://www.bbc.com/news/world-asia-china-52195034, April 7, 2020.
31. "How State Media and Censorship Took on Coronavirus 2020," *BBC*, https://www.bbc.com/news/world-asia-china-55355401, December 29, 2020.
32. Steven Borowiec, "Exits from Coronavirus Lockdown Split 'Wild' West from 'Cautious' East," *Asia Nikke*i, May 27, 2020, https://asia.nikkei.com/Spotlight/The-Big-Story/Exits-from-coronavirus-lockdown-split-wild-West-from-cautious-East.
33. Anne Symson, "Hong Kong Social Distancing Rules for COVID-19: What You Can and Can't Do," *Asia Tatler*, April 28, 2021, https://hk.asiatatler.com/life/hong-kong-social-distancing-covid-19.
34. "World Report 2019: Thailand," *Human Rights Watch*, https://www.hrw.org/world-report/2019/country-chapters/Thailand.

35. "World Report 2019: Thailand," *Human Rights Watch*, https://www.hrw.org/world-report/2019/country-chapters/Thailand.
36. Jonathan Head, "Thai Protests: Tens of Thousands Gather Again in Mass Defiance of Government," *BBC*, October 15, 2020, https://www.bbc.co.uk/news/world-asia-54548988.
37. Jiayun Feng, "More Than 240,000 Chinese Companies Declare Bankruptcy in the First Two Months of 2020," *SUP China*, April 29, 2020, https://supchina.com/2020/04/09/more-than-240000-chinese-companies-declare-bankruptcy-in-the-first-two-months-of-2020/.
38. "Hong Kong's Bankruptcy Filings Hit Four-Year High Amid Pandemic" *Caixin*, January 18, 2021, https://www.caixinglobal.com/2021-01-18/hong-kongs-bankruptcy-filings-hit-four-year-high-amid-pandemic-101652321.html.
39. Rajiv Narayan, "How COVID-19 Has Been Battering Human Rights: An Asia–Pacific Perspective," *Global Asia*, https://www.globalasia.org/v15no2/focus/how-covid-19-has-been-battering-human-rights-an-asia-pacific-perspective_rajiv-narayan, 15, 2, June 2020: 100–106.
40. Research Office Legislative Council Secretariat of Hong Kong, https://www.legco.gov.hk/research-publications/english/2021rb01-challenges-and-economic-impacts-arising-from-coronavirus-disease-2019-20201214-e.pdf, p. 11.
41. Phoonphongphiphat, Apornrat, "COVID Wave Crushes Thailand's Already Hobbled Tourism Sector," *Asia Nikkei*, January 29, 2021, https://asia.nikkei.com/Business/Business-trends/COVID-wave-crushes-Thailand-s-already-hobbled-tourism-sector2.
42. Athira Nortajuddin "Suicide: Thailand's Epidemic in a Pandemic," *The Asean Post*, March 18, 2021, https://theaseanpost.com/article/suicide-thailands-epidemic-pandemic.
43. *UNODC*, https://www.unodc.org/southeastasiaandpacific/en/what-we-do/anti-corruption/topics/covid-19.html.
44. "Social Protection Responses to COVID-19 in Asia and the Pacific: The Story so Far and Future Considerations," *ILO*, August 19, 2020, https://www.ilo.org/wcmsp5/groups/public/---asia/---ro-bangkok/documents/publication/wcms_753550.pdf.
45. *ILO*, August 19, 2020, https://www.ilo.org/asia/publications/WCMS_753550/lang--en/index.htm.

46. Vaishnavi Chaudhry, "The Impact of COVID-19 on Uighur Muslims: An Ignored Crisis," *LSE*, April 23, 2020, https://blogs.lse.ac.uk/humanrights/2020/04/23/the-impact-of-covid-19-on-uighur-muslims-an-ignored-crisis/.
47. Lee, "COVID Pandemic Pushes 75 Million More People into Poverty in India, Study Shows," *CNBC*, March 19, 2021, https://www.cnbc.com/2021/03/19/covid-pandemic-pushes-75-million-more-people-into-poverty-in-india-study.html.
48. "The Government Distributed Money to Help 26 Million People," *ThaiPublica,* May 1, 2020, https://thaipublica.org/2020/05/the-government-distributed-money-to-help-26-million-people/.
49. Usa Khiewrord, and Peter Morrison, "Thailand Needs to Do More to Support Older People from the Impact of the COVID-19 Pandemic," *Relief Web,* July 8, 2020, https://reliefweb.int/report/thailand/thailand-needs-do-more-support-older-people-impact-COVID-19-pandemic.

Bibliography

"CCSA Spokesman Clarifies Threat of Jail for not Using MorChana App." *The Nation Thailand,* January 7, 2021. https://www.nationthailand.com/news/30400869.

"Coronavirus Apps and Dashboard." *WebMD,* 2020. https://www.webmd.com/lung/coronavirus-apps#1.

"Coronavirus Disease (COVID-19): Small Public Gatherings." *World Health Organization,* August 6, 2020. https://www.who.int/emergencies/diseases/novel-coronavirus-2019/question-and-answers-hub/q-a-detail/coronavirus-disease-COVID-19-small-public-gatherings.

"COVID-19 Coronavirus Pandemic." *Worldometers,* March 19, 2021. https://www.worldometers.info/coronavirus/.

"COVID-19: How You Can Conveniently Help?." *Bangkok Post,* March 26, 2020. https://www.bangkokpost.com/life/social-and-lifestyle/1886775/COVID-19-how-you-can-conveniently-help.

"Expat Working in China." Interview by S. Sipim. November 15, 2020.

"KHN Morning Briefing." *KHN,* March 26, 2020. https://khn.org/morning-breakout/scientists-are-learning-hard-and-valuable-lessons-about-COVID-19-but-many-questions-are-still-unanswered/.

"Policy Brief: The Impact of COVID-19 on South-East Asia." *United Nations,* July 2020. https://www.unescap.org/sites/default/d8files/2020-07/SG-Policy-brief-COVID-19-and-South-East-Asia-30-July-2020.pdf.

"Raid on Junk Shop Suspected of Recycling Used Face Masks." *Thai PBS World,* March 2, 2020. https://www.thaipbsworld.com/raid-on-junk-shop-suspected-of-recycling-used-face-masks/.

"The Government Distributed Money to Help 26 Million People." *ThaiPublica,* 1 May, 2020. https://thaipublica.org/2020/05/the-government-distributed-money-to-help-26-million-people/.

"WHO Coronavirus (COVID-19) Dashboard." *World Health Organization,* March 17, 2021. https://COVID19.who.int.

"World Report 2019: Thailand." *Human Rights Watch.* https://www.hrw.org/world-report/2019/country-chapters/Thailand.

Arora, Prasant. "We Stand Together Recently Preparing to Consider Helping 1.7 Million People Who Have Failed to Register." *Thairath,* May 8, 2020. https://www.thairath.co.th/news/business/1860579.

Arunmas, Phusadee, Dumrongkiat Mala, and Penchan Charoensuthipan. "Mask Shortage 'Baffling.'" *Bangkok Post,* March 15, 2020. https://www.bangkokpost.com/thailand/special-reports/1878975.

Dunford, Daniel, Becky Dale, Nassos Stylianou, Ed Lowther, Maryam Ahmed, and Irene de la Torre Arenas. "Coronavirus: The World in Lockdown in Maps and Charts." *BBC,* April 7, 2020. https://www.bbc.com/news/world-52103747.

Gallagher, James. "Coronavirus Cure: What Progress Are We Making on Treatments?." *BBC,* January 13, 2021. https://www.bbc.com/news/health-52354520.

Ganguly, Meenakshi. "Sri Lanka Uses Pandemic to Curtail Free Expression." *Human Rights Watch,* April 3, 2020. https://www.hrw.org/news/2020/04/03/sri-lanka-uses-pandemic-curtail-free-expression.

Graham-Harrison, Emma, and Lily Kuo. "China's Coronavirus Lockdown Strategy: Brutal But Effective." *The Guardian,* March 19, 2020. https://www.theguardian.com/world/2020/mar/19/chinas-coronavirus-lockdown-strategy-brutal-but-effective.

Gunia, Amy. "Thailand's Future Forward Party Has the Support of Young Thais. A Court Could Disband It Entirely." *Time*, January 20, 2020. https://time.com/5756668/thailand-future-forward-party/.

Head, Jonathan. "Thai Protests: Tens of Thousands Gather Again in Mass Defiance of Government." *BBC,* October 15, 2020. https://www.bbc.co.uk/news/world-asia-54548988.

Higgins-Dunn, Noah. "Dr. Fauci Says New Data Shows COVID Vaccines Appear to be Less Effective Against Some New Strains." *CNBC,* January 22,

2021. https://www.cnbc.com/2021/01/21/dr-fauci-says-COVID-vaccines-appear-to-be-less-effective-against-some-new-strains.html.

Khiewrord, Usa, and Peter Morrison. "Thailand Needs to Do More to Support Older People from the Impact of the COVID-19 Pandemic." *Relief Web,* 8 July, 2020. https://reliefweb.int/report/thailand/thailand-needs-do-more-support-older-people-impact-COVID-19-pandemic.

Kitenge, Seleman Yusuph. "Globalization and the COVID-19 Pandemic: How Is Africa's Economy Impacted?." *Policy Center for the New South Publications* (April 2020). https://doi.org/10.13140/RG.2.2.34703.74404.

Le Page, Michael. "Coronavirus: How Well Prepared are Countries for a COVID-19 Pandemic?." *New Scientist,* February 12, 2020. https://www.newscientist.com/article/mg24532693-500-coronavirus-how-well-prepared-are-countries-for-a-COVID-19-pandemic/#ixzz6V71dC1S7.

Micklethwait, John, and Adrian Woolridge. *The Wake-Up Call: Why the Pandemic Has Exposed the Weakness of the West and How to Fix It.* New York: Harper Collins, 2020.

Saa, Lisa, and Kenneth Iwuji. "Coronavirus Disease 2019: A Threat to Global Health." *Southwest Respiratory and Critical Care Chronicles* (May 2020) https://doi.org/10.12746/swrccc.v8i34.673.

Siegel, Marc. *COVID: The Politics of Fear and the Power of Science.* Tennessee: Turner, 2021.

Sinha, Alex. "NSA Surveillance Since 9/11 and the Human Right to Privacy." *Loyola Law Review* (March 2014) https://dspace.loyno.edu/jspui/bitstream/123456789/121/1/Sinha.pdf.

Weintraub, Karen. "'Very inconsistent': 2 Allergic Reactions in the UK to COVID-19 Vaccine Puzzle Researchers." *USA Today News,* September 12, 2020. https://eu.usatoday.com/story/news/health/2020/12/09/COVID-pfizer-vaccine-allergic-reaction-uk/6505867002/.

Wingfield-Hayes, Rupert. "COVID-19: No Lockdown. Plus There Is a Very Old Age Population but Why Does Japan Have a Low Mortality?." *BBC,* July 7, 2020. https://www.bbc.com/thai/international-53307060.

Woo, Jun Jie. *Capacity Building and Pandemic: Singapore's Response to COVID-19.* Singapore: Palgrave Macmillan, 2020.

Yang, William, Marwaan Macan-Markar, Akane Okutsu and Cliff Venzon. "Coronavirus: Economic Contagion Is Already Rippling Through Asia." *Nikkei Asia,* January 29, 2020. https://asia.nikkei.com/Spotlight/The-Big-Story/Coronavirus-Economic-contagion-is-already-rippling-through-Asia.

CHAPTER 8

Europe and the New World Order

Alexandre Vautravers

Introduction

In 2020, the European Union looked like a ship without steam. Without power, it was reduced to hope for favorable currents, a puppet to volatile and contradictory winds and influences, to suffer the blows of the weather and the environment. Part of this is contextual, but some of it is self-inflicted. We will show that this situation is generated by insecurity, but also produces more insecurity, inside and outside of the continent.

The strategic posture of the EU has rarely been as fragmented and closer to irrelevance. Arguing at the outbreak of the COVID-19 epidemic that the health systems were primarily a national prerogative, the Union lost all legitimacy and all levers, both in the community and intergovernmental fields. It was further weakened with the Brexit-saga and internal divisions about the conservative stance of Central/Eastern members of the Union, not to mention divisions on migration issues. Europe has been confused by Macron's political and military bilateral promises to Germany. And it suffers from the weaknesses of Germany's economy and the *fin de regne* of its Chancellor.

A. Vautravers (✉)
Department of Security, Employment and Health (DSES), Geneva, Switzerland

C. Varin (ed.), *Global Security in Times of Covid-19*, New Security Challenges, https://doi.org/10.1007/978-3-030-82230-9_8

To top it off, by taking a moralizing and confrontational stance towards former US President Trump, several Western European leaders alienated their main ally and supporter. The 'rift' in EU–US relations has weakened the Washington Consensus and the international multilateral system, as demonstrated throughout the pandemic and once more at the 2021 G7 meeting. This has at the same time created mixed signals to Russia, with the consequence of exacerbating Putin's hybrid conflicts and influence.

Europe's weakness and lack of direction poses not only questions, it also creates threats—both internal and international. Any strategic void in Europe will naturally be filled. We will examine several possible hypotheses of this Aristotelian maxim.

First, the reasons for this lack of decision and capacities in strategic and defense matters will be explored. Then the chapter will turn to the EU–US relations and their new challenges in the wake of COVID-19. Next, the vulnerability of the EU to external threats, crisis and other factors will be highlighted. And finally, the internal divisions within the EU, some of which have been exacerbated by the recent terrorism, immigration and pandemic waves, will be addressed.

The State of European Defense and Cooperation

Europe's failure to get ahead of the COVID epidemic in 2020 or show any meaningful leadership in the crisis is arguably the result of a long period of diminishing unity and influence. The discourse on the European unification since the 1950s has been largely made up of three arguments: a historical one, a political one and, arguably and more recently, an economic one. The first argument comes from the experiences of the World Wars, the Holocaust, the loss of strategic influence and decolonization. This can be found in many of the speeches of the EU's founding fathers. It is still very much present, to this day, in the pro-European political rhetoric. The second argument is the political idea and hope of peace through cooperation, sharing and interdependence. European construction has taken place in a very empirical fashion, but in a highly idealized manner as well.[1]

The third argument, which may have been pragmatic and functionalist at first, has increasingly become the major argument of the European elite. Since the fall of the Berlin Wall, defense spending and security forces have been substantially reduced. With these reductions however, national European armies have faced increasing challenges—many of them due to reductions of numbers and budgets below a critical mass, creating capacity gaps in the forces and increasing the cost of materiel and infrastructure development, procurement and maintenance. A common defense has therefore conveniently been portrayed as a solution to improve both capacities and economies of scale. However, such economies have yet to materialize, given the many critiques against the development and procurement of 'European' armaments.[2] Is European common defense therefore a utopia? The challenges of a common European defense are many. And until these issues can be resolved, there may only be small, incremental, technical steps in the direction of common defense. These issues include:

First, the European Union project has been built on the ashes of the Second World War. This was at a time of incredible decline and weakness for most European nations. It also took place under the direct threat of the recurrence of war—one in which continental Europe would be a battleground, as it was both divided and subdued. It had no access to nuclear weapons. Finally, both extremist and traditional parties were excluded from the post-war political spectrum. Despite their marginal influence before the War, the 'catholic right' (CDU) and the 'socio-democrats' (SPD) became the main actors of the Bundesrepublik, and still are now. Of course, these two parties may be the two faces of the same coin: capitalism with a conscience and a socialist party accepting private propriety and the market economy. But this coalition is over. The emergence of new forces—in particular the development of neo-Marxist movements, the green parties and the resurgence of communism, not to mention the re-emergence of conservative right, nationalist or sovereigntist parties, have broken a carefully crafted, but somewhat 'politically correct' or 'neutralized' democratic machine.

Second, the European defense construction has been historically bogged down with constitutional issues. Germany's Grundgesetz imposes many limits to the use of its armed forces, while the French Constitution maintains an executive direct-line between the President's finger and the use of force—all the way up to the executive order of a nuclear strike. Several of the member-states are neutral, which challenges the traditional definition of the word, leading to another form of 'muted' or 'proxy' political debate. A more detailed analysis would, without a doubt, list as many issues as there are members in the EU with regards to their respective political straitjackets on the use of force and other matters. The creation of the EU has, arguably, added another switch in the form of the consensus-nature of its intergovernmental organization. The result has been that the only European consensus on the use of military force has been the twelve 'Petersberg missions,' defined in a 1992 Declaration. It is worth noting that these missions—humanitarian and rescue tasks, peace-keeping tasks, crisis management and peace-making—all take place below the threshold of war, because territorial defense remains in the hands of NATO.

Third, neutrality and foreign policy are not the only barriers to mutualized interventions and cooperation. Some European countries have a colonial past, which may sharply contrast with the contemporary foreign policy agenda of some, if not all EU members. This creates caveats, in which former colonial powers may push for interventions and exercise influence over their former protectorates, while others have limited themselves and will not deploy combat troops in their former colonies or areas of influence. These post-colonial relationships have also played out during the crisis, for example at the France-Africa summit in May 2021, meant to crystalize France's sphere of influence on the continent post-COVID.

Fourth, for many of the reasons listed above and then some, such as political or economic interest, in situations of international crisis EU leaders have repeatedly shown substantial disunity. The examples of the 1990s Balkans conflicts, the 2001 call to a Global War on Terror, the peace enforcement operation in Libya in 2011 or in Syria in 2016, or even the 2013 peacekeeping operation in Mali, show how divergent the positions of the EU intergovernmental leadership are, and how quiet the communitarian leadership is, in such cases. This begs the question of an EU strategic position on the Ukrainian conflict, *vis-à-vis* Russia, not to mention *vis-à-vis* the People's Republic of China. In several cases, a clear divide has even appeared between two sides—such as the 'coalition of the willing' after 9/11, the tenants of an Eastern-facing strategy versus those looking towards the Middle East and North Africa (MENA) at the Wales and Warsaw NATO summits of 2014 and 2016. Today, the positions are perhaps even more fragmented. This disunity in the face of external pressures—or crises—has again been visible during the Coronavirus 2019–2020 pandemic, with regards to vaccines distribution, travel regulations and so on, which may be revelatory to some but in view of Europe's history, appears to be an ongoing trend.

Fifth, the mutualization of overseas/projection operations is today challenged. Historically, the 1956 Suez operation 'Musketeer' showed the French and the British that combined or multinational operations had become a necessity, because of their increasingly limited forces and their lack of strategic autonomy. For this reason, 'interoperability' has become a prerequisite and a mantra for equipping, structuring and training military units in Europe and beyond—in both the North Atlantic Treaty Organization (NATO) and the United Nation's Department of Peacekeeping Operations (UN-DPKO). While we have discussed the political and macro issues above, it is evident that on a tactical and technical level, the trend of the two decades has been the search for autonomy, hence the definition of tactical 'modules,' regular training and the creation of standing bi-national or regional military units. A French military author[3] warns that 'the more multinational the military unit, the less likely it will be used.' Proof is in the pudding: the two EU 'battlegroups,' whose denomination is an ironic paradox in itself and were created in 2005, were declared operational two years later... but have yet to see any military action.

Last, the overlap and confusion that exists between NATO and the EU (and formerly, the Western European Union), in effect neutralize the latter and put most of Europe's security in the hands of the former. Different repartition models were tried. The 1992 Petersberg Declaration suggests that the EU handles primarily actions below the threshold of war, while NATO assumes the responsibility of 'defense.' It is perhaps the simplest and most successful model. This repartition also has its drawbacks, given that the EU assumes the more appealing and politically correct 'soft' missions, while NATO—and the US Government—are left with the 'harder' issues to resolve.[4]

To sum up, this overlap has little military or technical justification. It exists because of the inability to form a consensus, the lack of political courage and commitment, the lack of strategic autonomy, the subcritical nature of most European armies—so well illustrated by the term 'Bonsai armies.'[5] Furthermore, 'double dipping' as this practice has become known in the military, is a convenient political excuse, which has allowed governments to lower defense budgets and security preparedness throughout Europe. Some of the same argumentation has allowed borrowing and investment 'leveraging' to replace some of the fundamentals of our economies. Unfortunately, as we have experienced during the 2008–2010 economic crises, or more recently during the Coronavirus pandemic, the 'pooling and sharing' paradigm makes good political and economic sense only in peacetime. But owning a section of a shared blanket, falls uncomfortably short of having one in the closet when you need it.

A Growing Atlantic Rift and the Rise of Russia and China

The West has been, for the last century, a successful alliance between 'paradise' and 'power.' Robert Kagan's visionary book[6] explains how post-1945 Western Europe has turned away from war. It also explains how the alliance between 'soft' and 'hard' power, conviction and coercion, foreign investment and the imposition of rules and 'like-mindedness' have been so successful.

The same book, when discussing the relationship between the Western allies, is also original in designating it as a 'rift.' The term is not only correct in its geographical definition, given that the North American and Eurasian continental plates separate over the Mid-Atlantic ridge. More so, they are actually growing apart. And this fact as well, may also apply to transatlantic political relations.

Interestingly, the 2004 volume argued that the reason for this distancing was the increasing attention of the US towards the economic growth of Japan and the 'Asian Tigers.' Kagan warned that a strategic shift in focus from an Atlantic-based partnership to a Pacific-focused one, could strain and jeopardize the Western alliance. As Harold MacKinder could have argued, the geopolitical positioning of the US is both an opportunity as a global sea power, but also a curse in having to decide between the West and the East. Whereas Russia's geopolitical location has made it able to reach both seas, the House of Romanov and the battle of the Tsushima straits (1905) have long decided its European inclination. Meanwhile, the democratic decentralization of services, politics and the economy in the US, may have cultivated internal uncertainties and tensions, as well as differing worldviews on the West and the East coasts.

We can argue that the concept of the Atlantic rift describes well the present situation between the US and Western Europe, despite the fact that the economic driver today is China's economy, and no longer its neighbors. In addition, Kagan imagined a situation in which the US would focus on Asia in order to develop trade and partnerships, not in a situation where the US armed forces would need to perform an action of 'rebalancing' against a new competitor or foe.

Despite these differences between the vision and reality, we believe that a shift in focus of the US political leadership from Europe and the USSR or Russia, to the Asia–Pacific and China, accelerates the incomprehension, the division, the search for autonomy, and the strategic decline of

Europe. Indeed, while there still are possibilities for strategic cooperation on the European continent, in the MENA region and in Africa, the capabilities for such cooperation decrease with the combined augmentation of distance and costs. The deployment of NATO forces to the Balkans in 1995, by train, road or sea, is evidently cheaper than the strategic projection of forces by sea and air to the Persian Gulf in 2003, which in turn is less than half the price of the projection by air, sea and road to Afghanistan since 2001.[7] Notwithstanding inflation or political will, European nations are able to cooperate with the US forces when close to their bases. But their ability to do so decreases with distance and time.

The American policy refocusing on Russia and on NATO, under Presidents Obama and Trump, may therefore reassure their European security partners. Just like the choice of a fixed, land-based anti-missile defense installed in Eastern Europe was able to reassure these partners, much more than a naval-based, flexible and mobile system, which can be deployed and activated where and when the US commander-in-chief decides it—not to mention under what conditions, and at what cost to the US partner.

The liberty with which European leaders have criticized the Trump administration may be a passing epiphenomenon, one which focuses on the tone and the temporary, rather than the substance and long term. But the possibility that this may have caused deeper, and longer-lasting damage, must also be taken into consideration. Indeed, after the usual post-electoral excitement and traditional Western European race to Washington D.C. in early 2017, some of the most enthusiastic heads of state have also cooled down the quickest. After two memorable handshake moments in July and August 2017, Macron's April 2018 visit to Washington was the moment of a very public *retournement de veste* and the December 2019 NATO meeting shows how quickly the relationship has cooled down. The breakthrough positions by Macron on European defense mutualization, including France's nuclear arsenal, as well as the opening of discussions between Paris and Berlin regarding a possible future EU seat at the United Nations Security Council, have alienated Trump.

Conflict and Insecurity in a Multipolar World

Saying that our world is changing, becoming more multipolar, with volatile and emerging risks, has become a *lieu commun* in strategic documents, the world over. But it is perhaps useful to recall some of the major trends that have developed in the last decades.

Although it may be challenging and unpopular, we must accept that the traditional dialectic of 'peace' and 'war' is no longer sufficient to describe the complex dynamics between states and a number of non-state actors. The two definitions of international and non-international armed conflict, in the fourth Geneva Convention of 1949, give us a false sense of comprehension of these phenomena. They blind us, as well, to the hybridity of present conflicts, which may be due to the proximity or the influence of an armed conflict on neighboring areas or countries that host diasporas from the conflict regions, or political tensions due to foreign policy decisions, to intervene or not, unilaterally or in a coalition. Today, certain regions in conflict areas are safer than certain districts or regions in countries at peace. Some places officially in conflict are among the most praised touristic destinations. And we know that military action by the P5 may not be sanctioned by the UN—or indeed need to be.

The concept of 'soft power' coined in the 1990s by Joseph Nye[8] is now dead in the water.[9] This was an appealing theory, especially to the strategists of the Clinton presidential campaign of 1992 who were looking for a way to reduce defense spending without diminishing the global influence of the US. In practice however, the theory crashed twice in 1995 already, when two genocides were declared, in Rwanda and Bosnia & Herzegovina. The limits of 'soft power' became extremely apparent, especially in the face of leaders who were prepared to murder or have their own population murdered. This reality sprang in the face of those who denied it the strongest. It explains why the now renamed 'liberal interventionists'—chief among whom, some of the most influential members of the Clinton administration—became so prone to intervene under both the Republican and Democratic presidents who followed. While the use of force was limited by the threat of escalation and nuclear release under the Cold War, both the unipolar and the multipolar configurations that followed, have seen a 'banalization of the use of force in international relations.'[10]

Today, conflicts and insecurity are characterized by the multiplication of actors and the absence of reference or a proper international standard.

Some of these actors may be non-governmental organizations, but they may also be supranational or international. Conflicts of the fourth generation, after the end of the Cold War, are characterized by the presence of 'spoilers' [11] or parties to the conflict whose objective is not victory or peace, but who fight for the continuation of conflict. This notion has now percolated into the alliances, which may be interest—or objective-oriented, often motivated by reciprocal advantages, limited in time or by national political circumstances. All of this results in conundrums for which Syria's civil war may be a dangerous blueprint: officially, all of the states are acting at the request of one or more parties to the conflict on the ground, and their stated objective is the end of the fighting as well as the unity of the country. But in practice, we see that the objective 'endstate' of each of these international actors is different, sometimes conflictual. Given that all of these actors are part of one or more coalitions, conflicts today may ironically take place between self-proclaimed allies, in truth a form of geopolitical competition, rather than between enemies who have long ago renounced the use of force.

The question of sovereignty versus the right to interfere and the responsibility to protect is not resolved. But whereas the latter was allowed to become the paradigm of the 1990s in the West at least, today's growing influence of Russia and China in world affairs and in the UN Security Council has imposed a much more restrictive interpretation of R2P.

Over half a century of academic research and publication has not managed to find a single causality for conflicts. While the dominant explanation during the Cold War was political, the 'flat' world of the 1990s has tried to find the sources of war in poverty and competition for scarce resources. The fact that no single explanation is sufficient is probably closer to the truth. Sudden economic or political changes and fragile states—such as the fall of the Berlin Wall, but also the development of national or international jihadism—are probably a more suitable consensus on the causes of conflicts. The result is that many conflicts take place in failed states or regions. This, in turn, makes it harder to go back to a functional and sustainable peace, which may never have existed before.

These may take much longer to reconstruct than the buildings and crops destroyed by the shells and bullets of a century ago. We understand that a third of the conflicts today have started over thirty years ago. Such 'protracted' conflicts may be impossible to resolve with our conventional and legal means. 'Negative peace' may be easier to reach than Justice for all. And our contemporary tendency to judge the past, judge our ancestors, claim reparations for their losses, has made the resolution process perhaps more important and sustainable, than the fleeting dream of a hypothetical 'endstate'—if such a jargon still means anything.

European Disintegration in the Wake of COVID-19

On 23 June 2016, the UK EU referendum startled not only the British elites and Government, but all EU countries. A spin doctor's dream name—Brexit—so perfectly epitomized the coming chapter of the European integration. Indeed, this issue became so fundamental that the political attention and agendas have turned from construction to introspection, all matters ceasing.

The significant and strategic issues of the day have been instantly adjourned. The issue of terrorism, along with the actions in Libya and Syria, have been dropped, perhaps with a sigh of relief. The 'migrant crisis' is answered with denial and political correctness. The tensions deriving from it have received benign neglect. There are reactions only to the critiques, labeled as problem makers and egoists.

Germany and France have pursued their respective welcome policies and their Dublin agenda. Italy has tried to tame the waves. Central and Eastern European countries have erected walls. EU leaders have acted as if 'crisis management' had become the new political doctrine. The old adage '*gouverner c'est prévoir*' has definitely become '*ringard*.'

We have listed, above, historical reasons for the disunity of the EU. In the last few years, however, the discontinuity has focused on three main issues: the relationship with the US, a common or autonomous defense architecture as well as defense spending, the management of immigration from the South and its contested links with integration or fragmentation and terrorism respectively. While the first set of issues require the revisiting of the Constitutional Treaties, the latter refer to the Dublin and Schengen agreements, which pre-existed the EU. The frustration with the Dublin agreements and the management of mass immigration from North Africa and through Turkey, has alienated several Central European Governments. The threat of sanctions and the 'Alleingang' of Poland, the Czech Republic and progressively of the Visegrad countries, has already weakened the EU internally.

While each of these issues could potentially have open the way to institutional reforms within the Union and encourage an increase in centralization and prerogatives in the Community-system, the exact opposite has occurred. The context of Brexit and, more humbly, the renegotiations of the EU-Swiss 'bilateral' negotiations—most notably stumbling on the issues of freedom of movement and immigration—has led to a shutdown of all discussion on EU reform. While this gives the EU negotiators a temporary backing, all of these unsettled issues are piling up and will make the opening of future discussions more difficult.

Economic shocks and the recession have tested the core values and institutions of the EU. So far, these have well resisted—provided the main creditors continue to accept the financial burden, and provided the net debtors remember their place, when times come to vote.

COVID-19 has been a stress test for the EU in at least three ways. Firstly, the silence of the Commission on the pandemic, stating that healthcare is a national issue. This has not only surprised the public; it has upset both pro- and anti-Union partisans. Secondly, the lack of initiative and of clarity from the Commission has allowed tensions and competition to settle in between European member states. There have been cases of seizure of healthcare materials, the blocking of aircraft on national territory, accusations of blackmail, miscommunication and misinformation, mismatches of unilaterally decided sanitary measures, the closing of international, but also of internal borders between Schengen partners, and so forth.

European governments are accused of regularly producing reports, analyses, recommendations, but not acting upon them. The question of strategic reserves and supply dependencies, for example, shows how little action and budget has been invested in these areas.[12] The same, of course, holds true in the area of defense and security. While all NATO countries have pledged to devote two percent of the GDP to defense, only five have done so to this day. Germany in 2016 announced that it would honor its commitment... but gradually, and it will only reach this target in ten years.

Finally, after having taken an extremely lenient and cooperative approach with many of its partners and members, keeping to a 'soft' approach as noted before, the EU Commission and Council have gradually taken a tougher and tougher stance on political issues, such as enlargement, political and economic convergence criteria, bilateral agreements, in particular with regards to Turkey and other countries' adhesion requests, the negotiations and treatment of the UK Government in the context of Brexit, the treatment of the Swiss negotiators during the same period, to list a few cases.

This novel and harder stance naturally feeds into the Eurosceptic discourse. By not addressing these issues, it allows tensions to grow within the Union, between the member states and now, between groups of member states. The lack of clarity and process on issues such as Brexit, or Catalonia's separatism, echo into a process of political fragmentation of the EU and as long as there is no project, no objective, no economic incentive, this fragmentation process may be slow, but it is unchallenged. Worse, if countries outside of the EU show better balance sheets, and if they are better able to tackle issues such as migration or the pandemic, the EU may lose even more credit among the public, and may become even less representative and less unitary.

Conclusion

Has the Coronavirus pandemic changed the global balance of power? Not fundamentally, but it has accelerated the changes, made them more visible, and it may also have upset the multilateral system in the process. Some authors have called it an 'accelerator of conflicts.'[13] This bold and provocative title finds little in the way of proof and no demonstration, however.

It seems the most significant controversy, and the one that may produce the greatest changes in the long run, is the realization of Europe's de-industrialization and its dependency towards Chinese production. It will take some time to verify if the EU and its member's stance towards the People's Republic is affected by the crisis. Alas, it is possible however, that 're-industrialization,' 'reserves' or 'strategic autonomy'[14] may remain empty words—just as 'common defense,' 'European procurement' and 'battlegroups' still sound hollow in the EU's security rhetoric.

Russia has indeed renewed its aircraft inventory around the Western concept of high performance 'multirole' aircraft; on land, it has developed and introduced new families of light armored wheeled vehicles, for low-threat and low-intensity operations and in order to increase strategic mobility. Russia has also turned many of its divisions into a tactical organization closely resembling NATO's brigade system. The professionalization of its cadre is now the norm. It maintains its strategic forces in high readiness and at high cost.

Whereas the development of Russia's military capabilities has focused on a symmetric response to the US and NATO forces or capabilities,[15] China's military developments have taken another path. Beijing's efforts have, in the past three decades, centered upon the modernization of its air defenses and fighters, the development of new destroyers and anti-ship cruise missiles for the purpose of sea denial, and investment into many types of systems for export purposes. While clearly targeting US weapon systems, its forces and its allies, these efforts still fall short of assuming a clear and deliberate defense posture or area of influence in Asia. The construction of the People's Liberation Army's two aircraft carriers and a further four units, will not be able to challenge the US and its allies' sea power for a while longer.

Despite China's military weaknesses or shortcomings, it can be argued that it poses more of a strategic threat to US interests than Russia ever will.[16] It is however important, for the Western Alliance to be maintained, that Russia remains the number one opposition in the US Defense posture. It is also essential for Russia to receive this form of recognition. This reassures public opinion, in the West and in the East as well. And it stabilizes policies. This can be viewed as a form of Clausewitzian 'true war' for the purposes of the respective opinion and interests of all parties. It also makes a confrontation unlikely.

All this time, no one really wants or can imagine a 'true war' between the US and China. Such a denial encourages the paradoxes already mentioned: we may have more interests in common with our 'enemies,' while we may engage in competition and struggle, even conflict, with our closest 'allies.'

Those who look forward to a brighter future will cite Joe Biden's election in the US and the resuming of multilateral diplomacy, the pharmaceutical solution and potential resolution to the COVID-19 crisis. While idealists hope, ideologues believe. They may argue that the economic slowdown is a sign that the environment can be preserved; they may see a sign of the end of entrepreneurial capitalism. One may even think wishfully that international organizations, or the EU, may rise up to the challenge and become stronger as a result of it.

The realists will argue that none of these hopes have materialized. And in fact, the silence and absence of the EU in the times of COVID can be added to a list of previous failures in the face of danger or necessity. When the health crisis will have been resolved, the world will likely be more fragmented globally, and more focused on its national policies and economic interests.

Notes

1. René Schwok, *La construction européenne contribue-t-elle à la paix?* (Lausanne: EPFL Press, 2016).
2. The illustrations and publications on the failure, the issues or the higher-than-expected costs of multinational armament programs are many, ranging from the case of the distinction of France from the European Multi-Role Combat Aircraft (MRCA) Tornado program in the late 1970s and the Eurofighter in the 1990s, the stubborn reluctance of the British Government and armed forces to trade in their Chieftain and Challenger tanks for a common solution, the embarrassment of the Airbus A400M program, or the competing frigate/destroyer programs…

   For the sake of concision, we will singularly point to: Comptroller and Auditor General, "Ministry of Defence: Management of the Typhoon Project," *National Audit Office*, March 2, 2011, https://www.nao.org.uk/wp-content/uploads/2011/03/1011755.pdf, 28–33.
3. Michel Goya, French Colonel (ret.) and author.
4. Alexandre Vautravers, "La Défense européenne: divisions et perspectives," in *Quelles perspectives géopolitiques pour l'Europe?*, ed. Gyula Csurgai (Genève: L'Âge d'Homme, 2004); Alexandre Vautravers, "L'Europe au Coeur des choix stratégiques," in *Quel avenir pour l'OTAN?*, ed. Pierre Pascallon (Paris: L'Harmattan, 2007).
5. Christian Mölling, "Europe without Defence," *SWP-Aktuell* no. 56. (2011). https://www.swp-berlin.org/fileadmin/contents/products/comments/2011C38_mlg_ks.pdf.
6. Robert Kagan, *Of Paradise and Power: America and Europe in the New World Order* (New York: Vintage, 2004).
7. Linda Bilmes and Joseph Stiglitz, *The Three Trillion Dollar War* (New York: W.W. Norton, 2008).
8. Joseph Nye, *Soft Power: The Means to Success in World Politics* (New York: Ingram, 2005).
9. Alexandre Vautravers, "El poder blando es papel mojado," *el Orden Mundial en el S. XXI,* May 12, 2017, https://elordenmundial.com/el-poder-blando-es-papel-mojado/. Accessed 19 September 2020.

10. "Rapport sur la politique de sécurité de la Suisse (RAPOLSEC)," *Département de la Défense, de la Protection de la population et des sports (DDPS)*, 2016.
11. Rupert Smith. *The Utility of Force: The Art of War in the Modern World* (London: Penguin Books, 2005).
12. Olivier Zajec, "Prospective de défense: 'Prévoir ne suffit plus," *Défense et sécurité internationales (DSI)* no. 147, (May–June 2020), 18–19.
13. Holger Alish, and Stephan Maninger, "Corona als Konfliktbeschleuniger? Realistische Implikationen im Kontext der globalen sino-amerikanischen Rivalität," *Österreischiche Militärzeitschrift (ÖMZ)*, no. 4 (2020): 419–427.
14. Charles Michel, President of the E.U. Council. Cited in: Delphine Deschaux-Dutard, "La pandémie de COVID-19 aura-t-elle raison de la défense européenne?," *Défense et sécurité internationales (DSI)*, no. 148, (July–August 2020). 40–41.
15. Mark Galeotti, *The Modern Russian Army 1992–2016* (Oxford: Osprey, 2017).
16. Holger Alish, and Stephan Maninger, "Corona als Konfliktbeschleuniger? Realistische Implikationen im Kontext der globalen sino-amerikanischen Rivalität," *Österreischiche Militärzeitschrift (ÖMZ)*, no. 4 (2020): 419–427.

Bibliography

"Rapport sur la politique de sécurité de la Suisse (RAPOLSEC)." *Département de la Défense, de la Protection de la population et des sports (DDPS)*. 2016.

Alish, Holger, and Stephan Maninger. "Corona als Konfliktbeschleuniger? Realistische Implikationen im Kontext der globalen sino-amerikanischen Rivalität." *Österreischiche Militärzeitschrift (ÖMZ)*, no. 4 (2020): 419–427.

Bilmes, Linda, and Joseph Stiglitz. *The Three Trillion Dollar War.* New York: W.W. Norton, 2008.

Comptroller and Auditor General. "Ministry of Defence: Management of the Typhoon Project." *National Audit Office*, March 2, 2011. https://www.nao.org.uk/wp-content/uploads/2011/03/1011755.pdf, 28–33.

Deschaux-Dutard, Delphine. "La pandémie de COVID-19 aura-t-elle raison de la défense européenne?." *Défense et sécurité internationales* (DSI) no. 148 (July–August 2020): 40–41.

Galeotti, Mark. *The Modern Russian Army 1992–2016*. Oxford: Osprey, 2017.

Kagan, Robert. *Of Paradise and Power: America and Europe in the New World Order*. New York: Vintage, 2004.

Mölling, Christian. "Europe without Defence." *SWP-Aktuell* no. 56. (2011). https://www.swp-berlin.org/fileadmin/contents/products/comments/2011C38_mlg_ks.pdf.

Nye, Joseph. *Soft Power: The Means to Success in World Politics*. New York: Ingram, 2005.

Schwok, René. *La construction européenne contribue-t-elle à la paix?*. Lausanne: EPFL Press, 2016.

Smith, Rupert. *The Utility of Force: The Art of War in the Modern World*. London: Penguin Books, 2005.

Vautravers, Alexandre. "El poder blando es papel mojado." *el Orden Mundial en el S. XXI,* May 12, 2017. https://elordenmundial.com/el-poder-blando-es-papel-mojado.

Vautravers, Alexandre. "L'Europe au Coeur des choix stratégiques." in *Quel avenir pour l'OTAN?,* edited by Pierre Pascallon. Paris: L'Harmattan, 2007.

Vautravers, Alexandre. "La Défense européenne: Divisions et perspectives." In *Quelles perspectives géopolitiques pour l'Europe?*, edited by Gyula Csurgai. Genève: L'Âge d'Homme, 2004.

Zajec, Olivier. "Prospective de défense: 'Prévoir ne suffit plus." *Défense et sécurité internationales (DSI)* no. 147, (May–June 2020). 18–19.

CHAPTER 9

The Social Contract and Civil Unrest: The Tenuous Balance Between Freedom and Security

George E. Richards

Introduction

Extremism is the nursemaid of violence. In the crucible of time and ecology of space, it nestles a cradle of discontent where animosity mutates into hate with that hate, then metamorphosing into a legacy of brutality.

When hindsight permits, this past year may well serve as an allegorical representation of the failure of societies to contain the dissatisfaction of certain citizens who believe the systems of social order, both formal and informal, continue to both marginalize and victimize them. An analogy often used to describe the setting of race relations in the United States has been that of a tea kettle. A kettle is designed to contain boiling water; that is its purpose. Likewise, a healthy society should contain and curb

G. E. Richards (✉)
Edinboro University, Edinboro, PA, USA
e-mail: grichards@edinboro.edu

PROWIBO Online, London, UK

C. Varin (ed.), *Global Security in Times of Covid-19*, New Security Challenges, https://doi.org/10.1007/978-3-030-82230-9_9

fractious elements within it. When the pressure inside a kettle is too great, the roiling steam seeks a violent escape. The same is true for any society when the toll one segment experiences becomes too great to bear. The pressure within erupts when they simply cannot take anymore.

Global Considerations

Civil unrest has not been limited in recent years to any particular country's geographic borders. Across the globe, there was a confluence of conflict marked by extremism and violence. In 2019, 47 jurisdictions witnessed a growth in the intensity of protests, which carried over into 2020. Protests were commonplace in locations as diverse as Belarus, Hong Kong, Nigeria, Sudan, and Lebanon, serving as precursors to those dividing citizens and classes in the United States.

As 2020 began, civil unrest was quickly becoming a global rule, rather than the exception. Variables influencing protests could be limited in number or a combination of several. The four most prevalent were:

- Racial Discrimination,
- COVID-19,
- Economic Downturn/Stagnation, and
- Political Oppression.

Belarus

There have been ongoing political protests in Belarus since late May 2020. The impetus for these has been the mass disapproval of President Alexander Lukashenko's authoritarian regime. This series of protests, the largest in Belarusian history, were the result of the 2020 presidential election that Lukashenko, seeking his sixth term in office, ostensibly won. On 9 August 2020, Lukashenko claimed victory. His main challenger, Svetlana Tsikhanouskaya, rejected the incumbent's claims of victory as falsified, stating she had garnered 60% to 70% of the popular vote. A factor contributing to Lukashenko's lack of popularity had much to do with his stance regarding the COVID-19 pandemic, which he regarded as not being a serious threat. It was at this time the protests intensified.[1]

Five days after the election, Tsikhanouskaya announced the creation of the Coordination Council. Membership in the council was granted to all

Belarusians who believed Lukashenko's election was bogus. The Coordination Council issued a ukase to the president to order the government to cease all oppression, free detainees, and leave the office by 25 October 2020. Lukashenko did not comply. Subsequently national strikes began the day after. In late September, the European Union (EU) published a statement denying the legitimacy of the election while calling for a new one. Those protesting have been met with violence by government forces. The United Nations (UN) Human Rights Office claims over 450 detainees have been subjected to torture and violence. Sexual abuse and rape were also claimed to be commonplace in detention centers.[2]

Chile

Recent protests in Chile, known there as *estollido social* or *social outburst*, were characterized by violent rioting and mass demonstrations that began in October 2019. Originating in Santiago, the protests turned to rioting and quickly spread to other major urban centers. Initially, these were protests against increases in subway fares in Santiago. However, the ire of protesters was also fueled by perceptions of government corruption, increases in the cost of living, and growing privatization of services.[3]

On 18 October 2019, groups began vandalizing sections of Santiago's infrastructure. This included burning down 17 subway stations with 81 being damaged.[4] President Sebastián Piñera quickly declared a state of emergency at which time Chilean Army troops were mobilized to control crowds to stem mob violence and looting. It is estimated roughly 3.5 billion dollars in damage to property was done and over 300,000 jobs lost.[5]

In the best of times, the economic conditions of Chileans can be described as meager. The COVID-19 pandemic, coupled with the aforementioned incendiary conditions, served to further magnify these circumstances and the confrontations between protesters and law enforcement. During protests over lack of food and other basic necessities, police fired tear gas rounds to disperse the crowds. These conditions have led to a continuous circle of violence. "It's getting worse," said Ana Piquer, executive director of Amnesty International Chile. "More people are out of work, more people are protesting, so there is more repression. It's a very direct relation."[6]

China

It is estimated over a million people marched in the streets of Hong Kong on 9 June 2019 protesting the Chinese government's proposed law allowing extraditions to the mainland. One particular concern for Hong Kong residents was that they would be subject to the Chinese legal system. Although this march was mostly peaceful, there were some limited clashes with police officers. However, three days later, when protesters blocked a major highway in the city, police responded directly by firing tear gas canisters into the crowd. This police reaction may have broken up that demonstration, but their response is credited with contributing to a larger march that saw in excess of two million taking to the streets a few days later. This was followed by protesters breaking into the legislative chambers on 1 July with sporadic outbreaks of confrontation and violence continuing throughout the Fall.

The protests continued even though the proposed extradition legislation was withdrawn in September. The marches were continually fueled by calls for a democratic Hong Kong. New Year's Day 2020 was marked with more protests with demonstrators forming human chains stretching for miles through the downtown shopping district. This, too, resulted in clashes between protesters and police[7] which have been sporadically occurring since then.

Unlike other protests, those in Hong Kong during 2019 and 2020 have been described as "leaderless".[8] Organic in nature, they have cropped up with relatively little overall planning. If there is an identifying philosophical perspective at work in articulating the tactical aspects of the protests, it is Bruce Lee's "Be Like Water" which characterizes the flowing and shapeless organization of these protests. This approach has stymied law enforcement due to a lack of ability to gather intelligence.

France

In early December 2020, what began as a peaceful demonstration in Paris against COVID-legislation considered by some to be an assault on civil liberties degenerated into a riot. Protestors, many of whom were youths, committed arson, smashed shop windows, and hurled rocks and Molotov cocktails at police. Officers of the Préfecture de Police de Paris (Paris Police Prefecture) responded as police are often expected to do in situations such as these: with water cannons and tear gas. "France is facing a number of explosive factors—a bitterly contested law, a debate over police violence, fears of terrorism after the beheading of a school teacher and the ongoing COVID-19 crisis—combining to provide what one commentator called 'the wood, the petrol and the matches' to set the country alight."[9]

Russia

Responses to the arrest of opposition leader Alexei Navalny and the perceived excesses of President Vladimir Putin led to protests in nearly 200 towns across Russia in 2021.[10] Beginning on 23 January 2021, an estimated 40,000 people gathered to protest in Moscow. While not as large, similar protests occurred in St. Petersburg, Perm, and Yekaterinburg. As a result, some 4,000 people were detained.[11]

On 4 February 2021, Navalny's Chief of Staff announced there were no protests planned in the immediate future as the focus of Navalny supporters needed to be concentrated on the coming parliamentary elections. Yet this changed in mid-April as Navalny's office released a statement calling for new protests in the wake of the imprisoned Navalny's deteriorating health.[12] Concerned for his well-being, Navalny supporters started to organize and take to the streets again. Protests against the Putin administration's treatment of Navalny were not limited to the former Soviet Union. Support grew internationally with protests in Australia, Israel, Italy, Serbia, the United Kingdom, and the United States.

The United Kingdom

The United Kingdom also saw protests, some of which did take violent turns. For the most part, these protests were peaceful in nature. Black Lives Matter (BLM) protests took place in June 2020 in London, Coventry, and Newcastle. While no violence took place, these were in direct violation of Coronavirus lockdown rules and government warnings against assembly.[13] However, bands of what were thought to be right-wing groups episodically clashed with police and other groups with some degree of violence during this same time period.[14] London Metropolitan Police also found themselves under pressure for charges of excessive force during a vigil for a woman a police officer was accused of murdering. During the March 2021 protest, police were seen physically engaging with the crowd with woman pinned to the ground by officers. Officials later stated the force was necessary as the crowd was violating public order and not following regulations in place due to COVID-19.[15]

The United States

As I will discuss later in this chapter, protests against racial discrimination at the hands of police were commonplace in the United States in 2020. The factors that fed civil unrest in the United States were generally limited to Black Lives Matter and COVID-19. With one exception, it was the issue of race that fueled the most vociferous protests and civil unrest during this pivotal year. "… the United States finds itself in a unique position with levels of social unrest not experienced since the 1960s."[16] The aforementioned exception was the storming of the United States Capitol Building considered to be one of the most catastrophic breakdowns of security in American history.

On 6 January 2021, supporters of President Donald Trump stormed the Capitol Building protesting the election of former Vice-President Biden. Unlike the "leaderless" protests in Hong Kong, this protest, quickly turning into a riot, had been carefully planned. Various social media platforms were used to coordinate groups of what has been described as being made up of white supremacists and militia adherents. These groups, organized by what Beam referred to as "leaderless resistance," have traditionally been organized along the lines of cells that restrict interaction with outsiders. The ability to coordinate these "cells" was a significant logistical and technological feat.[17]

Congress, in a joint session, had gathered to count the electoral votes that cemented Biden's victory over Trump.[18] Earlier that day in a park near the White House, President Trump reiterated his claims of election irregularities before a crowd of his supporters. The president rhetorically threw gasoline on the fire of political suspicion when he stated, "If you don't fight like hell, you're not going to have a country anymore."[19]

During Trump's speech, certain members of the crowd started making their way towards the Capitol Building. The United States Capitol Police had a long-standing plan in place for how to deal with peaceful protests. However, peace was not what they were confronted with as thousands of Trump supporters soon swarmed the steps of the houses of Congress in the early afternoon of 6 January.[20]

At roughly 2:00 p.m., the protest reached the fever pitch associated with rioting when the building was breached and the ransacking of offices and defacing of property began. However, this was minor in light of the loss of life and injuries due to what Senate Majority Leader Mitch McConnell referred to as a "failed insurrection".[21] Officials later claimed there was no viable intelligence that the protest would turn violent. The police present that afternoon were significantly understaffed due to a lack of intelligence regarding the threat and not able to withstand attacks by those wielding pipes and using chemical agents. Further proof of careful planning by insurgents was obvious by the military-style apparel and tactics used. Nearly 140 police officers were injured as were an unknown number of the crowd present. Five people died as a result of the storming of the Capital. One officer died shortly thereafter as a direct result of wounds sustained during the breach.[22]

Institutionalized Discrimination and Routinization of Violence

It is an understatement to refer to 2020 as a seminal year regarding race relations in the United States. Although minorities have long dealt from various forms of discrimination, events of the past year have accentuated the misuse of force by police against members of these communities. The historical record of police violence against minorities everywhere is a substantive one. In recent years, this record has been added to by incidents of African-Americans shot by police in the United States in circumstances that can only be described as questionable. Prior to 2020, Ferguson, Missouri, Cleveland, Ohio, New York City, New York, and North Charleston, South Carolina were recent examples of cities in which public attention was galvanized around the perception of institutional racism perpetuated by over-zealous officers killing African-Americans.

Criminologist Samuel Walker[23] developed the "Wedding Cake Model" of the criminal justice system to address societal perceptions of crime seriousness and prevalence. The bottom layer of this four-layer conceptual cake is made up of misdemeanors, which constitute the majority of the workload of police and the courts. The next two layers involve first minor felonies and then those felony crimes considered especially serious. It is the top layer of the cake that Walker emphasizes. The smallest layer of a wedding cake, the one at the top, attracts the most attention as it is the most ornamented.

As with a wedding cake, Walker contended certain crimes, because of their graphic and extraordinary circumstances, become celebrated. These are the ones society becomes fixated upon. The early Spring and Summer of 2020 saw two of these celebrated cases: the killing of Breonna Taylor in Louisville, Kentucky and George Floyd in Minneapolis, Minnesota. Taylor and Floyd were Black. The officers involved were White. The exception to the Walker model here is his contention that celebrated crimes are rare. African-Americans would contend cases like Taylor and Floyd, regardless of the immense media coverage they generated, are routine. However, the influence these cases had on American society was not routine.

Two "Celebrated" Cases

On 13 March 2020, Breonna Taylor, a 26-year-old African-American female, was shot and killed by Louisville Metro Police Department, Louisville, Kentucky police officers. Using a "No Knock" warrant that does not require officers to announce themselves to occupants prior to entry, three Caucasian officers forced their way inside Taylor's apartment. Taylor's boyfriend, Kenneth Walker, the subject of the warrant, fired at what he said he thought were intruders. His shot hit one of the officers in the leg. The three officers then opened fire. Thirty-two shots were fired by police. Six shots hit Taylor, killing her. Walker was unharmed.

There were inconsistencies between the statements of Walker and the officers at the scene. Officers claimed that although they had a no-knock warrant that they still announced themselves after knocking on Taylor's apartment door. Walker has stood by his initial account when he said there was no warning prior to police entry. Neighbors of Taylor's were also mixed as to their recollections. Some said the police announced themselves before entering Taylor's residence. Others claimed no announcement was made.

One officer was terminated in June as it was found he fired through a covered door and window into Taylor's apartment. On 15 September 2020, the city of Louisville agreed to pay Taylor's family $12 million dollars and committed to reforming police practices. None of the officers involved were charged with homicide of any sort. The one officer who was dismissed for reckless firing of his weapon was charged with the considerably lesser penalty of wanton endangerment.[24]

Breonna Taylor's death made national news and angered the minority community within Louisville, Kentucky. However, it would take the death of George Floyd a few months later to galvanize the resentment and anger of the marginalized or those tired of seeing other Americans discriminated against into a full-blown social crusade. This "crusade" would soon grow to become a national and international movement, with Floyd and

Taylor being viewed as the latest additions in the litany of martyrs for this movement.

On 24 May 2020, Minneapolis, Minnesota police responded to a call from a convenience store clerk who claimed a customer, George Floyd, tried to purchase cigarettes using a counterfeit $20 bill. Upon arriving at the scene, officers took Floyd into custody. He was handcuffed and placed face down in the street. One of the four officers at the scene, Derek Chauvin, knelt on Floyd's neck for eight minutes, 46s to subdue him. Two other officers assisted in pinning Floyd down and the fourth kept onlookers from intervening. During the final two minutes of Floyd's detainment at the scene, he was motionless without a pulse. It was later determined his death was caused by asphyxia due to neck and back compression.[25] While officers called for medical assistance, none was offered to him at the scene.

Throughout the Summer of 2020, protests against police brutality and the marginalization of the minority community were commonplace in every major American city. There were moments of silence that lasted eight minutes and 46 s: the same amount of time Officer Chauvin's knee was on Floyd's neck. Some protests though, such as those in Louisville following the shooting of Breonna Taylor, evolved into riots which required police intervention, adding still more fuel to the perceptual flame of racial injustice. There were over 140 protests in the wake of George Floyd's death. At least six people were killed.[26]

Racial discrimination on the part of law enforcement against minority communities was not the only societal pathology that arose during 2020. The Black Lives Matter movement has not only contended with inequities in the justice system, but in health care systems as well. Similar to how the Taylor and Floyd cases drew attention to the discrimination against Black Americans by police, COVID-19 illuminated the stark contrast in the quality of health care between White and Black communities.

To understand the conditions leading to racial unrest in 2020, one must first appreciate that minorities consider victimization by the justice system routine. The lack of access to quality health care is also expected. The abysmal economic conditions in which many African-Americans find themselves are the norm, not the exception. When a Black man or woman is charged with a crime, it is quite probable they cannot afford the services of a defense attorney and will have to depend on an overworked, underpaid public defender.[27] Thus, the two victimization variables here influencing the precarious position of minorities in society (the justice system and lack of economic opportunities) have a symbiotic relationship.

COVID-19, the Social Contract, and Agenda Setting

In times of crisis, it is a necessity for the members of any society that identify themselves as citizens to assist with the mitigation of the crisis and help to assuage its impact. It is common in a democratic state for people to consider the relationship between the citizen and the government that rules them to generally be a one-sided arrangement where the government is the service provider and the citizen the recipient of these services. The obligations we have to obey traffic laws or serve on juries are routine and citizens do not generally consider them an intrusive hardship to be suffered.

However, crises, especially those impacting a significant number of people, require more of an active commitment on the part of the citizen to curb their behaviors for the greater good. The cost each of us pay to live in a society where the government does an effective job in providing security for citizens is that we relinquish certain "freedoms" to enjoy that security. Our compliance in concert with the government is essential in achieving this and is one of the central tenets of the Social Contract. Locke maintained the State of Nature existed prior to the creation of mechanisms of rule, The Social Contract was the result of when people recognized the threats to their security inherent in the State of Nature and surrendered some of their liberties to escape the brutality by which the State of Nature was known. Certain events derived from disaster and characterized by its subsequent chaos can become microcosmic States of Nature mirroring Thomas Hobbes' description of this theoretical state as being "… nasty, brutish, and short".

In times of war, the mechanisms of vanquished governments that had once maintained order can be destroyed leaving the populace without the security previously provided to them. Germany in the aftermath of World War II and the sectarian violence that broke out in Iraq after the fall of Saddam Hussein are examples of the bedlam which may lead to the victimization of citizens by lawless elements. Natural disasters may also usher in a temporary State of Nature. Public and private entities that may be overwhelmed by community may simply no longer be capable of providing the support and structure citizens have come to expect. The pitiable conditions in the New Orleans Louisiana Superdome during Hurricane Katrina is another instance where a society, without the protections of an active government response, can break down. During Katrina, there were reports of murder and rape taking place within the Superdome as there was no active police presence there.

The current pandemic is another in a long line of crises that have required citizens in every country to restrict their movements and behaviors to stem the spread of infection. Restricting travel, obeying mandatory curfews, staying home during lockdowns, wearing protective masks, and social distancing are among those dictates citizens have been expected to follow. While they are restrictive and inconvenient, these have largely been endured with most understanding the situation is temporary and government is acting as a *parens patriae* protector. There are some who have suffered internal ontological crises, but these have not been reported as widespread. For them government is still an overall agent for good. However, there have been a number of governments that have been accused of using the COVID-19 crisis to further agendas of oppression. The "New Normal" in some countries describes the changed behaviors of citizens as a result of the pandemic and may also show how those governing have taken advantage of a crisis to further their own ends.

In their report sponsored by Freedom House, Repucci and Slipowicz[28] discussed how the circumstances surrounding COVID-19 have led to a global decline in the democratic process. They cite the example of Sri Lankan Prime Minister Mahinda Rajapaska's efforts to control comments critical to his government's response to COVID-19 through widespread arrests and intimidation. Cuba has also sought to restrict the accurate reporting of conditions there by arrest and imprisonment. Turkey has also been targeted as using COVID to suppress dissent. A respondent from Turkey stated, "the Coronavirus was used as an excuse for the already oppressive government to do things that it has long planned to do, but had not been able to."[29] Like Sri Lanka and Cuba, Turkish officials quickly realized that control of the media was essential in furthering their agenda.

While lockdowns were common throughout the world at the beginning of the pandemic, certain people, long considered marginalized, were subjected to more intense and obtrusive control. The Roma peoples in Bulgaria and Slovakia have been historically subjected to police intimidation and harsher treatment than other ethnic groups living in these countries. Entire Roma neighborhoods were cordoned off with the excuse being made that it was done for the protection of the greater community. Jobs were lost as a result and the ability to obtain medical treatment for those infected by the Coronavirus was severely curtailed.[30]

The First Amendment to the Constitution of the United States guarantees American citizens the right of assembly. This is considered a fundamental human right as recognized in the International Covenant on Civil and Political Rights.[31] Recognizing this Constitutional protection, the question becomes how does a government reconcile (1) protecting the rights of all to protest peacefully with (2) the necessary restrictions to avoid the spread of contagion? This question has not been fully answered yet. However, Constitutional protections have been ignored before by American presidents. During the American Civil War, Abraham Lincoln suspended *habeas corpus* to quell the efforts of Confederate sympathizers criticizing his administration. Theoretically, the same could be done to enforce policies targeting those in defiance of virus protection compliance.

The Black Lives Matter protests occurring during the height of the COVID-19 pandemic were a significant concern for protesters, police, and health care workers. The tactics associated with each were in obvious conflict with the other. A protest is dependent upon the strength of a large, energetic crowd with people in close proximity to others. This runs directly counter to one of the chief dictates of disease infection prevention which is social distancing. The obvious concern here was the bifurcation of purpose and corresponding tactics to achieve these purposes could lead to a surge in COVID-19 infections.[32] Yet, while recognizing this risk, some health care experts believed protesting to change police treatment of minorities was worth the gamble.[33]

Heroes have emerged during the pandemic. Health care providers, emergency medical service workers, police, and teachers are now part of those professions that are seen as providing an essential service in times of crisis and doing it selflessly. There are others as well who deserve credit for their dedication. Yet, the trust in and appreciation for front line workers during the pandemic has not necessarily translated to those agents of government that have set the policies regarding the Coronavirus.

The Problem with a Micro-Level Perspective

The vast majority of police in the United States are employed by municipal and county law enforcement agencies. Thus, what law enforcement has done in the wake of the Coronavirus pandemic is to generally implement tactical responses at the micro-level. What works for one department may work for another and replication of programs may yield the same results. However, the perspective behind the creation of programming is usually limited to the department's jurisdiction. The adage "Necessity is the mother of invention" is an appropriate descriptor for departmental policies and procedures quickly created to cope with the added burdens of pandemic management in an order maintenance setting. President Franklin D. Roosevelt put it succinctly when he stated, "It is common sense to take a method and try it. If it fails, admit it frankly and try another. But above all, try something."[34]

COVID-19 is not the first global pandemic. It will not be the last. It is thought over 50,000,000 lives were lost in the Spanish Flu pandemic of 1918 and there have been others since. Each of these has helped public officials to develop best practices learned from the successes and failures of previous public-health strategies. Perhaps the best example of this has been mandated requirements for social distancing currently being used. Yet, those lessons learned from previous crises have not necessarily prepared first responders, particularly police, for the challenges of social unrest under the aegises of Black Lives Matter.

A pandemic causes fear. The obvious root of that trepidation is the fear of death. However, most will not suffer physical illness as a result of the Coronavirus. The reality is more the simple inconvenience of distance and travel and associations due to lockdowns. There are few people on the globe who have not been impacted by the inconvenience of the effects of COVID-19. Infections are not limited to a specific population. This is where it differs from the protests and riots that have accompanied the Black Lives Matter movement in 2020. COVID-19 does not discriminate.

Protests, Responses by Police, and Organizational Change in Law Enforcement

A guarantee of the First Amendment of the Constitution of the United States is the right of citizens to peacefully assemble. It can be curtailed, but these instances are relatively rare. In the past year, people have gathered *en masse* to call for police reform in the wake of the Taylor and Floyd shootings. Balancing the protections afforded civil liberties by the Constitution against the safeguards against disease transmission due to assembly, peaceful or otherwise, has been a challenging tightrope for law enforcement to walk.

There is no dearth of examples of clashes between BLM supporters and law enforcement, especially during the pivotal year of 2020. A simple web-based search string will reveal a multitude of instances. However, what is not as frequently mentioned is how the protests and the evolving nature of societal attitudes have transformed how the development of strategies and implementation of tactics towards members of the minority communities has been transformed. Three particular areas of police administration that have been changed as a result of BLM protests are:

- Training,
- Defunding, and
- Department Organization.

Training

In his article addressing racism in the American criminal justice system, Balko[35] discussed the concept of "systemic racism." According to Balko, it is not the individual within the system that is necessarily racist, but the system itself. "… often wrongly interpreted as an accusation that everyone in the system is racist. In fact, systemic racism means almost the opposite. It means that we have systems and institutions that produce racially disparate outcomes, regardless of the intentions of the people who work within them."[36]

If the systems of justice are racist, the question then becomes how is this eventually overcome? A common response to this in recent years has been training in "implicit bias". Implicit bias is centered around a psychological theory that unconscious bias will lead people to make immediate judgments about others in error. "For instance, unconscious associations of African Americans with crime might make cops quicker to see them as suspects."[37] Implicit bias enables heuristic reasoning functions that occur when we have incomplete information on which to make an informed decision.

While the popularity around the use of implicit bias training continues to gain in acceptance in police departments across the United States, there is no firm evidence that it produces the desired effect of changing how officers on the street perform their duties. Trainers maintain that although behaviors on the street may not be changing to the extent as management would like, officers are becoming more *aware* of bias. In a similar vein, there is no indication that diversity training or what Glaser refers to as "de-biasing" training[38] have any overall effect on officer behavior. However, the popularity of "de-biasing" training promises to be a fixed part of police instruction for at least the immediate future.

Defunding

The two deaths of Taylor and Floyd pushed the debate beyond police behaviors towards minorities to also include how the police should view their innate mission. There are some who believe the mission of policing in the United States should be dramatically changed. A recommendation as to what may change their worldview concerning minorities is through defunding.

Defunding entails reallocating a portion of monies in the annual police budget to other public agencies serving the general community, especially minorities. The logic here is that if you have an entity that is inherently or systematically biased and if you reduce its power to exact that bias you will lessen the opportunities for minority victimization by that body. The confusion over defunding comes from the impression all funding will be taken from police. This is not the case. "Defund does not mean abolish policing. And, even some who say abolish, do not necessarily mean to do away with law enforcement altogether. Rather, they want to see the rotten trees of policing chopped down and fresh roots replanted anew."[39]

An argument against defunding is how citizens will defend themselves against violent threats. Some members of the black community do not see this as a valid argument. "McHarris grew up in a neighborhood where there were 'real, discernible threats of gun violence,' and he said he never thought to call the police—that was for his own safety. Instead, he relied on neighbors who helped him navigate threats of danger."[40] Cities that have either begun to defund police or are openly considering it are Minneapolis, Minnesota, Los Angeles, California, San Francisco, California, and Baltimore, Maryland.

Department Organization

Closely related to the prospects of defunding is through changes in police department organizational structures. Proponents of defunding advocate for the reallocation of funds to be directed to social service programs such as mental health, drug addiction, and homelessness. It has been a traditional part of the police mission to assist with public service agencies with these types of social issues. However, their role has generally been limited to one of warehousing and segregation instead of participating in active treatment.

On 25 May 2020, New York Governor Andrew M. Cuomo issued Executive Order 203 that mandated all police departments within the state review current practices involving police relations with minorities (No. 203 2020). If cities do not comply, they risk losing future state funding. In response to this, Ithaca, New York Mayor Svante Myrick unveiled a plan to dissolve the current police structure and replace it with a bifurcated public service model. The revamped agency will be made up of armed public safety workers and unarmed community solution workers trained in mental health issues.[41]

Myrick's proposal, titled "Reimagining Public Safety," had the unanimous support of the Ithaca City Council in a March 31, 2021 vote. It calls for an expansion beyond public safety to that of public service. In explaining the rationale behind the proposal, Myrick stated, "You have to have law enforcement officers who are armed. It's a reality of American life, but when all you have is a hammer, every problem looks like a nail."[42]

As it has yet to be implemented, the level of success Ithaca, New York's reorganized public safety department will enjoy remains to be seen. One thing for certain though is that this experiment will be watched closely by those advocates who believe policing needs to dramatically change and traditionalists who maintain the current model of order maintenance is a necessary one.

Conclusion

Confronting the schizophrenic arrangement of challenges posed by the Coronavirus, political protests, and racial unrest has proved challenging for law enforcement agencies across the globe. While COVID-19 has forced police in the United States to adjust their organizational responses, the pandemic also served in some ways to further oppressive political agendas that use law enforcement as their enforcement arm by governments throughout the world. As mentioned earlier, the concerns for the social distancing required by COVID-19 are in direct conflict with how crowds gathered for protests assemble. Thus, COVID-19 has been used to suppress political dissent.

Chilean police were able to use this as a pretext for quashing protests targeting the actions of the Piñera Administration. The lockdown imposed by the police across Chile was severe with little sympathy shown for victims. One woman who went to police to report being raped was arrested herself for breaking curfew.[43] One expert on Egyptian politics stated, “The military regime has used COVID-19 as an opportunity to further repress political activists, rights defenders, lawyers, journalists, and doctors, arresting dozens, denying them basic assistance in places of detention, and placing several on terrorist lists.”[44] Referring to post-COVID conditions in Zimbabwe, one critic of the government there shared, “COVID-19 has also been used to arrest, abduct, rape, assault, and intimidate human rights activists, opposition party leaders/supporters, civil society leaders, journalists, and other dissenting voices on ‘allegations of violating lockdown conditions.’”[45]

It is easy enough to identify a problem. The first step to solving that problem is determining what causes it. While COVID-19 has stretched police resources and required new and innovative policies be implemented to manage the pandemic, the response of law enforcement has largely been tactical and, as a result, limited. Creating a viable vaccine for the Coronavirus is a responsibility for medical researchers, not the police. When a specific issue caused by COVID-19 arose in their jurisdiction, police handled it with the resources they have. Their worldview in this regard is restricted.

The challenges for law enforcement in dealing with racial issues, political oppression, and economic marginalization long predated the December 2019 COVID-19 outbreak. The causal variables behind these concerns are also considerably more varied than those associated with COVID-19 and, consequently, much more difficult to identify. The lack of faith in the American street-level bureaucracy to fairly serve them has festered in the minority community and these resulting cleavages within society have not narrowed over time. It is not necessarily that the minority community doubts the ability of law enforcement to serve them. It is rather their lack of faith in the willingness of police to do so. The deaths of Breonna Taylor and George Floyd have served to widen the gap of understanding and this loss of confidence. We have had a response. What we have lacked is sensitivity.

Lack of faith in the motives and abilities of law enforcement to serve every member of their community is not restricted to any one country. Regardless of mission or geographic area, the one absolute necessity police must have in order to accomplish their mission of protecting and serving all members of the community is trust. All must have confidence that police will enforce the law equitably in a competent manner. Patrol cars in the United States routinely have the phrase “To Protect and Serve” stenciled prominently on the vehicle. Without that confidence and expectation on the part of the public that all are entitled to protection by (and from) police, this promise of justice is a hollow one.

Notes

1. "Belarus Election: Exiled Leader Calls Weekend of 'Peaceful Rallies'," *BBC*, August 14, 2020, https://www.bbc.com/news/world-europe-53780685; Ivan Nechepurenko, "Europe's 'Last Dictator,' Facing Re-Election, Is Increasingly in Peril," *The New York Times*, August 7, 2020, https://www.nytimes.com/2020/08/07/world/europe/belarus-election-aleksandr-lukashenko.html.
2. "Human Rights Situation in Belarus in 2020," *Viasna*, January 8, 2021, http://spring96.org/en/news/101223.
3. "Chile Protests: Cost of Living Protests Take Deadly Toll," *BBC*, October 21, 2019, https://www.bbc.com/news/world-latin-america-50119649.
4. "Metro de Santiago: 80 estaciones dañadas o destruidas durante protestas." *BN Americas,* October 21, 2019. https://www.bnamericas.com/es/noticias/metro-de-santiago-80-estaciones-danadas-o-destruidas-durante-protestas.
5. Matías Vega, "General Iturriaga Decreta Toque De Queda En Santiago Para Afrontar Graves Disturbios," *BioBioChile*, October 20, 2019, https://www.biobiochile.cl/noticias/nacional/region-metropolitana/2019/10/19/general-iturriaga-anuncia-toque-de-queda-en-santiago-para-afrontar-graves-disturbios.shtml.
6. "Chile Police Using Covid-19 Quarantine as Pretext to Crush Protest, Activists Say," *The Guardian,* August 26, 2020, https://www.theguardian.com/global-development/2020/aug/26/chile-police-covid-19-quarantine-protest.
7. "Hong Kong Kicks Off 2020 with Fresh Protests," *BBC,* January 1, 2020, https://www.bbc.com/news/world-asia-china-50964278
8. "How Hong Kong's Leaderless Protest Army Gets Things Done." *Bloomberg*, August 22, 2019. https://www.bloomberg.com/graphics/2019-hong-kong-airport-protests/.
9. Kim Willsher, "Thousands March over Police Violence and Security Bill in Paris." *The Guardian*, December 5, 2020, https://

www.theguardian.com/world/2020/dec/05/thousands-march-over-police-violence-and-security-bill-in-paris.

10. Uliana Pavlova, "Protests for Jailed Kremlin Critic Navalny Sweep Russia," *The Moscow Times*, January 25, 2021, https://www.themoscowtimes.com/2021/01/23/protests-for-jailed-kremlin-critic-navalny-sweep-russia-a72708.
11. "Right Now He Is Being Killed in the Colony, and You Can't Wait Any Longer. Navalny's Team Announced a Rally without Waiting for the Gathering of Half a Million Participants," *Meduza*, April 18, 2021, https://meduza.io/news/2021/04/18/storonniki-navalnogo-anonsirovali-miting-v-podderzhku-politika-ne-dozhidayas-sbora-polumilliona-uchastnikov.
12. Ibid.
13. "Black Lives Matter Protests Held across England," *BBC*, June 20, 2020, https://www.bbc.co.uk/news/uk-england-53120735
14. "London Protests: Demonstrators Clash with Police," *BBC*, June 13, 2020, https://www.bbc.com/news/uk-53031072.
15. "London Police Under Pressure Over Clashes at Women's Protest," *Voice of America*, March 14, 2021, https://www.voanews.com/europe/london-police-under-pressure-over-clashes-womens-protest.
16. Kevin Drew, "Amid a Pandemic and Social Unrest, America Appears Unrecognizable to Its Allies," United States *News*, August 28, 2020, https://www.usnews.com/news/best-countries/articles/2020-08-28/amid-a-pandemic-and-social-unrest-america-appears-unrecognizable-to-its-allies
17. Morris Dees, and James Corcoran, *Gathering Storm: America's Militia Threat* (New York: Harper Collins, 1997).
18. Jay Reeves, Lisa Mascaro, and Calvin Woodward, "Capitol Assault a More Sinister Attack than First Appeared," *AP News*, January 11, 2021, https://apnews.com/article/us-capitol-attack-14c73ee280c256ab4ec193ac0f49ad54.
19. Calvin Woodward, "AP FACT CHECK: Trump's Call to Action Distorted in Debate," *AP News*, January 13, 2021, https://apnews.com/article/fact-check-trump-us-capitol-remarks-221518bc174f9bc3dd6e108e653ed08d.
20. Jeff Seldin, "US Capitol Police Overrun by Mob After Declining Help," *Voice of America*, January 8, 2021, https://www.voanews.

com/2020-usa-votes/us-capitol-police-overrun-mob-after-declin ing-help.
21. Richard Cowan, "'Mob Was Fed Lies': Mitch McConnell Accuses Trump of 'Provoking' Riot," *The Sydney Morning Herald*, January 19, 2021, https://www.smh.com.au/world/north-america/mob-was-fed-lies-mitch-mcconnell-accuses-trump-of-provoking-riot-20210120-p56vew.html.
22. Jemima McEvoy, "Woman Possibly 'Crushed to Death': These Are The Five People Who Died Amid Pro-Trump Riots," *Forbes*, January 10, 2021, https://www.forbes.com/sites/jem imamcevoy/2021/01/08/woman-possibly-crushed-to-death-these-are-the-five-people-who-died-amid-pro-trump-riots/?sh=d5b1e04737c6.
23. Samuel Walker, *Sense and Nonsense about Crime and Drugs: A Policy Guide* (Belmont: Thomson/Wadsworth, 2006).
24. Richard A. Oppel, Derrick Bryson Taylor, and Nicholas Bogel-Burroughs, "What to Know About Breonna Taylor's Death," *The New York Times,* May 30, 2020, https://www.nytimes.com/art icle/breonna-taylor-police.html.
25. Evan Hill et al., "How George Floyd Was Killed in Police Custody," *The New York Times*, June 1, 2020, https://www.nyt imes.com/2020/05/31/us/george-floyd-investigation.html.
26. Derrick Bryson Taylor, "George Floyd Protests: A Timeline," *The New York Times*, May 30, 2020, https://www.nytimes.com/art icle/george-floyd-protests-timeline.html.
27. Theodore Schoneman, "Overworked and Underpaid: America's Public Defender Crisis," *Fordham Political Review*, February 1, 2021, http://fordhampoliticalreview.org/overworked-and-und erpaid-americas-public-defender-crisis/.
28. Sarah Repucci and Amy Slipowicz, "Democracy under Lockdown: The Impact of COVID-19 on the Global Struggle for Freedom," *Freedom House*, October 2020, https://freedomhouse.org/sites/default/files/2020-10/COVID-19_Special_Report_Final_.pdf.
29. Ibid.
30. "Roma Persecution Intensifies during the Coronavirus Pandemic in Europe," *The World*, August 14, 2020, https://www.pri.org/stories/2020-08-24/roma-persecution-intensifies-during-corona virus-pandemic-europe.

31. "International Covenant on Civil and Political Rights," *OHCHR*, https://www.ohchr.org/EN/ProfessionalInterest/Pages/CCPR.aspx.
32. John Bacon, "Coronavirus Updates: George Floyd Protests Could Fuel COVID Cases, Trump Postpones G7 Summit," *USA Today*, May 31, 2020, https://www.usatoday.com/story/news/health/2020/05/31/coronavirus-update-donald-trump-g-7-summit-church-reopenings-cuomo/5293061002/.
33. Mallory Simon, "Over 1,000 Health Professionals Sign a Letter Saying, Don't Shut down Protests Using Coronavirus Concerns as an Excuse," *CNN*, June 5, 2020, https://www.cnn.com/2020/06/05/health/health-care-open-letter-protests-coronavirus-trnd/index.html.
34. Aiken, Debbie, "Remembering FDR's Commencement Speech at Oglethorpe," *The Source*, September 12, 2018, https://source.oglethorpe.edu/2012/05/22/remembering-fdrs-commencement-speech-at-oglethorpe/.
35. Radley Balko, "Opinion|There's Overwhelming Evidence That the Criminal Justice System Is Racist. Here's the Proof.," *The Washington Post*, June 10, 2020, https://www.washingtonpost.com/graphics/2020/opinions/systemic-racism-police-evidence-criminal-justice-system/.
36. Ibid.
37. Martin Kaste, "NYPD Study: Implicit Bias Training Changes Minds, Not Necessarily Behavior," *NPR*, September 10, 2020, https://www.npr.org/2020/09/10/909380525/nypd-study-implicit-bias-training-changes-minds-not-necessarily-behavior.
38. "Cracking the Code: Implicit Bias and Racial Profiling," *Cal Alumni Association*, September 12, 2016, https://alumni.berkeley.edu/events/california-live/cracking-the-code-jack-glaser.
39. Rashawn Ray, "What Does 'Defund the Police' Mean and Does It Have Merit?" *Brookings*, May 3, 2021, https://www.brookings.edu/blog/fixgov/2020/06/19/what-does-defund-the-police-mean-and-does-it-have-merit/.
40. Scottie Andrew, "There's a Growing Call to Defund the Police. Here's What It Means," *CNN*, June 17, 2020, https://www.cnn.com/2020/06/06/us/what-is-defund-police-trnd/index.html.
41. Andrew Donovan, "Ithaca's Mayor Wants to Abolish Police Department, Apologizes to Officers for Telling GQ First," *WSYR*,

February 25, 2021, https://www.localsyr.com/news/local-news/ithacas-mayor-wants-to-abolish-police-department-apologizes-to-officers-for-telling-gq-first/.

42. Zach Wheeler, "Ithaca Common Council Unanimously Approves Ambitious Police Reform Plan," *My Twin Tiers*, April 1, 2021, https://www.mytwintiers.com/news-cat/top-stories/ithaca-common-council-unanimously-approves-ambitious-police-reform-plan/.
43. "Chile Protests: Cost of Living Protests Take Deadly Toll," *BBC News*, October 21, 2019, https://www.bbc.com/news/world-latin-america-50119649.
44. Sarah Repucci and Amy Slipowicz, "Democracy under Lockdown: The Impact of COVID-19 on the Global Struggle for Freedom," *Freedom House*, October 2020, https://freedomhouse.org/sites/default/files/2020-10/COVID-19_Special_Report_Final_.pdf.
45. Ibid.

Bibliography

"CA Police Chief Joins 'Black Lives Matter' Protest, Scolded by Police Union." *Newstex Trade & Industry Blogs*, December 13, 2014.

"Right Now He Is Being Killed in the Colony, and You Can't Wait Any Longer. Navalny's Team Announced a Rally without Waiting for the Gathering of Half a Million Participants." *Meduza*, April 18, 2021. https://meduza.io/news/2021/04/18/storonniki-navalnogo-anonsirovali-miting-v-podderzhku-politika-ne-dozhidayas-sbora-polumilliona-uchastnikov.

"Belarus Election: Exiled Leader Calls Weekend of 'Peaceful Rallies'." *BBC*, August 14, 2020. https://www.bbc.com/news/world-europe-53780685.

"Belarus Opposition Protests End in Arrests." *BBC*, June 20, 2020. https://www.bbc.com/news/world-europe-53115921.

"Black Lives Matter Protests Held across England." *BBC*, June 20, 2020. https://www.bbc.co.uk/news/uk-england-53120735.

"Metro de Santiago: 80 estaciones dañadas o destruidas durante protestas." *BN Americas,* October 21, 2019. https://www.bnamericas.com/es/noticias/metro-de-santiago-80-estaciones-danadas-o-destruidas-durante-protestas.

"Chile Police Using Covid-19 Quarantine as Pretext to Crush Protest, Activists Say." *The Guardian,* August 26, 2020. https://www.theguardian.com/global-development/2020/aug/26/chile-police-covid-19-quarantine-protest.

"Chile Protests: Cost of Living Protests Take Deadly Toll." *BBC*, October 21, 2019. https://www.bbc.com/news/world-latin-america-50119649.

"COVID Jan 6 21." *Police Executive Research Forum*. https://www.policeforum.org/covidjan621.

"Cracking The Code: Implicit Bias and Racial Profiling." *Cal Alumni Association*, September 12, 2016. https://alumni.berkeley.edu/events/california-live/cracking-the-code-jack-glaser.

"Critical Issues Oct 26." *Police Executive Research Forum*. https://www.policeforum.org/criticalissuesoct26.

"Freedom to Navalny!" *ОВД-Инфо*, January 23, 2021. https://ovdinfo.org/news/2021/01/23/akcii-svobodu-navalnomu-23-yanvarya-2021-goda-onlayn.

"George Floyd: What Happened in the Final Moments of His Life." *BBC*, July 16, 2020. https://www.bbc.com/news/world-us-canada-52861726.

"Hong Kong kicks off 2020 with fresh protests." *BBC*, January 1, 2020. https://www.bbc.com/news/world-asia-china-50964278

"How Hong Kong's Leaderless Protest Army Gets Things Done." *Bloomberg*, August 22, 2019. https://www.bloomberg.com/graphics/2019-hong-kong-airport-protests/.

"In 2020, 47 Countries Witness surge in civil unrest." *Security Magazine,* January 29, 2020. https://www.securitymagazine.com/articles/91622-in-2020-47-countries-witness-surge-in-civil-unrest

"International Covenant on Civil and Political Rights." *OHCHR*. https://www.ohchr.org/EN/ProfessionalInterest/Pages/CCPR.aspx.

"Janesville Police Department." *Everbridge Nixle,* March 23, 2020. https://local.nixle.com/alert/7888560/https://local.nixle.com/alert/7888560/.

"London Protests: Demonstrators Clash with Police." *BBC*, June 13, 2020. https://www.bbc.com/news/uk-53031072.

"No. 203: New York State Police Reform and Reinvention Collaborative." *New York State Police Reform And Reinvention Collaborative,* June 12, 2020. https://www.governor.ny.gov/news/no-203-new-york-state-police-reform-and-reinvention-collaborative.

"Novel Coronavirus COVID-19." *Multnomah County*, March 12, 2021. https://multco.us/novelcoronavirus-covid-19.

"Pillar Six—Officer Safety and Wellness:" *Evesham Police*. http://eveshampd.org/index.php/en/component/sppagebuilder/?view=page&id=94.

"Responding to COVID-19." *Police Executive Research Forum*. https://www.policeforum.org/covid-19-response.

"The Most Significant Criminal Justice Policy Changes from the COVID-19 Pandemic." *Prison Policy Initiative*, May 18, 2021. https://www.prisonpolicy.org/virus/virusresponse.html.

"The Real-Life Changes to Policing Won by Black Lives Matter Protests." *Axios*, June 12, 2020. https://www.axios.com/black-lives-matter-protest-police-reform-64c6efb2-31a5-463a-bc1d-2db7b24360d5.html.

"Topeka Police Reveal Changes to Response Protocols." *The Topeka Capital-Journal*, March 19, 2020. https://www.cjonline.com/news/20200319/topeka-police-reveal-changes-to-response-protocols.

"Training & Information Results." *IADLEST*. https://www.iadlest.org/search-results/search/cancelled?search=cancelled.

Aiken, Debbie. "Remembering FDR's Commencement Speech at Oglethorpe." *The Source*, May 22, 2012. https://source.oglethorpe.edu/2012/05/22/remembering-fdrs-commencement-speech-at-oglethorpe/

Andrew, Scottie. "There's a Growing Call to Defund the Police. Here's What It Means." *CNN*, Cable News Network, June 17, 2020. https://www.cnn.com/2020/06/06/us/what-is-defund-police-trnd/index.html.

Balko, Radley. "There's Overwhelming Evidence That the Criminal Justice System Is Racist. Here's the Proof." *Washington Post*, June 10, 2020. https://www.washingtonpost.com/graphics/2020/opinions/systemic-racism-police-evidence-criminal-justice-system/.

Barry, John M. *The Great Influenza: The Epic Story of the Deadliest Plague in History*. New York: Viking, 2004.

Barry, Orla. "Roma Persecution Intensifies during the Coronavirus Pandemic in Europe." *The World*, August 24, 2020. https://www.pri.org/stories/2020-08-24/roma-persecution-intensifies-during-coronavirus-pandemic-europe.

Bell, Monica. "Police Reform and the Dismantling of Legal Estrangement." Essay, *The Yale Law Journal*. https://www.yalelawjournal.org/essay/police-reform-and-the-dismantling-of-legal-estrangement.

Cowan, Richard. "'Mob Was Fed Lies': Mitch McConnell Accuses Trump of 'Provoking' Riot." *The Sydney Morning Herald*, January 19, 2021. https://www.smh.com.au/world/north-america/mob-was-fed-lies-mitch-mcconnell-accuses-trump-of-provoking-riot-20210120-p56vew.html.

Dees, Morris, and James Corcoran. *Gathering Storm: America's Militia Threat*. New York: Harper Collins, 1997.

Donovan, Andrew. "Ithaca's Mayor Wants to Abolish Police Department, Apologizes to Officers for Telling GQ First." *WSYR*, February 25, 2021. https://www.localsyr.com/news/local-news/ithacas-mayor-wants-to-abolish-police-department-apologizes-to-officers-for-telling-gq-first/.

Drew, Kevin. "Amid a Pandemic and Social Unrest, America Appears Unrecognizable to Its Allies." *U.S. News*, August 28, 2020. https://www.usnews.com/news/best-countries/articles/2020-08-28/amid-a-pandemic-and-social-unrest-america-appears-unrecognizable-to-its-allies

Effron, Lauren. "Arizona Police Chief Says Meditation Should Be a Key Piece of Officer Development." *ABC News*, March 8, 2017. https://abcnews.go.

com/Health/arizona-police-chief-meditation-key-piece-officer-development/story?id=45966480.

Ferdinand, Keith C., and Samar A. Nasser. "African-American COVID-19 Mortality: A Sentinel Event." *Journal of the American College of Cardiology* 75, no. 21 (2020): 2746–48. https://doi.org/10.1016/j.jacc.2020.04.040.
Ferdinand, Keith C., and Samar A. Nasser. "African-American COVID-19 Mortality: A Sentinel Event." *Journal of the American College of Cardiology* 75, no. 21 (2020): 2746–48. https://doi.org/10.1016/j.jacc.2020.04.040.
Griffin, Oliver. "Death Toll from Colombia Protests Rises as Cities Brace for COVID Fallout." *Reuters*, May 11, 2021. https://www.reuters.com/world/americas/colombian-cities-brace-more-covid-infections-after-protests-2021-05-11/.

Heaslip, Vanessa, and Jonathan Parker. "The Hidden Impact of Coronavirus on Gypsy, Roma Travellers." *The Conversation*, January 14, 2021. https://theconversation.com/the-hidden-impact-of-coronavirus-on-gypsy-roma-travellers-141015.

Hill, Evan, Ainara Tiefenthaler, Drew Jordan, Haley Willis, and Robin Stein. "How George Floyd Was Killed in Police Custody." *The New York Times*, May 31, 2020. https://www.nytimes.com/2020/05/31/us/george-floyd-investigation.html.

Kaste, Martin. "NYPD Study: Implicit Bias Training Changes Minds, Not Necessarily Behavior." *NPR*, September 10, 2020. https://www.npr.org/2020/09/10/909380525/nypd-study-implicit-bias-training-changes-minds-not-necessarily-behavior.

Kramer, Andrew E. "In Russia, a Virus Lockdown Targets the Opposition." *The New York Times*, March 19, 2021. https://www.nytimes.com/2021/03/19/world/europe/russia-covid-opposition.html.

Krawatzek, Felix, and Gwendolyn Sasse. "Belarus Protests: Why People Have Been Taking to the Streets—New Data." *The Conversation*, February 4, 2021. https://theconversation.com/belarus-protests-why-people-have-been-taking-to-the-streets-new-data-154494.

McEvoy, Jemima. "Woman Possibly 'Crushed To Death': These Are The Five People Who Died Amid Pro-Trump Riots." *Forbes*, January 10, 2021. https://www.forbes.com/sites/jemimamcevoy/2021/01/08/woman-possibly-crushed-to-death-these-are-the-five-people-who-died-amid-pro-trump-riots/?sh=d5b1e04737c6.

Miah, Malik. "Justice Requires The Legal System Be Abolished And Replaced." *International Viewpoint,* October 7, 2020. https://internationalviewpoint.org/spip.php?article6845.

Nechepurenko, Ivan. "Europe's 'Last Dictator,' Facing Re-Election, Is Increasingly in Peril." *The New York Times*, August 7, 2020. https://www.nytimes.

com/2020/08/07/world/europe/belarus-election-aleksandr-lukashenko.html.

Oppel, Jr., Richard A, Derrick Bryson Taylor, and Nicholas Bogel-Burroughs. "What to Know About Breonna Taylor's Death." *The New York Times*, January 6, 2021. https://www.nytimes.com/article/breonna-taylor-police.html.

Pavlova, Uliana. "Protests for Jailed Kremlin Critic Navalny Sweep Russia." *The Moscow Times*, January 25, 2021. https://www.themoscowtimes.com/2021/01/23/protests-for-jailed-kremlin-critic-navalny-sweep-russia-a72708.

Bacon, John. "Coronavirus Updates: George Floyd Protests could Fuel COVID Cases, Trump Postpones G7 Summit." *USA Today*, May 31, 2020. https://eu.usatoday.com/story/news/health/2020/05/31/coronavirus-update-donald-trump-g-7-summit-church-reopenings-cuomo/5293061002/.

Price-Haywood, Eboni G., Jeffrey Burton, Daniel Fort, and Leonardo Seoane. "Hospitalization and Mortality among Black Patients and White Patients with COVID-19." *New England Journal of Medicine* (June 2020): 2534–2543. https://www.doi: https://doi.org/10.1056/NEJMsa2011686.

Ramzy, Austin, and Mike Ives. "Hong Kong Protests, One Year Later." *The New York Times*, June 9, 2020. https://www.nytimes.com/2020/06/09/world/asia/hong-kong-protests-one-year-later.html.

Ray, Rashawn. "What Does 'Defund the Police' Mean and Does It Have Merit?" *Brookings*, May 3, 2021. https://www.brookings.edu/blog/fixgov/2020/06/19/what-does-defund-the-police-mean-and-does-it-have-merit/.

Reeves, Jay, Lisa Mascaro, and Calvin Woodward. "Capitol Assault a More Sinister Attack than First Appeared." *AP News*, January 11, 2021. https://apnews.com/article/us-capitol-attack-14c73ee280c256ab4ec193ac0f49ad54.

Repucci, Sarah, and Amy Slipowicz. "Democracy under Lockdown: The Impact of COVID-19 on the Global Struggle for Freedom." *Freedom House,* October 2020. https://freedomhouse.org/sites/default/files/2020-10/COVID-19_Special_Report_Final_.pdf.

Rohan, Annie J., and Kathleen Rice Simpson. "Black Lives Matter." *MCN: The American Journal of Maternal/Child Nursing* 46, no. 1 (2021): 5–5. https://doi.org/10.1097/nmc.0000000000000680.

Schoneman, Theodore. "Overworked and Underpaid: America's Public Defender Crisis." *Fordham Political Review*, November 20, 2018. http://fordhampoliticalreview.org/overworked-and-underpaid-americas-public-defender-crisis/.

Seldin, Jeff. "US Capitol Police Overrun by Mob After Declining Help." *Voice of America*, January 8, 2021. https://www.voanews.com/2020-usa-votes/us-capitol-police-overrun-mob-after-declining-help. September 12, 2018.

Simon, Mallory. "Over 1,000 Health Professionals Sign a Letter Saying, Don't Shut Down Protests Using Coronavirus Concerns as an Excuse." *CNN*

Health, June 5, 2020. https://edition.cnn.com/2020/06/05/health/health-care-open-letter-protests-coronavirus-trnd/index.htmlN.

Taylor, Derrick Bryson. "George Floyd Protests: A Timeline." *The New York Times*, March 9, 2021. https://www.nytimes.com/article/george-floyd-protests-timeline.html?

Taylor, Jamila. "Racism, Inequality, and Health Care for African Americans." *The Century Foundation*, May 7, 2020. https://tcf.org/content/report/racism-inequality-health-care-african-americans/?session=1.

"Human Rights Situation in Belarus in 2020." *Viasna*, January 8, 2021. http://spring96.org/en/news/101223.

Vega, Matías. "General Iturriaga Decreta Toque De Queda En Santiago Para Afrontar Graves Disturbios." *BioBioChile*, October 20, 2019. https://www.biobiochile.cl/noticias/nacional/region-metropolitana/2019/10/19/general-iturriaga-anuncia-toque-de-queda-en-santiago-para-afrontar-graves-disturbios.shtml.

Walker, Samuel. *Sense and Nonsense about Crime and Drugs: A Policy Guide*. Australia: Wadsworth, 2006.

Wheeler, Zach. "Ithaca Common Council Unanimously Approves Ambitious Police Reform Plan." *My Twin Tiers*, April 1, 2021. https://www.mytwintiers.com/news-cat/top-stories/ithaca-common-council-unanimously-approves-ambitious-police-reform-plan/.

Willsher, Kim. "Thousands March over Police Violence and Security Bill in Paris." *The Guardian*. Guardian News and Media, December 5, 2020. https://www.theguardian.com/world/2020/dec/05/thousands-march-over-police-violence-and-security-bill-in-paris.

Woodward, Calvin. "AP FACT CHECK: Trump's Call to Action Distorted in Debate." *AP News*, January 13, 2021. https://apnews.com/article/fact-check-trump-us-capitol-remarks-221518bc174f9bc3dd6e108e653ed08d.

Yu, Elaine, and Yan Zhao. "In Pictures: 'Flow like Water'—Hong Kong Protesters Converge on Police HQ after Day of Wildcat Road Occupations." *Hong Kong Free Press HKFP*, June 19, 2020. https://hongkongfp.com/2019/06/21/pictures-flow-like-water-hong-kong-protesters-converge-police-hq-day-wildcat-road-occupations/.

CHAPTER 10

The Impact of COVID-19 on the Landscape of Terrorism

Lewis Herrington

Introduction

On Wednesday 20 January 2021, the UK reported 1,820 COVID-19 related deaths.[1] In just one day, the virus killed three times more people than 20 years of domestic terrorism across the whole of Europe. Reflecting on such monumental humanitarian devastation and economic disruption, the threat of terrorism seems almost irrelevant. Therefore, before proceeding any further, allow us to briefly consider the fundamental question of whether the global pandemic has significantly downgraded the strategic importance of terrorism. How can Al-Qaeda be a threat to national security at a time when policymakers face a virus with the power to wipe out an entire generation? Can there be anything more terrifying than an enemy who cannot be negotiated with and refuses to accept formal terms of surrender? In May 2021, India's world-famous health care system collapsed under the strain of trying to oxygenate

L. Herrington (✉)
Regent's University, London, UK

C. Varin (ed.), *Global Security in Times of Covid-19*, New Security Challenges, https://doi.org/10.1007/978-3-030-82230-9_10

tens of thousands of patients dying from coronavirus.[2] Patients literally suffocated to death on the pavement outside hospitals.

In some respects, COVID-19 and conventional terrorism are similar. Both represent acts of violence that are indiscriminate, unpredictable, and almost impossible to prevent. Yet, the virus has achieved what generations of terrorists could only fantasize about—death, disruption, and economic suicide on a global scale. Primarily, terrorism is designed to coerce policymakers by creating fear amongst the target population. During the 2nd intifada, suicide bombers in Israel often targeted buses. Yet Israelis were resilient and defied their attackers. Similarly, the 7 July 2005, bombing of the London Transport network had very little impact on passenger numbers. Dramatically contrast this with the significant decline in the use of public transport throughout 2020. Aside from the tremendous economic, social, and psychological impact, COVID-19 has created genuine fear amongst the population. Even the vaccinated have struggled to resume the same kind of close, tactile relationships they once enjoyed before the pandemic. Due to national lockdowns, isolation has increased significantly. Worryingly, we may be on the precipice of a global mental health crisis. In summary, the implication of this 'new normal' is that strategically, terrorism, counterterrorism and counterextremism are no longer a priority and should therefore be significantly downgraded in respect of national security.

Is a continued war on terrorism justified when there appears to be no end in sight for the global pandemic? We believe so. In May 2021, reports emerged that COVID-19 originated in a laboratory in Wuhan, China.[3] The following month, writing in the Wall Street Journal, two US scientists claimed that genome sequencing almost certainly proves the virus was man-made.[4] Assuming these claims are true, COVID-19 may represent the first generation of bioweapons with the potential to disrupt international peace and security. Critically, the world may be on the verge of a new age of terrorism in which biological weapons dominate the landscape. A man-made bioweapon is a potential game changer for asymmetric warfare. For the first time in history, terrorists have in their sights a magic elixir that terrifies both policymakers and the public. Recognizing the economic and humanitarian destruction of bioweapons, it is hardly unreasonable to believe that terrorists of all ideological persuasions are today actively seeking to develop or obtain a second generation of coronavirus. Importantly, given the nature of COVID-19, terrorist actors need only smuggle variants from A to B. Should a new version of coronavirus emerge, the race may be on to spread it across Europe and the US. If western nations are tied up fighting another global pandemic, they will have less time, energy, and resources to fight international terrorist groups. On that basis, it is entirely rational for us to explore the impact of COVID-19 on the terrorism landscape since it first emerged in January 2020.

Radicalization

COVID-19 has increased the legitimacy of extremist groups resulting in widespread recruitment. The ratio between extremists to terrorists is roughly 10,000:1. Inevitably, when the extremist fellowship increases, so do the number of potential terrorists. This is supported by McCauley and Moskalenko who note that 'because terrorists are few in relation to all those who share their beliefs and feelings, the terrorists may be thought of as the apex of a pyramid'.[5] By applying this model, one could assume that a more politicized population at the base could increase the number of extremists in the middle and ultimately the number of potential terrorists at the Apex. We suggest this is likely true of all forms of extremism including the far-right, anarchist, and Islamist. However, we urge caution against authoritarian measures designed to shut down political movements in response to the heightened threat. There will always be extremists, and a minority who are willing to carry out acts of terrorism. Perhaps this is a structural cost that liberal democracy must accept. Only history can decide what the relationship is between extremism and legitimate political struggle. In the absence of political extremism, would the anti-slavery or anti-apartheid movements have emerged? Recognizing the connection between extremism and terrorism, it is important to understand how COVID-19 has impacted radicalization during 2020.

Notwithstanding key differences between far-right terrorists in the US, militants in Syria and lone actor terrorists in Europe, the process of radicalization appears relatively similar. In each case, the gradual adoption of an ideology facilitates an incubatory environment of like-minded individuals. In social psychology, an *in-group* is a social group with which a person identifies. For example, the far-right or Islamism. By contrast, an *out-group* is a social group with which an individual does not identify. For example, immigrants or non-Muslims. Unification within the in-group helps propel individuals to adopt an increasingly extremist position. Within this milieu, followers compete to become the most respected and revered. Narcissists are especially vulnerable to this increasingly dangerous competition. For a tiny minority, the final stage is the willingness to carry out an act of terrorism as a martyr. In this scenario, the individual sacrifices his life to satisfy his desire for infamy. The need to champion over all other extremists outweighs any consequences. Norwegian far-right extremist, Anders Breivik, was so determined to be recognized as the spearhead of the anti-immigration movement that he murdered children attending a left-wing summer school on the island of Utøya in 2011. COVID-19 has provided space and time for conspiracy theorists to fuel extremist narratives across the entire spectrum. The remainder of this section is divided in two parts. First, we will consider how militant groups have utilized the virus as propaganda to increase their overall support base (top down). Secondly, we will look at how government measures to defeat the virus have fueled interest in extremist ideology amongst the population (bottom up).

Propaganda (Top-Down Supply)

We begin our exploration of radicalization during a global pandemic by examining how extremist groups have capitalized on the distraction of COVID-19 to consolidate their resources. Throughout 2020, while governments around the world frantically re-directed their energies, resources, and military capabilities to contain the spread of contagion, both ISIS and Al-Qaeda stepped up their social media propaganda to spread their ideology in the hope of attracting new followers.[6] In this respect, the use of disinformation or propaganda is an important part of the radicalization process. Extremism is, to some extent, the acceptance of 'conspiracy theories' as truth such that an individual becomes completely obsessed with his or her validation and acceptance by others. In a minority of cases, the fixation becomes so great that they come to believe they have a divine obligation to sacrifice their life for 'the cause'. Disinformation is effective as it addresses the emotional insecurity that often arises during a time of crisis due to uncertainty. COVID-19 has caused tremendous uncertainly on a global scale. Even the most advanced western governments have struggled to provide accurate information. In 2020, critics heavily attacked UK Prime Minister Boris Johnson for providing seemingly contradictory guidance during lockdown. Propaganda can quickly attract new followers to a political movement. More followers lead to wider dissemination and potentially more candidates for the radicalization pipeline. Although some governments attempted to provide a counternarrative, especially around the vaccine, much of the responsibility for addressing this situation has fallen to the private sector.[7] It has led some observers to ask who is really in charge of the fight against COVID-19, the state or the multinational corporation.

In early 2020, at the beginning of global pandemic, extremist groups seized on the opportunity to frame COVID-19 as part of their own political narrative. Islamists exploited COVID-19 for multiple purposes, placing it within a larger eschatological framework in which God is punishing western infidels by destroying their societal infrastructure and economy they built. Within Jihadist circles, the pandemic has been interchangeably described as the 'wrath of God' and 'divine retribution'.[8] The Islamic State's (ISIS) narrative around COVID-19 has gradually transformed over time. For instance, when the contagion first broke out in the Chinese city of Wuhan, IS termed it God's punishment on 'communist China' for oppressing the Uyghur Muslims.[9] Subsequently, when the contagion entered Iran, the terror group termed it God's anger on the Shiites for polytheistic practices. Finally, when the coronavirus hit Europe, IS adjusted its narrative to present the pandemic as God's revenge against the 'infidels' and 'crusaders' for attacking the 'mujahideen' in Syria. On the 28th March 2020, ISIS spokesman Abu Hamza Al-Qurashi compared the pandemic to the biblical story of Moses cursing the Pharaoh with ten plagues until he relented and released God's people.[10] Suggestions that COVID-19 is divine punishment deeply resonate with Muslims who have witnessed Russia's carpet bombing of Chechnya, China's oppression of Uighurs, Myanmar's rape and genocidal killing of Rohingya, and the US coalition attacks on Muslim civilian populations in Syria and Iraq. Al-Qaeda have used the pandemic to invite westerners to reflect on the alleged perils of capitalism and the failure of global governance to contain the virus.[11] William Avis has suggested that Al-Qaeda's statement on COVID-19 is a PR-exercise, primarily targeting Western audiences.[12]

While Islamists have suggested COVID-19 is divine retribution, other far-right groups have unsurprisingly forwarded their own racial explanations of the pandemic. Swedish neo-Nazi group, 'Nordic Resistance Movement' claimed that COVID-19 is a Jewish made virus designed to impact the international stock market.[13] According to the United Nations, conspiracy theories of social control (e.g. microchips vaccines) are bolstered by government responses to the COVID-19 crisis, including mass surveillance and use of the military in domestic policing.[14] Lockdowns, contact tracing, and vaccinations have allowed the far-right to emerge from the depths of the internet to congratulate themselves for having known the truth, that 'an evil cabal of Zionist elites have been planning to survey and ultimately destroy ordinary citizens in pursuit of a New World Order'.[15] Belgian intelligence services have identified left-wing and right-wing extremists trying to raise tensions between sections of the population and questioning the authority of the government to create chaos in society. Both sides want to see the downfall of the current system, paving the way for the realization of their own ideological objectives. The links between COVID-19, extremist ideology and terrorism were made clear in the case of Timothy Wilson. During the height of the pandemic, this alleged Neo Nazi was fatally wounded while on the verge of trying to detonate a car bomb at a Kansas City medical center. It is alleged that before the attack, he stated: 'the Zionist operated government is using it COVID-19 as an excuse to destroy our people. They scar people and have society break down. Mark my words, it is coming. I hope people are ready'.[16]

Politicization (Bottom-Up Demand)

It is human nature to seek answers, but most humans only believe truths they have discovered for themselves. In this second part of our analysis on radicalization during a global pandemic, we will consider how COVID-19 has helped facilitate the socialization of individuals towards extremist movements. An understanding of this process is vital, since it is within these enabling environments that new identities are forged and terrorism occasionally emerges. Officially, there is no shortage of recognition that COVID-19 has likely increased the amount of traffic directed towards extremism. According to a UN report, 'a captive audience harboring anxieties and uncertainties during social distancing potentially provides a fertile ground for radicalization'.[17] During 2021 when national lockdowns peaked, worldwide internet data usage surged between 50 and 70%. Globally, over 1.5 billion students in 191 countries were spending more time online. Amongst these, around 400 million had been directly affected by conflict and were thus vulnerable and receptive to extremist ideology'.[18] Of significance to counterradicalization policymakers, the 'incel' ideology (which overlaps a great deal with far-right extremism), was born and propagated almost entirely online. Canadian authorities recently classified the misogynistic brand of violence attributed to the movement as terrorism.[19]

'Big tech' has subsequently come under tremendous pressure to regulate misinformation and remove extremist content from online platforms. In June 2019, police arrested the UK's youngest far-right Neo-Nazi.[20] Aged just 14 years old, the boy had self-radicalized entirely online. Throughout 2019, he posted messages on chat forums in which he incited others to kill members of the Jewish and LGBT + community using nail bombs, firearms, and various other methods. Fortunately, neither he nor his followers were able to act out these fantasies. Previously, in an unrelated case, another 14-year-old boy from the U.K. conspired with a friend in Australia to carry out a terrorist attack against police officers. These are both examples of vulnerable teenagers who forged online extremist identities which give them a sense of purpose. With the significant rise of 'home schooling' throughout the West during lockdown, it is easy to believe that there will be an increase in the number of young individuals seeking to entertain themselves by engaging in 'dangerous' but 'exciting' activities that offer a distraction from the monotony of isolation. For most, engagement in extremism will likely end when lockdown ends. The desire to reunite with real friends will outweigh shallow acquaintances. However, statistically, it is almost certain that when lockdown ends, a minority will seek to act out the violent narratives that constitute their newly adopted identities.

Poverty does not directly cause terrorism yet provides the conditions in which terrorism may emerge. For example, most Islamist terrorists in Europe are poor young migrants from North Africa, especially Morocco, Tunisia, and Algeria. Magnus Ranstorp has argued that in the developing world, COVID-19 has resulted in millions of children falling into extreme poverty.[21] This is compounded by the fact that wealthy countries have cut their humanitarian aid budgets as a direct result of the pandemic. Moreover, fewer employment opportunities for the MENA region's large youth population coupled with protests that persist due to deep political and socio-economic grievances are likely to add fuel to pre-existing extremist narratives in the Middle East and beyond. Audrey Cronin suggests that the inability of the west to respond effectively to COVID-19 has significantly fueled political violence including riots, hate crimes, inter-communal tensions, and the rise of criminal governance. She adds, 'terrorism is just one element of the growing political instability as people find themselves suffering economically, unable to recreate their pre-COVID lives'.[22] Speckhard further argues that 'during lockdowns, people feel alone and disempowered… and looking for belonging and answers; this makes them perfect prey for terrorist recruiters who already have the skills to develop close bonds over the Internet and to incite people to violence without ever meeting in person'.[23]

Terrorist Attacks

To what extent has COVID-19 impacted the landscape of terrorist attacks? In June 2020, the UNCTED suggested that the imposition of lockdowns and travel restrictions had disrupted terrorist operations.[24] Challenging this finding, Kruglanski et al. claimed that despite the world's overwhelming preoccupation with the COVID-19 pandemic, all the indications were that terrorism was increasing.[25] To understand these two competing narratives, we must recognize that each may be referring to a different terrorist landscape. While one region (for example Europe) may be completely locked down and thus terrorism has been largely disrupted, another region (e.g. Nigeria) may be mostly free of COVID-19 and therefore terrorism is thriving as government forces have been diverted to delivering PPE and vaccines. It is difficult to reliably evaluate the impact of COVID-19 on terrorist attacks. Ordinarily, it takes months if not years of planning before a terrorist attack takes place. A spike or decline in terrorist attacks should not automatically lead us to conclude that COVID-19 is responsible. Correlation is not causation. In exploring the landscape of terrorist attacks, we are concerned with three distinct actors. Firstly, classic insurgents. Typically, Islamist insurgents fighting against local governments supported by western special forces. For example, Al-Qaeda in Iraq and ISIS in Syria, Boko Haram in Nigeria and the Taliban in Afghanistan. Secondly, Islamist extremists in Europe who are willing to carry out terrorism either on their own initiative or at the direction of foreign insurgents. Examples include the men responsible for the 2004 Madrid bombing, the 2005 London bombing, and the Manchester 2017 attack. Lastly, there is the potential for terrorist attacks by non-Islamist extremists. This includes far-right nationalists and various other new groups that have emerged during the COVID-19 pandemic. Let us begin our analysis by examining classic insurgents who have largely continued to operate in Iraq, Syria and Afghanistan despite calls for a humanitarian ceasefire to focus on the pandemic.

Classic Insurgency

Commenting at the start of the COVID-19 pandemic, UNCTED suggested that insurgents would likely be limited in their ability to carry out attacks. Firstly, restrictions on freedom of movement would mean fewer crowded spaces. This assumption makes sense given that insurgent groups in Iraq are renowned for using truck bombs against civilian markets in Iraq. Second, restrictions on the movement of goods would likely cut the supply of food, medicine, finance, and weapons. Presumably, insurgents would be inclined to preserve their supplies until logistics returned to normal. In Afghanistan, the Taliban rely on the sale of narcotics to fund their operations. During COVID-19, the flow of drugs into Europe has declined. A reduced income would presumably limit the ability to fund offensive operations against the Afghan government. Third, the global focus on COVID-19 has reduced media attention given to terrorist attacks. Add to this a general redirection of money to help pay for medical supplies and the net income for terrorists' groups has likely declined significantly since late 2019. Despite these problems, evidence suggests that in 2020, insurgents have not merely continued to carry out attacks but in some regions, intensified their efforts.

The Armed Conflict Location and Event Data Project (ACLED) provides a useful tool for the analysis of terrorist events around the globe. Between January 2019 and December 2019, ACLED recorded 577 acts of violence against civilians by insurgents in the Middle East.[26] Despite the global pandemic, between January 2020 and December 2020, that number increased by 16.5%, to 672. Unsurprisingly, most attacks took place in Syria, Iraq, and Yemen. In April 2020 alone, ISIS launched over 100 attacks in Iraq.[27] Despite the tragedy of COVID-19, the Taliban have continued to demonstrate their willingness to carry out crimes against humanity in Afghanistan. Twenty years fighting the US military has seemingly done little to change the group's antiquated ideas regarding gender quality and the right of girls to pursue education. ISIS and its affiliated groups have been equally devastating in their terrorist operations against innocent civilians. Communiques issued by ISIS in March 2020 directed followers to exploit the weakness caused by COVID and show no mercy against western crusaders. Perhaps viewed as a gift from God against the enemies of Islam, COVID-19 has led militant groups in Egypt, Niger, Nigeria, Philippines, Syria, and Pakistan to significantly increase their attacks.[28]

Islamist Terrorism in Europe

Observers have presumed that social distancing and lockdowns would significantly reduce the potential for terrorist attacks in the parts of Europe most devastated by COVID-19. For example, Madrid 2004 and London 2005 both relied on packed commuter trains. Similarly, Paris 2015 and London Bridge 2017 relied on bustling nightlife on the streets or inside pubs, clubs and restaurants. However, not all terrorism in Europe 2001–2019 relied on crowded locations. At least 35% of attackers used of knives which subsequently resulted in a smaller number of victims.[29] During the pandemic, lengthy queues were regularly seen outside large supermarkets and small groups of friends and family continued to meet in local parks. For the determined terrorist, there was no shortage of potential targets throughout 2020.

According to Europol, during the height of the 2020 European lockdown, only six Islamist terrorist attacks took place in the EU.[30] However, significantly, the modus operandi of five of these incidents was mass stabbings. In each case, the individual used knives, except for a November incident when the attacker made used of firearms and a fake suicide vest. According to Speckhard, there are approximately 1,000 ISIS terrorists in Europe ready to act.[31] Recognizing that the predicted number of knife-based attacks took place, we suggest it is only due to the absence of large crowds that the predicted vehicle and explosive based attacks were not carried out. As lockdown restrictions begin to lift in 2021, we anticipate there will be a significant rise in terrorist attacks towards the end of the year.

Non-Islamist Terrorism

The final group to consider are non-Islamist extremists. According to Jones, the far-right extremists have not been 'sitting idle' during the COVID-19 pandemic. The Center for Strategic and International Studies explain that 'white supremacists and other like-minded extremists conducted two-thirds of the terrorist plots and attacks in the United States in 2020 (…). Anarchists, anti-fascists, and other extremists orchestrated twenty percent of the plots and attacks, though the number of incidents grew from previous years as these extremists targeted law enforcement, military, and government facilities and personnel'.[32] During 2020 there were at least fifty vehicle ramming attacks targeting protestors.[33]

Inthe US alone, the far-right, anti-vaccine, anti-lockdown and various other extremists groups have intensified their attacks, feeding off protests against police brutality.[34] In 2020, the far-right was responsible for 90% of terrorist attack, compared to 66% in 2019.[35] Furthermore, Michael Negata highlights how dissatisfaction with the US government response to the pandemic has resulted in a substantial increase in domestic terrorism. On the first day of lockdown in March 2020, the FBI disrupted a plot in Missouri to attack a hospital. The attacker had allegedly been inspired by the rhetoric of the loosely organized far-right anti-government extremist movement known as the 'boogaloo boys'. In the UK, extremist conspiracies have dramatically increased during lengthy periods of house arrest. One such conspiracy around the 5G telecommunication network resulted in the destruction of equipment by extremists. What is clear is that COVID-19 has significantly fueled domestic extremism. However, radicalization is an incubation process—an increase in extremism takes time to translate into an increase in terrorism. As the world gradually returns to normal in early 2022, amidst an economic depression, the conditions will be ripe for a wave of domestic terrorism.

Bioterrorism

In May 2021, US President Joe Biden announced an urgent investigation into the origins of COVID-19.[36] This announcement followed increasing reports the virus 'leaked' from a virology lab in Wuhan, China.[37] A classified US intelligence report claims that three researchers from that lab were treated in hospital in November 2019, just before the virus began infecting humans in the city.[38] If we assume that COVID-19 was entirely man-made, then we are now in an age where states and eventually non-state actors can engineer biological weapons of mass destruction. What might a world look like where terrorists are constantly seeking to develop or gain access to second or third generation coronavirus bioweapons? Although there is no suggestion that the Wuhan lab was part of any military programme, the weaponization of nature is hardly unprecedented. Throughout history, rudimentary forms of biological warfare have been widely pursued. In 1975, the Biological Weapons Convention (BWC) came into force, prohibiting the development, production and use of biological weapons. As of March 2021, 183 states have signed the treaty.[39]

Historically, terrorist groups have used and continue to seek out chemical and biological weapons. Terrorists are not party to the BWC and have a long history of pursuing the acquisition of weapons of mass destruction. In 2019, researchers at the International Center for the Study of Violent Extremism (ICSVE) interviewed doctoral-level scientists who had been recruited by ISIS to study scientific journals about biological and chemical advancements and from these, compile instructions on what to buy and how to create weapons of mass destruction in a lab they were running in Erbil, Iraq.[40] During the first few months of 2020, when the devastation of COVID-19 became clear, the Islamic State and Al-Qaeda touted the destructive effects of the virus on the West, and white supremacist groups called for their adherents to use the virus in spray bottles to infect specific targets.[41] In May 2020, the sixth edition of Voice of Hind, a pro-Islamic State propaganda magazine, encouraged Muslims to become infected with the virus in order to spread it to security forces and disbelievers.[42] For their part, right-wing extremist groups in the US have encouraged those of their followers on social networks who contracted COVID-19 to spread the disease to law enforcement, non-Whites, and Jews, for example, by spreading saliva on door handles at FBI offices or synagogues.[43]

Has bioterrorism become more attractive to modern day terrorist groups? The inability of even highly developed countries to effectively stop the spread of the virus has hardly gone unnoticed. Based on these experiences, Ackerman and Peterson have suggested that 'particularly vicious terrorist groups might attempt to build new biological weapons to achieve their extremist goals'.[44] Juan Zarate concurs when he writes, 'the severity and extreme disruption of a novel coronavirus will likely spur the imagination of the most creative and dangerous groups and individuals to reconsider bio-terrorist attacks'.[45] Ali Soufan warned that 'although the barriers to entry for terrorists to get their hands on bioweapons remain high, they are gradually being lowered due to technological advances and the democratization of science'.[46] In 2020, the Council of Europe felt the need to issue a warning when intelligence services raised concerns about extremist groups seeking to capture the coronavirus for possible use as a bioweapon.[47] In terms of lethality, COVID-19 is not in the same league as chemical weapons such as VX Gas, Sarin or even Chlorine. Evidence gathered during the COVID-19 pandemic suggests it has a mortality rate of about 1%.[48] However, as a weapon of mass disruption, COVID appears to be the most devastating virus to impact the planet in over one hundred years.

COVID-19 has demonstrated the power of biological agents to disrupt, disable, and deny the most powerful nations in the world from pursuing their national interests. During the height of the pandemic in 2020, western nations including the US, Britain, France, Germany, and Australia were almost entirely shut down as near total lockdown restricted the movement of entire populations. No witness to the global economic, sociological, and humanitarian devastation caused by COVID-19, could possibly deny its attractiveness to non-state actors engaged in asymmetric warfare against a technologically superior adversary. Since 9/11, the hallmark of Islamist terrorism has been mass casualty attacks. No conventional method of suicide terrorism comes anywhere close to the number of casualties that can be achieved using a biological weapon. Historically, WMD has always been out of reach of terrorist groups due to the significant technicalities involved in production and distribution. Despite having the state level capabilities, the Iranians and North Koreans have struggled to create viable nuclear weapons. Notwithstanding the unlikely scenario in which they gain access to the technical knowledge required, the suggestion that Al-Qaeda or ISIS might develop a nuclear device in a tent in Iraq or Afghanistan is farcical—although stealing it is a different matter. Yet with COVID-19 and its variants running wild throughout the world, the possibilities for bioterrorism are endless. Critically, if intelligence reports are correct and COVID-19 was engineered in a lab in Wuhan, we can reasonably assume the technical knowledge necessary to create a new variant will eventually enter the public domain.

Does coronavirus represent the next generation of terrorism? The answer to this question is not straightforward because we are dealing with several variables that are unpredictable and uncontrollable. First, the pandemic is unprecedented in modern history and therefore global governance on this issue is still very much in its infancy. How powerful states react to COVID-19, will likely determine whether terrorists' groups consider bioweapons a viable alternative to conventional attacks. While the US allegedly adopted a liberal approach and allowed nature to take its course, European states have been far more authoritarian in protecting citizens ahead of their economies. The opportunity to shut down Europe is highly attractive to both ISIS and Al-Qaeda. Second, the effectiveness of treatment and immunization varies considerably. If vaccines eliminate the harm caused by current and future variants of coronavirus, it is unlikely that any form of bioterrorism connected to the virus will emerge. Third, COVID-19 variants threaten to completely derail efforts to eradicate or at least bring the virus under control. Fourth, there are long-term side effects of having COVID-19. There is evidence of secondary disease caused by COVID including lung damage, long COVID, and black fungus. Even if coronavirus only injures a population, it will remain a dangerous risk to the state and therefore attractive to terrorist groups.

Generally, whether terrorists will pursue bioterrorism will likely depend on the target country in terms of current infection level, variant types, treatment capabilities and appetite for risk. For example, consider India in early 2021 when the daily infection rate had reached approximately 200,000 per day. In this scenario, a terrorist group threatening to spread the virus would be of diminished concern. Compare this with New Zealand in June 2020 when daily new cases were zero. Is it plausible that in this scenario, far-right extremists might seek to spread COVID-19 amongst ethnic minority communities? Let us consider another potential scenario. In May 2021, the 'Indian variant' of COVID-19 threatened to derail the UK roadmap out of lockdown. Consequently, the government intensified its efforts to vaccinate areas where people had tested positive. Recognizing how significant the global pandemic has been in forcing western military forces to disengage from Africa, Afghanistan, Syria, and Iraq, is it possible that insurgent groups encouraged followers in the UK to deliberately spread variants along with misinformation about the vaccine? If the West is tied up fighting COVID-19, insurgents are free to regroup, consolidate and rebound against territory lost to government forces. Although insurgent groups might encourage the spread of COVID-19 against a distant enemy, it is unlikely they would seek to use such bioweapons domestically. Any attempt to disrupt government forces would almost certainly result in 'blowback'. First, against the civilian population that may support the insurgents. Second, against the insurgent forces themselves. That said, ISIS are highly apocalyptic in their outlook. It is not entirely implausible that they view COVID as a weapon from God and therefore are willing to ravage the entire state of Syria in the expectation that God would determine the outcome in their favor.

Counter Terrorism

Counterterrorism strategies seek to prevent non-state actors from accomplishing their terrorist goals. Strategic and tactical operations can include everything from educating school children on the dangers of extremism to military led targeted assassinations of terrorist leaders. In the front-line war on terror, there are roughly four main agents. First, civil servants. Across government, a range of specialist units are responsible for tracking and intercepting terrorist finance, education, policy development, and co-ordination of activities designed to counterideologies known to fuel violent extremism. One such agency in the UK is the Office for Security and Counter Terrorism (OSCT). Second, intelligence agencies. It is the responsibility of organizations like the FBI and MI5 to investigate and disrupt terrorist plots before they come to fruition. Third, police officers. Front line services are necessary to execute arrest warrants for individuals suspected of engaging in terrorist activity. Fourth, preventative military engagements abroad. In this section, we consider how COVID-19 has impacted these various agencies in the short, medium, and long term.

Short-Term View

The global pandemic has significantly reduced the ability of western states to fully participate in the war on terrorism. According to Kruglanski and Speckhard, coalition allies have been so concerned about the spread of COVID-19 in Iraq that they have proactively removed troops from front line duties.[49] At the tactical level, Colin Clarke notes how 'the coronavirus has forced US special forces commandos to begin withdrawing from conflict zones around the world'.[50] In a COVID-19 special edition of West Point's CTC Sentinel, Ali Soufan highlights how US-led global coalition troops have drawn down following the suspension of training. Confined to their bases to prevent transmission of the disease, troops are no longer performing the kind of counterinsurgency operations necessary to prevent insurgents from regaining lost territory. Furthermore, knowledge that troops are concentrated in a single location has likely increased the level of attacks directed at them. While deteriorating political and military conditions in Iraq predate the global pandemic, the US withdrawing its attention and resources from the region has exasperated the challenges faced by the fragile Iraqi government. Domestically, there has also been an impact on counterterrorism, including a shift from community policing to lockdown enforcement. Fewer officers have been available to carry out routine checks on individual extremists suspected of planning a terrorist attack. In the March 2020 issue of Al-Naba magazine, ISIS emphasized that coalition forces were 'stretched to the maximum' in efforts to curb the pandemic and therefore followers should use this opportunity to strike at the enemy.[51] Laitith Al-Khouri suggests that ISIS will try to take advantage of the pandemic by launching attacks where there are fewer security measures.[52]

Medium-Term View

Tactical shielding of western forces is intermittent. Insurgent groups may be reluctant to act given the uncertainty of troop movements. However, the medium-term reallocation of military forces to health emergencies, may result in an overall strategic change of direction. In Afghanistan, the Taliban long understood that the US could not remain in the country indefinitely and that it was simply a matter of time before they would regain power. Although a peace deal had been brokered long before COVID-19, the global pandemic accelerated the US departure. Consequently, the Afghan government had less time to handle the transition in 2021. More generally, the focus on tackling COVID-19 has created an opening for insurgent groups to regain lost territory and potentially expand into areas not previously explored. This in turn may result in an increase in both financial support and new recruits. Abdul Basit highlights that in several developing countries fighting insurgency, COVID-19 is forcing them to reallocate their human and financial capital to relief activities including the distribution of PPE and vaccines.[53] Consequently, the reserve military forces needed to guard installations, secure terrorist prisoners, and provide an emergency troop surge are simply not available. Magnus Ranstorp has suggested that ISIS will intensify its efforts during the global pandemic to liberate prisoners held in Syria, Iraq, and other detention facilities.[54]

Long-Term View

The global pandemic will likely have a severe long-term impact on the global war on terrorism. Former US president George W Bush claimed that the purpose of occupying Afghanistan and Iraq was to remove ungoverned space used by terrorist groups to train resources and plan attacks against the West. This objective has arguably been successful. Both Al-Qaeda in Afghanistan and ISIS in Iraq have mostly been denied the space and time needed to effectively organize and execute large scale terrorist attacks. Islamist insurgents in the Middle East have been reduced to inciting followers in Europe and the US to carry out small scale operations. This may change over the next five years. A long-term strategic change in priorities from counterterrorism to counterpandemic, may allow these groups to regroup, re-occupy, and re-emerge more powerful than before. This fear is shared by the Financial Action Task Force (FAFF) who have commented that the expected long-term reallocation of military and financial resources away from tackling groups like Al-Qaeda and ISIS and towards health emergencies, could significantly weaken the global war on terror.[55] In June 2020, the UN reported that some member states had already announced the reallocation of resources including withdrawal of foreign armies involved in operations against ISIS.[56] Furthermore, Campbell highlights how the UK has delayed military deployments to Africa to focus on fighting the COVID-19 virus.[57] Without the tremendous intelligence and military resources of powerful western nations, local government forces in Africa are ill equipped to prevent a resurgence of Islamist extremists.

Conclusion

What might we expect the landscape of terrorism to look like in the post COVID era? This is a difficult question to answer because it depends on variables beyond our control. Logically, there seem to be several possible scenarios. First, total eradication. COVID-19 ends completely. Consistent with the Spanish Flu 1918–1920, by 2022 there are no more reported cases of COVID-19 and its variant strains anywhere in the world. Second, the disease becomes manageable, like influenza. COVID-19 continues to circulate in the same way as an 'ordinary' flu but is easily managed and no longer presents a public health emergency. Third, new vaccine resistant variants of COVID-19 result in a continued war against nature. Regardless of how COVID-19 plays out, there has and will continue to be a devastating impact on the world economy. Observers suggest two possible outcomes. First, as Audrey Cronin says, 'as often happens in history, the terrorist threat will likely be gradually overshadowed by bigger problems as economies fail and we face the prospect of a global depression'.[58] This scenario assumes that bioterrorism never materializes. Alternatively, terrorism may surge due to the expansion of extremist ideology during the pandemic. Olympic levels of resentment towards capitalism and global governance could result in a world-wide 'Arab Spring'.

Extremism has flourished during the global pandemic and the foundations for revolution may have been laid during the lockdowns of 2020. Unable to leave home, millions of people sought unity and new political ideologies in chat rooms, internet websites and on various social media platforms. Ironically, the resources needed to 'de-radicalize' these individuals may no longer be available. Pantucci has suggested that even if COVID-19 is eradicated or becomes manageable, the pressure on government budgets could lead to pressure to cut national counterterrorism and CVE budgets.[59] Lockdown disrupted activities that are often critical to the success of long-term counterradicalization efforts, and it is unlikely these programmes will resume when the pandemic eventually ends.[60] Budget cuts to counterextremism will likely begin when they are needed the most. Large numbers of disillusioned and unemployed people, especially youths, present an opportunity for terrorist groups and the operational consequences of increased recruitment and radicalization are likely to be felt then.[61] In the post-COVID-19 world, some new forms of violence such as anti-establishment protest movements, violent environmental activism and anti-technology groups may also emerge.[62] In terms of countering violent extremism, researchers have suggested that states may realign, rather than reduce funding, including prioritizing 'dual-use' hard security measures (such as digital surveillance) at the expense of long-term programmes focused on tackling the root causes of terrorism.[63]

Notwithstanding the likely decline in domestic counterextremism, will the same be true for the global war on terrorism? Can the US and the UK continue to afford and justify low intensity conflicts waged against insurgents in Iraq, Syria, and North Africa? One study in 2020 concluded that 'COVID-19 will almost certainly handicap domestic security efforts and international counter-ISIS cooperation'.[64] Even if COVID-19 is completely eradicated and Western states return to pre-2020 normality, there will almost certainly be a long-term impact on military campaigns against ISIS, Al-Qaeda, and various other Islamist insurgent groups. Persistent challenges to international cooperation and multilateralism may be exacerbated by the pandemic, negatively impacting contributions to multinational forces involved in counterterrorism or peacekeeping operations. This will likely be compounded by a reduction in the funding of technical assistance and capacity-building.[65] Lieutenant General (Ret) Michael Nagata, has remarked, 'I believe the aftermath of today's pandemic will be characterized by terrorism finding a more hospitable global environment for recruitment, growth, and action than before'.[66] We agree. In the best-case scenario, COVID-19 is completely eradicated. However, the financial impact of the global pandemic means that it is unlikely the global war on terrorism will easily regain medium-term losses. In Afghanistan, we anticipate the Taliban will have completely regained power by the end of 2022. In the worst-case scenario, new mutations of COVID-19 or second-generation coronavirus will continue to have an impact on national security policy and force western nations to completely withdraw from overseas deployment. Should this be the case, insurgent groups in Iraq and Syria will continue to rebound and there will be nobody to challenge them. Of great concern is that in this final scenario, where variants remain in the wild, ISIS will have the time and space needed to develop the kind of bioterrorism capabilities discussed above. Whatever the outlook in 2022 is for the global pandemic, it is unlikely the War on Terror will ever be the same.

Notes

1. Sarah Marsh, "UK Reports 1,820 More Covid Deaths, the Most Recorded in One Day", *The Guardian*, January 20, 2021, https://www.theguardian.com/world/2021/jan/20/uk-reports-1820-covid-deaths-in-record-daily-high.
2. Peter Beaumont, "Covid: India Posts Global Record Deaths After State Revises Data", *The Guardian*, June 10, 2021, https://www.theguardian.com/world/2021/jun/10/covid-india-posts-global-record-deaths-after-state-revises-data.
3. Peter Beaumont, "Did Covid Come from a Wuhan Lab? What We Know So Far", *The Guardian*, May 27, 2021, https://www.theguardian.com/world/2021/may/27/did-covid-come-from-a-wuhan-lab-what-we-know-so-far.
4. Steven Quay, and Richard Muller, "The Science Suggests a Wuhan Lab Leak", *The Wall Street Journal*, June 15, 2021, https://www.wsj.com/articles/the-science-suggests-a-wuhan-lab-leak-11622995184.
5. Clark McCauley, and Sophia Moskalenko, 'Mechanisms of Political Radicalization: Pathways Toward Terrorism', *Terrorism and Political Violent* 20 no. (2008): 417, https://doi.org/10.1080/09546550802073367
6. Arie Kruglanski et al., "Terrorism in Time of the Pandemic: Exploiting Mayhem", *Global Security: Health, Science and Policy*

5 no.1 (2020): 121–132, https://doi.org/10.1080/23779497.2020.1832903

7. Kate Starbird, "How to Cope with an infodemic", *Brookings*, April 27, 2020, https://www.brookings.edu/techstream/how-to-cope-with-an-infodemic/.
8. James Gordon Meek, "Terrorist Groups Spin COVID-19 as God's 'Smallest Soldier' Attacking West", *ABC News*, 2 April, 2020, https://abcnews.go.com/International/terrorist-groups-spin-covid-19-gods-smallest-soldier/story?id=69930563.
9. "Contending with ISIS in the Time of Coronavirus", *International Crisis Group*, March 31, 2020, https://www.crisisgroup.org/global/contending-isis-time-coronavirus.
10. Arie Kruglanski et al., "Terrorism in Time of the Pandemic: Exploiting Mayhem", *Global Security: Health, Science and Policy* 5 no.1 (2020): 121–132, https://doi.org/10.1080/23779497.2020.1832903
11. Andrew Hanna, "What Islamists Are Doing and Saying on COVID-19 Crisis", *Wilson Center*, May 14, 2020, https://www.npr.org/2020/06/21/880963592/vehicle-attacks-rise-as-extremists-target-protesters.
12. William Avis, "The COVID-19 Pandemic And Response On Violent Extremist Recruitment And Radicalization", *Applied Knowledge Services*, May 4, 2020, https://gsdrc.org/publications/the-covid-19-pandemic-and-response-on-violent-extremist-recruitment-and-radicalisation/.
13. Matt Katz, "Jewish Americans Say They Are Scapegoated for The Coronavirus Spread", *NPR*, May 13, 2020, https://www.npr.org/2020/05/13/854852779/jewish-americans-feel-scapegoated-for-the-coronavirus-spread.
14. "The Impact of the COVID-19 Pandemic on counter-terrorism and Countering Violent Extremism", *United Nations Counter-Terrorism Committee Executive Directorate (UN-CTED),* June 2020, https://www.un.org/securitycouncil/ctc/sites/www.un.org.securitycouncil.ctc/files/files/documents/2021/Jun/cted-paper-the-impact-of-the-covid-19-pandemic-on-counter-t_0.pdf.
15. Chris McGreal, "A Disgraced Scientist And A Viral Video: How a COVID Conspiracy Theory Started", *The Guardian*, May 14, 2020, https://www.theguardian.com/world/2020/may/14/coronavirus-viral-video-plandemic-judy-mikovits-conspiracy-theories.

16. Associated Press, "FBI Agents Kill Man Allegedly Plotting Bomb Attack On Hospital Amid Coronavirus Pandemic", *The Guardian*, Match 26, 2020, ttps://www.theguardian.com/us-news/2020/mar/26/hospital-bomb-attack-man-killed-fbi-agents-missouri.
17. "The Impact of the COVID-19 Pandemic on Counterterrorism and Countering Violent Extremism", *United Nations Counter-Terrorism Committee Executive Directorate (UN-CTED),* June 2020, https://www.un.org/securitycouncil/ctc/sites/www.un.org.securitycouncil.ctc/files/files/documents/2021/Jun/cted-paper-the-impact-of-the-covid-19-pandemic-on-counter-t_0.pdf.
18. Ibid.
19. "Teenage Boy Charged in Canada's First 'incel' Terror Case", *BBC News*, May 20, 2020, https://www.bbc.co.uk/news/world-us-canada-52733060.
20. Damien Gayle, "Britain's Youngest Convicted Terrorist Avoids Jail", *The Guardian*, Feb 8, 2021, https://www.theguardian.com/uk-news/2021/feb/08/britains-youngest-convicted-terrorist-avoids-jail.
21. Audrey Cronin et al., "Special Issue: COVID-19 & Counter Terrorism", *Combating Terrorism Center at West Point* 13, no. 6 (June 2020): 1–53, https://ctc.usma.edu/wp-content/uploads/2020/06/CTC-SENTINEL-062020.pdf.
22. Ibid.
23. Anne Speckhard, and Molly Ellenberg, "ISIS in Their Own Words", *Journal of Strategic Security* 13, no.1 (2020): 82–127, https://doi.org/10.5038/1944-0472.13.1.1791.
24. "The Impact of the COVID-19 Pandemic on Counterterrorism and Countering Violent Extremism", *United Nations Counter-Terrorism Committee Executive Directorate (UN-CTED),* June 2020, https://www.un.org/securitycouncil/ctc/sites/www.un.org.securitycouncil.ctc/files/files/documents/2021/Jun/cted-paper-the-impact-of-the-covid-19-pandemic-on-counter-t_0.pdf.
25. Arie Kruglanski et al., "Terrorism in Time of the Pandemic: Exploiting Mayhem", *Global Security: Health, Science and Policy* 5 no.1 (2020): 121–132, https://doi.org/10.1080/23779497.2020.1832903.

26. Armed Conflict Location and Event Data Project (ACLED), ACLED collects real-time data on the locations, dates, actors, fatalities, and types of all reported political violence and protest events across the world.
27. Colin Clarke, "Yesterday's Terrorists Are Today's Public-Health Providers", *Foreign Policy,* April 8, 2020, https://foreignpolicy.com/2020/04/08/terrorists-nonstate-ungoverned-health-providers-coronavirus-pandemic/.
28. SITE Intelligence Group, "Weekly in SITE on Islamic State", *SITE Enterprise*, July 9, 2020.
29. Lewis Herrington, *Understanding Islamist Terrorism in Europe* (London: Routledge, 2021).
30. Ibid.
31. Anne Speckhard, and Molly Ellenberg, "ISIS in Their Own Words", *Journal of Strategic Security* 13, no.1 (2020): 82–127, https://doi.org/10.5038/1944-0472.13.1.1791.
32. Seth Jones, "The War Comes Home: The Evolution of Domestic Terrorism in the US", *Center for Strategic & International Studies*, October 22, 2020, https://www.csis.org/analysis/war-comes-home-evolution-domestic-terrorism-united-states.
33. Hannah Allam, 'Vehicle attacks rise as extremists target protesters', *NPR*, June 21, 2020, https://www.npr.org/2020/06/21/880963592/vehicle-attacks-rise-as-extremists-target-protesters
34. Seth Jones et al., "The Escalating Terrorism Problem in the US. The Escalating Terrorism Problem in the US", *Center for Strategic and International Studies*, June 17, 2020, https://www.npr.org/2020/06/21/880963592/vehicle-attacks-rise-as-extremists-target-protesters.
35. Ibid.
36. "Statement by President Joe Biden on the Investigation into the Origins of COVID-19", *The White House*, May 26, 2021, https://www.whitehouse.gov/briefing-room/statements-releases/2021/05/26/statement-by-president-joe-biden-on-the-investigation-into-the-origins-of-covid-19/.
37. Peter Beaumont, "Did COVID Come from a Wuhan Lab? What we Know So Far", *The Guardian,* May 27, 2020, https://www.theguardian.com/world/2021/may/27/did-covid-come-from-a-wuhan-lab-what-we-know-so-far.

38. Michael Gordon, "Intelligence on Sick Staff at Wuhan Lab Fuels Debate on COVID-19 Origin", *The Wall Street Journal,* May 23, 2021, https://www.wsj.com/articles/intelligence-on-sick-staff-at-wuhan-lab-fuels-debate-on-covid-19-origin-11621796228.
39. The Biological Weapons Convention (BWC), which effectively prohibits biological and toxin weapons, was opened for signature on 10 April 1972 and entered into force on 26 March 1975, See; Seth Carus, "The History of Biological Weapons Use: What We Know and What We Do Not", *Health Security* 13, no. 4 (2015): 219–55, https://doi.org/10.1089/hs.2014.0092.
40. Anna Speckhard, and Ardian Shajkovci, "ISIS Chemical-Weapons Expert Speaks." *The Daily Beast*, March 11, 2019, https://www.thedailybeast.com/isis-chemical-weapons-expert-speaks-in-exclusive-interview.
41. Josh Margolin, "White Supremacists Encouraging Their Members To Spread Coronavirus to Cops, Jews, FBI Says." *ABC News*, March 23, 2020, https://abcnews.go.com/US/white-supremacists-encouraging-members-spread-coronavirus-cops-jews/story?id=69737522.
42. Chelsea Daymon, and Meili Criezis, "Pandemic Narratives: Pro-Islamic State Media and the Coronavirus," *Combating Terrorism Center at West Point* 13, no. 6 (June 2020): 31, https://ctc.usma.edu/pandemic-narratives-pro-islamic-state-media-and-the-coronavirus/.
43. Gary Ackerman, and Hayley Peterson, "Terrorism and COVID-19: Actual and Potential Impacts", *Perspectives on Terrorism* 14, no.3 (2020): 65, https://www.universiteitleiden.nl/perspectives-on-terrorism/archives/2020#volume-xiv-issue-3.
44. Ibid.
45. Audrey Cronin et al., "Special Issue: COVID-19 & Counter Terrorism", *Combating Terrorism Center at West Point* 13, no. 6 (June 2020): 1–53, https://ctc.usma.edu/wp-content/uploads/2020/06/CTC-SENTINEL-062020.pdf.
46. Ibid.
47. "Covid-19 Pandemic: The Secretariat of the Committee on Counter-Terrorism Warns Against the Risk of Bioterrorism", *Council of Europe Newsroom*, 6 May, 2020.
48. Sabine Elsland, "COVID-19 Deaths: Infection Fatality Ratio is About 1% says New Report", Imperial College London, October

29, 2020, https://www.imperial.ac.uk/news/207273/covid-19-deaths-infection-fatality-ratio-about/.
49. Arie Kruglanski et al., "Terrorism in Time Of The Pandemic: Exploiting Mayhem", *Global Security: Health, Science and Policy* 5 no.1 (2020): 121–132, https://doi.org/10.1080/23779497.2020.1832903.
50. Colin Clarke, "Yesterday's Terrorists Are Today's Public-Health Providers", *Foreign Policy,* April 8, 2020, https://foreignpolicy.com/2020/04/08/terrorists-nonstate-ungoverned-health-providers-coronavirus-pandemic/.
51. Mina Al-Lami, "Jihadists See COVID-19 as an Opportunity. The Global Network on Extremism and Technology", *Global Network on Extremism & Technology*, 1st June 2020, https://gnet-research.org/2020/06/01/jihadists-see-covid-19-as-an-opportunity/.
52. Mia Bloom, "How Terrorist Groups Will Try to Capitalize on the Coronavirus Crisis", *Just Security*, April 3, 2020, https://www.justsecurity.org/69508/how-terrorist-groups-will-try-to-capitalize-on-the-coronavirus-crisis/.
53. Abdul Basit, "COVID-19: A Challenge Or Opportunity For terrorist Groups?", *Journal of Policing, Intelligence and Counter Terrorism* 15, no.3 (2020): 263–275, https://www.tandfonline.com/doi/full/10.1080/18335330.2020.1828603.
54. Audrey Cronin et al., "Special Issue: COVID-19 & Counter Terrorism", *Combating Terrorism Center at West Point* 13, no. 6 (June 2020): 1–53, https://ctc.usma.edu/wp-content/uploads/2020/06/CTC-SENTINEL-062020.pdf.
55. "Covid-19-Related Money Laundering And Terrorist Financing: Risk And Policy Response", *FATF*, 2020, https://www.fatf-gafi.org/media/fatf/documents/COVID-19-AML-CFT.pdf, 3.
56. "The Impact of the COVID-19 Pandemic on Counterterrorism and Countering Violent Extremism", *United Nations Counter-Terrorism Committee Executive Directorate (UN-CTED),* June 2020, https://www.un.org/securitycouncil/ctc/sites/www.un.org.securitycouncil.ctc/files/files/documents/2021/Jun/cted-paper-the-impact-of-the-covid-19-pandemic-on-counter-t_0.pdf.
57. John Campbell, "How Jihadi Groups in Africa will Exploit COVID-19", *Council on Foreign Relations*, April 3, 2020, https://www.cfr.org/blog/how-jihadi-groups-africa-will-exploit-covid-19.

58. Audrey Cronin et al., "Special Issue: COVID-19 & Counter Terrorism", *Combating Terrorism Center at West Point* 13, no. 6 (June 2020): 1–53, https://ctc.usma.edu/wp-content/uploads/2020/06/CTC-SENTINEL-062020.pdf.
59. Raffaello Pantucci, "Key Questions for Counter-Terrorism Post-COVID-19", *Counter Terrorist Trends and Analyses* 12, no.3 (2020):1–6, https://www.jstor.org/stable/26915443.
60. Eric Rosand et al., "Preventing Violent Extremism During and After the COVID-19 Pandemic", *Brookings*, April 28, 2020, https://www.brookings.edu/blog/order-from-chaos/2020/04/28/preventing-violent-extremism-during-and-after-the-covid-19-pandemic/.
61. Gary Ackerman, and Hayley Peterson, "Terrorism and COVID-19: Actual and Potential Impacts", *Perspectives on Terrorism* 14, no. 3, (2020): 59–73. https://www.universiteitleiden.nl/perspectives-on-terrorism/archives/2020#volume-xiv-issue-3.
62. Raffaello Pantucci, "Key Questions for Counter-Terrorism Post-COVID-19", *Counter Terrorist Trends and Analyses* 12, no.3 (2020):1–6, https://www.jstor.org/stable/26915443.
63. Ibid.
64. "Contending with ISIS in the Time of Coronavirus", *International Crisis Group*, March 31, 2020, https://www.crisisgroup.org/global/contending-isis-time-coronavirus.
65. Reed Wood, "Pandemics and Political Violence", *Political Violence at a Glance*, April 8, 2020, https://politicalviolenceataglance.org/2020/04/08/pandemics-and-political-violence.
66. Audrey Cronin et al., "Special Issue: COVID-19 & Counter Terrorism", *Combating Terrorism Center at West Point* 13, no. 6 (June 2020): 1–53, https://ctc.usma.edu/wp-content/uploads/2020/06/CTC-SENTINEL-062020.pdf.

Bibliography

"Afghanistan: Deadly Suicide Attack Targets Funeral in Nangarhar." *Al-Jazeera*, May 12, 2020. https://www.aljazeera.com/news/2020/5/12/afghanistan-deadly-suicide-attack-targets-funeral-in-nangarhar.

"Contending with ISIS in the Time of Coronavirus." *International Crisis Group*, March 31, 2020. https://www.crisisgroup.org/global/contending-isis-time-coronavirus.

"Covid-19 Pandemic: The Secretariat of the Committee on Counter-Terrorism Warns Against The Risk of Bioterrorism." *Council of Europe Newsroom*, 6th of May 2020

"Covid-19-Related Money Laundering And Terrorist Financing: Risk And Policy Response." *FATF*, 2020. https://www.fatf-gafi.org/media/fatf/documents/COVID-19-AML-CFT.pdf

"London Police Under Pressure Over Clashes at Women's Protest." *Voice of America*, March 14, 2021. https://www.voanews.com/europe/london-police-under-pressure-over-clashes-womens-protest.

"Statement by President Joe Biden on the Investigation into the Origins of COVID-19." *The White House*, May 26, 2021. https://www.whitehouse.gov/briefing-room/statements-releases/2021/05/26/statement-by-president-joe-biden-on-the-investigation-into-the-origins-of-covid-19/

"Teenage Boy Charged in Canada's First 'Incel' Terror Case." *BBC News*, May 20, 2020. https://www.bbc.co.uk/news/world-us-canada-52733060

"The Impact of the COVID-19 Pandemic on Counter-Terrorism and Countering Violent Extremism." *United Nations Counter-Terrorism Committee Executive Directorate (UN-CTED)*, June 2020. https://www.un.org/securitycouncil/ctc/sites/www.un.org.securitycouncil.ctc/files/files/documents/2021/Jun/cted-paper-the-impact-of-the-covid-19-pandemic-on-counter-t_0.pdf.

Ackerman, Gary, and Hayley Peterson. "Terrorism and COVID-19: Actual and Potential Impacts." *Perspectives on Terrorism* 14, no. 3, (2020): 59–73. https://www.universiteitleiden.nl/perspectives-on-terrorism/archives/2020#volume-xiv-issue-3.

Al-Lami, Mina. "Jihadists see COVID-19 as an opportunity. The Global Network on Extremism and Technology." *Global Network on Extremism & Technology*, 1st June 2020. https://gnet-research.org/2020/06/01/jihadists-see-covid-19-as-an-opportunity/.

Allam, Hannah. "Vehicle attacks rise as extremists target protesters." *NPR*, 21st June 2020. https://www.npr.org/2020/06/21/880963592/vehicle-attacks-rise-as-extremists-target-protesters.

Associated Press. "FBI Agents Kill Man Allegedly Plotting Bomb Attack On Hospital Amid Coronavirus Pandemic." *The Guardian*, 26th March 2020. https://www.theguardian.com/us-news/2020/mar/26/hospital-bomb-attack-man-killed-fbi-agents-missouri.

Avis, William. "The COVID-19 Pandemic and Response on Violent Extremist Recruitment and Radicalisation." *Applied Knowledge Services*, 4 May, 2020. https://gsdrc.org/publications/the-covid-19-pandemic-and-response-on-violent-extremist-recruitment-and-radicalisation/.

Bacon, John. "Coronavirus Updates: George Floyd Protests Could Fuel COVID Cases, Trump Postpones G7 Summit." *USA Today*, May 31, 2020. https://

www.usatoday.com/story/news/health/2020/05/31/coronavirus-update-donald-trump-g-7-summit-church-reopenings-cuomo/5293061002/.

Barenblatt, Daniel. *A Plague upon Humanity*. London: Harper Collins, 2005.

Basit, Abdul. "COVID-19: A Challenge or Opportunity for Terrorist Groups?" *Journal of Policing, Intelligence and Counter Terrorism* 15, no. 3, (2020): 263–275. https://doi.org/10.1080/18335330.2020.1828603

Beaumont, Peter. "Covid: India posts Global Record Deaths After State Revises Data." *The Guardian*, June 10, 2021, https://www.theguardian.com/world/2021/jun/10/covid-india-posts-global-record-deaths-after-state-revises-data.

Beaumont, Peter. "Did Covid Come from a Wuhan lab? What We Know so Far." *The Guardian Online*, May 27, 2021. https://www.theguardian.com/world/2021/may/27/did-covid-come-from-a-wuhan-lab-what-we-know-so-far.

Bloom, Mia. "How Terrorist Groups Will Try to Capitalize on the Coronavirus Crisis." *Just Security*, April 3, 2020. https://www.justsecurity.org/69508/how-terrorist-groups-will-try-to-capitalize-on-the-coronavirus-crisis/.

Campbell, John. "How Jihadi Groups in Africa Will Exploit COVID-19." *Council on Foreign Relations*, April 3, 2020. https://www.cfr.org/blog/how-jihadi-groups-africa-will-exploit-covid-19

Carus, Seth. "The History Of Biological Weapons Use: What We Know And What We Do Not." *Health Security* 13, no. 4 (2015): 219–55. https://doi.org/10.1089/hs.2014.0092.

Clarke, Colin. "Yesterday's Terrorists Are Today's Public-Health Providers." *Foreign Policy,* April 8, 2020. https://foreignpolicy.com/2020/04/08/terrorists-nonstate-ungoverned-health-providers-coronavirus-pandemic/.

Cronin, Audrey, Michael Nagata, Magnus Ranstorp, Ali Soufan, and Juan Zarate. "Special Issue: COVID-19 & Counter Terrorism." *Combating Terrorism Centre at West Point* 13, no. 6 (June 2020): 1–53. https://ctc.usma.edu/wp-content/uploads/2020/06/CTC-SENTINEL-062020.pdf.

Daymon, Chelsea, and Meili Criezis. "Pandemic Narratives: Pro-Islamic State Media and the Coronavirus." *Combating Terrorism Centre at West Point* 13, no. 6 (June 2020): 1–53. https://ctc.usma.edu/pandemic-narratives-pro-islamic-state-media-and-the-coronavirus/.

Gayle, Damien. "Britain's youngest convicted terrorist avoids jail." *The Guardian*, February 8, 2021. https://www.theguardian.com/uk-news/2021/feb/08/britains-youngest-convicted-terrorist-avoids-jail.

Gordon, Michael. "Intelligence on Sick Staff at Wuhan Lab Fuels Debate on Covid-19 Origin." *The Wall Street Journal,* May 23, 2021. https://www.wsj.com/articles/intelligence-on-sick-staff-at-wuhan-lab-fuels-debate-on-covid-19-origin-11621796228.

Guarrieri, Thomas R., and Collin J. Meisel. "Extremists and Unconventional Weapons: Examining the Pursuit of Chemical and Biological Agents."

Behavioural Sciences of Terrorism and Political Aggression 13, no. 1 (2021): 23-42. https://doi.org/10.1080/19434472.2019.1698633

Hanna, Andrew. "What Islamists Are Doing and Saying on COVID-19 Crisis." *Wilson Centre*, May 14, 2020. https://www.wilsoncenter.org/article/what-islamists-are-doing-and-saying-covid-19-crisis.

Herrington, Lewis. *Understanding Islamist Terrorism in Europe*. London: Routledge, 2021.

Jones, Seth. "The Escalating Terrorism Problem in the United States. The Escalating Terrorism Problem in the United States." *Centre for Strategic and International Studies*, June 17, 2020. https://www.csis.org/analysis/escalating-terrorism-problem-united-states.

Jones, Seth. "The War Comes Home: The Evolution of Domestic Terrorism in the United States." *Centre for Strategic & International Studies*, October 22, 2020. https://www.csis.org/analysis/war-comes-home-evolution-domestic-terrorism-united-states.

Katz, Matt. "Jewish Americans Say They Are Scapegoated for The Coronavirus Spread." *NPR*, May 13, 2020. https://www.npr.org/2020/05/13/854852779/jewish-americans-feel-scapegoated-for-the-coronavirus-spread.

Kruglanski, Arie, Rohan Gunaratna, Molly Ellenberg, and Anne Speckhard. "Terrorism in Time of the Pandemic: Exploiting Mayhem." *Global Security: Health, Science and Policy* 5, no. 1 (2020): 121-132. https://doi.org/10.1080/23779497.2020.1832903.

Makoii, Akhtar. "Taliban Declare Three-Day Eid Ceasefire as 11 Killed in New Bombing." *The Guardian*, May 10, 2021. https://www.theguardian.com/world/2021/may/10/taliban-declares-three-day-eid-ceasefire-after-afghanistan-school-bomb-attacks.

Margolin, Josh. "White Supremacists Encouraging Their Members to Spread Coronavirus to Cops, Jews, FBI says." *ABC News*, March 23, 2020. https://abcnews.go.com/US/white-supremacists-encouraging-members-spread-coronavirus-cops-jews/story?id=69737522.

Marsh, Sarah. "UK Reports 1,820 More Covid Deaths, the Most Recorded in One Day." *The Guardian*, January 20, 2021. https://www.theguardian.com/world/2021/jan/20/uk-reports-1820-covid-deaths-in-record-daily-high.

McCauley, Clark and Sophia Moskalenko. "Mechanisms of Political Radicalization: Pathways Toward Terrorism." *Terrorism and Political Violent* 20, no. 3 (2008):415-433. https://doi.org/10.1080/09546550802073367.

McGreal, Chris. "A Disgraced Scientist and a Viral Video: How a Covid Conspiracy Theory Started." *The Guardian*, May 14, 2020. https://www.theguardian.com/world/2020/may/14/coronavirus-viral-video-plandemic-judy-mikovits-conspiracy-theories.

Meek, James. "Terrorist Groups Spin COVID-19 as God's 'Smallest Soldier' Attacking West." *ABC News*, April 2, 2020. https://abcnews.go.com/Int

ernational/terrorist-groups-spin-covid-19-gods-smallest-soldier/story?id=69930563.

Mowatt-Larssen, Rolf. "Al-Qaeda's Pursuit of Weapons of Mass Destruction." *Foreign Policy*, January 25, 2010. https://foreignpolicy.com/2010/01/25/al-qaedas-pursuit-of-weapons-of-mass-destruction/.

Ong, Kyler and Nur Azman. "Distinguishing Between the Extreme Far-right and Islamic State's (IS) Calls to Exploit COVID-19." *Counter Terrorist Trends and Analyses* 12, no.3 (2020):18–21. https://www.jstor.org/stable/26915446.

Pantucci, Raffaello. "Key Questions for Counter-Terrorism Post-COVID-19." *Counter Terrorist Trends and Analyses* 12, no.3 (2020):1–6. https://www.jstor.org/stable/26915443.

Pearson, Alex. "Germany: Man Charged with Producing Biological Weapon at Home in Cologne." *DW*, June 14, 2018. https://www.dw.com/en/germany-man-charged-with-producing-biological-weapon-at-home-in-cologne/a-44214079.

Quay Steven Quay and Richard Muller. "The Science Suggests a Wuhan Lab Leak." *The Wall Street Journal*, June 15, 2021. https://www.wsj.com/articles/the-science-suggests-a-wuhan-lab-leak-11622995184.

Rosand, Eric, Khalid Koser, and Lilla Schumicky-Logan. "Preventing Violent Extremism During and After the Covid-19 Pandemic." *Brookings*, April 28, 2020. https://www.brookings.edu/blog/order-from-chaos/2020/04/28/preventing-violent-extremism-during-and-after-the-covid-19-pandemic/.

Rosenau, William. "Aum Shinrikyo's Biological Weapons Program: Why Did it Fail?" *Studies in Conflict & Terrorism* 24, no.4 (2001): 289–301. https://doi.org/10.1080/10576100120887.

SITE Intelligence Group. "Weekly in SITE on Islamic State." *SITE Enterprise*, July 9, 2020.

Speckhard, Anna, and Ardian Shajkovci. "ISIS Chemical-Weapons Expert Speaks." *The Daily Beast*, March 11, 2019. https://www.thedailybeast.com/isis-chemical-weapons-expert-speaks-in-exclusive-interview.

Speckhard, Anne and Molly Ellenberg. "ISIS in Their Own Words." *Journal of Strategic Security* 13, no. 1 (2020): 82-127. https://doi.org/10.5038/1944-0472.13.1.1791.

Starbird, Kate. "How to Cope with an infodemic." *Brookings*, April 27, 2020. https://www.brookings.edu/techstream/how-to-cope-with-an-infodemic/.

Wood, Reed. "Pandemics and Political Violence." *Political Violence at a Glance*, April 8, 2020. https://politicalviolenceataglance.org/2020/04/08/pandemics-and-political-violence/.

CHAPTER 11

Organized Crime During and After the Pandemic

Virginia Comolli

Introduction

COVID-19 and its subsequent restrictions have impacted most, if not all, aspects of public and private life. As such, it is no surprise that illicit activities, criminality and its by-products, have been as affected by the pandemic as legal businesses and trade. The impact has not been entirely negative for criminal groups. This crisis has shown the level of adaptability that criminal enterprises possess. This chapter assesses how COVID-19 has changed the way of conducting illicit business, with a focus on organized forms of criminality that have significant economic impacts and often transnational connections. It also looks at how permanent those changes are likely to be in the coming years. The chapter then concludes with reflections on how law enforcement must contend with the changing criminal landscape.

To note, there is no universally agreed definition of organized crime. However, the term is commonly used to refer to a serious crime planned

V. Comolli (✉)
The Global Initiative against Transnational Organized Crime, London, UK

C. Varin (ed.), *Global Security in Times of Covid-19*, New Security Challenges, https://doi.org/10.1007/978-3-030-82230-9_11

and executed by a group of three or more individuals working together on a continuing basis. Organized crime is almost always perpetrated for financial gains, often involves the use and/or threat of violence, and can span across international boundaries. These activities take place both in the physical and digital domains and it is common for organized criminal groups to run, or be involved in, legitimate as well as illicit businesses. Among the activities that fall under the category of organized crime are drug, human and arms trafficking, migrant smuggling, money laundering, extortion, counterfeit goods, wildlife and cultural property smuggling, and cybercrime.[1]

Adaptable Criminal Entrepreneurs

Crime and organized crime are ubiquitous. Many in the Western world might spend their entire lives without ever knowingly encountering organized crime, but it is as present in the City of London as in the favelas of Rio the Janeiro or in conflict-ridden Sahel. The reason being that criminal actors are, by definition, opportunistic, willing and able to adapt to different environments in developed and developing countries, in peaceful as well as fragile or unstable contexts. Additionally, evidence shows they are often quick to exploit opportunities brought about by new technologies, ease of movement, weaknesses in law enforcement and governance systems, as well as by economic and other types of crises. For instance, in the aftermath of the 2008 financial crisis, there was a clear uptick in fraud and financial crime.[2] In many conflict zones past and present, from Colombia to Iraq, criminal groups have taken advantage of war economies and disruptions in the supply chain to make money on the black market by supplying weapons as well as foodstuff, to mention just two examples.[3] The European migration crisis of the 2010s created lucrative opportunities, i.e. an almost endless supply of victims, that people smugglers and traffickers were quick to exploit.[4] The 2014–2016 Ebola outbreak in West Africa facilitated the expansion of illegal, unreported and unregulated (IUU) fishing in the Gulf of Guinea, a business that results in billions of dollars' worth of losses for the region's economy each year.[5] With these past experiences in mind, it is easy to conclude that the COVID-19 pandemic and its secondary effects are unlikely to be any different, and indeed are (and will be) opening up avenues for criminal exploitation.

COVID-19's Impact on Crime

The lockdown that first started in Wuhan, China, and was extended to virtually every part of the world, the closure of borders and marketplaces, travel and supply chain disruptions, and declining consumer demand for many goods have all undermined economic activities across all regions. The United Nations estimated a 27% fall, year on year, in global trade growth in the second quarter of 2020—a rate worse than during the 2008 financial crisis.[6] In the face of this crisis, legitimate businesses had to develop creative solutions to stay afloat, such as expanding their online offerings. Similarly, some criminal activities such as street dealing, trafficking using commercial flights and property theft have been curtailed by social distancing measures and travel restrictions and, as a result, criminal groups have doubled their efforts in cybercrime, fraud and counterfeiting, especially of medical supplies and medicines, to survive and even expand.[7] All of these have registered a spike during the pandemic.

Cybercrime

Cyber-enabled crimes have been flourishing in recent years, both on the open Internet and the so-called Dark Net (or Dark Web), a part of the Internet that is only accessible through the anonymized search browser Tor and is not picked up through regular searches. Whilst not all activities and fora are illegal, the Dark Net is a marketplace for stolen documents and identities, drugs, weapons, counterfeit money and the likes.[8]

In 2020, millions of potential crime victims have been home-bound for several weeks or months, representing the ideal targets for cyber criminals who take advantage of people's vulnerability, loneliness, boredom and general increasing reliance on online services—a combination of factors that makes them more likely to click on malicious links, purchase from unsafe websites and fall prey to romance and business email compromise (BEC) scams. Indeed, in its April 2020 COVID-19 global threat assessment, Interpol highlighted a marked increase in the number of malicious domains, malware and ransomware targeting both individuals and organizations. This was accompanied by a spike in drug sales taking place online using social media, the Dark Net and encrypted messaging apps.[9]

Disturbingly, online sexual exploitation, especially of children, rose during the pandemic. Warnings issued by the American Federal Bureau of Investigation (FBI) indicate that children who are home-schooled for protracted periods of time might be vulnerable to grooming for sexual exploitation.[10] Additionally, regular consumers of pornographic and pedo-pornographic material have had more time in their hands, and those who might have thought of accessing such content in the past and never acted upon those desires might, during lockdown, have had the time and curiosity to experiment and enter into contact with like-minded online communities. These factors are likely to have led to a spike in demand, prompting criminals to coerce even more vulnerable adults and children into live or recorded sexual acts to meet that demand for more and new content.[11]

Fraud

A second area criminals have been quick to exploit during the pandemic is fraud, often conducted online. Europol has identified 'fraud schemes, supply scams and decontamination scams' as key concerns during the pandemic, with the expectation that old and new fraudulent schemes would proliferate in the course of 2020 as the pandemic continued.[12] The agency reported that criminals had 'adapted investment scams to elicit speculative investments in stocks related to COVID-19 with promises of substantial profits'.[13] These activities have significant financial costs for individuals, businesses and institutions. Supply scams have proved particularly lucrative. Notably, authorities in Germany, Ireland and the Netherlands were able to uncover a complicated fraud scheme centred around EUR 1.5 million worth of face masks. In March 2020, scrambling to find masks, Germany's health authorities tried to source a large consignment via Germany-based companies that, in turn, reached out to Spanish suppliers. Unbeknown to the Germans, and despite appearing legitimate, the Spanish company's website was fake. It was in the course of email interactions, and following the Spaniards claiming to be unable to source such a large number of masks (10 million) that an Irish middleman came into the scene. This individual brokered a deal between the German companies and a Dutch supplier, which required advanced payment of EUR 1.5 million. Just before delivery was due, the Dutch supplier claimed not to have received the payment and requested a EUR 880,000 emergency transfer. At this stage, the victims became suspicious, contacted local authorities and an investigation was launched in partnership with Interpol. As a result, it was possible to freeze the EUR 1.5 million transaction and recall the transfer of EUR 880,000 from a British bank that was about to reach a Nigerian bank account. It was revealed that the Dutch company's website had been cloned and criminals had posed as representatives of what was in fact a legitimate business. Needless to say, the company had no record of the order for masks.[14]

Counterfeiting and Sales of Sub-standard Goods

As the example mentioned above anticipates, ever-entrepreneurial criminal entities have been eager to exploit the opportunities presented by the pandemic. The health sector has been one of their targets. It should be noted, however, that criminal infiltration of the health system in many countries predates the COVID-19 pandemic and has made them even more vulnerable during this crisis. In the often-cited case of Italy, which incidentally was one of the worst-hit countries in 2020, the mafia's involvement in healthcare and the running of hospitals is a long-standing plague. Analysis by the Italian Parliamentary Antimafia Commission points to the mafia controlling procurement processes to ensure only companies linked to the clans would win contracts. This is both lucrative and creates new avenues for money laundering. Additionally, in a number of hospitals, mafia groups have made sure that management and medical positions were filled by often unqualified affiliates and supporters as a way to control usually large health care budgets but also to consolidate their support-base by offering job opportunities. A further way to win favours, including from corrupt police officers and politicians, is to facilitate access to medical treatments (effectively avoiding what are often months-long waiting lists). Finally, trusted doctors would discreetly treat criminals and produce fake medical certificates.[15]

This level of corruption and mafia involvement have resulted in the dissolution of a number of local health units in Italy, which have then been placed under administration.[16]

The by-products of situations like the one described are very severe and have large health implications. Corruption and related mismanagement of funds have reduced resources to purchase essential supplies leaving some hospitals and ambulance services without life-saving equipment and forcing patients to seek treatment outside their regions, as exemplified by a 2018 operation against the 'Ndrangheta in the southern region of Calabria.[17] These shortcomings are bound to undermine any health system's resilience in the face of crises.[18]

The mafia has also long been involved in waste management. Evidence indicates that Italian groups have become involved in contracts for disposing of the ever-growing medical waste produced in the pandemic such as personal protective equipment (PPE).[19] As pre-COVID-19 investigations indicate, in addition to the corruption and extortion that accompany the illicit waste disposal, the environmental and public health impacts are severe. The infamous 'eco-mafias' are known for burying toxic waste, resulting in high cancer incidence in the affected areas, and to ship waste to emerging and developing countries lacking adequate disposal and recycling facilities.[20] During the pandemic, Operation Pangea XIII, which was conducted by law enforcement, custom and regulatory authorities from 90 countries, resulted in the seizure of over USD 14 million worth of potentially dangerous pharmaceuticals and 121 arrests worldwide in March 2020. The agencies involved recovered thousands of counterfeit and substandard masks, 'corona spray', 'coronavirus packages' or 'coronavirus medicine'.[21] Notwithstanding the financial loss—this is a business worth an estimated USD 431 billion annually[22]—counterfeit and fake medicines and vaccines carry health risks for those taking them. They often contain the wrong amount of active ingredients and, when they are legitimate, they are likely to have been stolen, hence they could be expired or have been poorly stored by the time they reach the user.

This trend and associated risk have further consolidated throughout the pandemic. As European countries faced a second wave of the virus in late 2020 and the development of vaccines was making good progress, Europol warned that as vaccines entered the market, counterfeit versions would no doubt follow suit to meet the high demand. Criminals are expected to circulate fake information, posing as legitimate pharmaceutical companies, in an attempt to sell fake vaccines in licit and illicit physical markets as well as on the Dark Web and the open internet.[23]

The above is likely to have an additional side effect. In the era of fake news and amidst the spread of misinformation surrounding COVID-19 vaccines—ranging from claims that Western vaccines are not effective all the way to deep-state conspiracy theories—there is the risk that hearing about fake COVID-19 medicines will undermine public faith in legitimate vaccines and, consequently, uptake.[24]

COVID-19's Impact on Law Enforcement

Members of law enforcement agencies around the world have not been immune to the adverse effects of the virus. The epidemic has affected staff shortages with officers falling sick or being placed in self-isolation. The resources available for intelligence and investigative work have shrunk with police officers in many countries having to focus on public order policing such as enforcing lockdown restrictions and responding to civil unrest in some places. Notably, in the first weeks of March 2020, Europol recorded a 30% decrease in the number of messages exchanged between individual member-states and the agency—a reflection that national authorities were, albeit only temporarily, focusing their attention elsewhere. Fortunately, by May of that year, the agency confirmed the return to pre-pandemic levels of exchanges.[25]

Deployments to enforce restrictions of movement—which in a number of cases have been supplemented by the military—have also meant that officers assigned to rural areas have been reallocated to cities, i.e. areas of higher population density. As ever, criminals are quick to take advantage of new opportunities and there is the risk, as Vanda Felbab-Brown argues, that these police redeployments to cities would leave the countryside more vulnerable to illicit activities. In parts of Africa and Asia, this might reduce law enforcement pressure on poachers and wildlife traffickers whereas reduced police presence may result in an uptick in drug crop cultivation in Mexico and methamphetamine production in rural United States.[26]

In view of potential staff shortages, but also to limit the risk of contagion and prison overcrowding, police forces have had to re-think the ways they respond to and prioritize calls. Police departments in the United States instructed officers to deal with certain crimes with misdemeanour summons and citations rather than arrests. In a similar vein, guidelines were issued to avoid incarceration for minor violations of parole.[27] As prisons around the world have been identified as COVID-19 hotspots owing to their often-crowded conditions and poor hygiene, thousands of prisoners in Iran and Afghanistan have been set free either temporarily or permanently (following pardon). Whereas those inmates also included innocents, e.g. victims of rape and political dissidents, the release of actual criminals is not without risk. Whilst out of prison they might try to abscond and therefore it is yet to be seen whether it would be possible to re-incarcerate convicts once the health emergency is over.[28]

Criminals or Local Heroes?

Aside from the financial loss and the violence that accompanies organized crime, arguably the most detrimental impact that criminal groups have had on states and societies has to do with their role in undermining governance and state authority and weakening the social contract between the authorities and the populations they are mandated with governing and protecting. This process comes in many forms from full-blown state capture, such as in Guinea-Bissau,[29,30] to milder types of corruption. Many studies have been produced documenting the different relationships (including for instance collaboration and cooption) between state authorities and criminals in different regions of the world. Highly disturbing, yet not uncommon, are scenarios in which criminal actors establish almost parallel states, becoming service-providers and filling gaps that the state is unable or unwilling, for a variety of reasons, to fill. These include the provision of security, access to utilities such as water, electricity, housing and waste management, jobs and even some rudimentary justice and dispute resolution. Reporting during the pandemic shows that this also applied to healthcare provision and the implementation of safeguarding methods.

Examples of Criminal Service-Provision During the Pandemic

The COVID-19 pandemic has created opportunities for both organized criminal organizations and less sophisticated gangs in countries as diverse as, for instance, Brazil, Italy, Japan and South Africa to impose or expand their informal control and governance systems in the affected areas by distributing supplies and helping local communities during lockdowns as a way to build their political capital.

Evidence from Italy shows how different mafia syndicates have adapted to the pandemic. In purely business terms, they temporarily abandoned trafficking routes through European ports affected by travel restrictions in favour of others less affected by disruptions, and they also relied on 'emergency' cocaine stocks to keep their business going.

Yet, a key aspect of the mafiosi's strategy, and arguably the one with the longest-term impact, was to exploit the crisis to consolidate their hold on territory and boost popular support. In parts of Calabria, where the '*Ndrangheta* originates, it was the *mafiosi* who enforced the lockdown, whereas in Sicily the *Cosa Nostra* distributed food parcels.[31] Similar but more ostentatious scenes were seen in Mexico. Here, armed criminals in the state of Michoacán supervised the distribution of groceries to local citizens whilst competing groups would instruct local municipalities to set up food banks from which they would then source hand-outs.[32]

In South Africa, where lockdown measures were particularly stringent and the government banned the sale of alcohol and cigarettes, local gangs that would normally battle each other reached a truce in April. Mediated by an evangelical pastor in Cape Town, the terms of the truce also involved collaboration between rival gangs to distribute food, soap and other essential goods to people in the neighbourhood, making use of their rather efficient distribution network (although normally it is used for drugs and arms).[33] Whereas this felt like a miracle to local residents, gangs also took advantage of the situation to sell alcohol and tobacco on the black market.

As fears of the virus deepened and the Bolsonaro administration was late to intervene, Brazil's criminal gangs proved very active in the *favelas* (slums) they control in the main cities. In Rio de Janeiro, the Red Command group went around the Cidade de Deus (City of God) *favela* with loudspeakers enforcing the lockdown:

> We are imposing a curfew because nobody is taking [coronavirus] seriously. It's best to stay at home and chill. The message has been given.[34]

In the Santa Marta slums, they reportedly distributed soap and placed signs asking people to wash their hands before entering the area.[35] Similar to their 'colleagues' in Mexico, Brazilian criminals did not swap crime for charitable actions altogether during the pandemic. Narcotic trafficking and extortion continued broadly unabated.[36] The infamous Japanese Yakuza gangs also adopted a dual approach of humanitarian support and exploitation. On the one hand, they offered to help those in need and distributed face masks, on the other they became involved in coronavirus-related fraud, taking advantage of a new loan scheme introduced by the government to see people through the health (and economic) crisis.[37]

The instances from Europe, Africa, the Americas and Asia listed above are among the many examples of criminals, from different geographies and with different levels of organization and sophistication, *partly* behaving as forces of good by somewhat alleviating the hardship endured by the population during the lockdown and by enforcing measures to contain the spread of the virus. Many other similar cases could be cited, but despite the temporary ceasefires and the food donations, these groups are neither heroes nor modern Robin Hoods. As already discussed, organized criminal groups around the world have been exploiting the 'opportunities' created by COVID-19 and in deprived areas they have used their charitable work for less than altruistic reasons. In Mexico, to mention one instance, the Jalisco New Generation Cartel and the Sinaloa Cartel have used donated food boxes for propaganda purposes by printing images of their historical and current leaders on them.[38] The Gulf Cartel would put its branded stickers on hand sanitizers gifted to locals.[39]

It can be argued that these actions are aimed at securing (additional) public support and highlighting the inadequacy of state responses. This, in turn, consolidates groups' legitimacy and feeds the sadly widespread (and in some cases broadly accurate) notion that in many countries, criminal actors and the state-within-the-state that they have put in place are the only ones capable of delivering services to communities and offering protection. This scenario represents a setback for any progress made towards good governance in many emerging and developing countries and it indeed has implications for the consolidation of democracy. Specifically, the deepening of support and gratitude for crime groups in countries where political parties are openly affiliated to them would give those political entities an advantage at the time of elections, and result in the strengthening of territorial control by the cartels (or other criminal groups) in question.[40] It is important to note that these challenges are not simply the prerogative of emerging, fragile or unstable regions. Italy, a G7 economy, has been facing a similar predicament during the pandemic with mafia groups giving gifts of hundreds of euros to people in need whose state benefits were delayed, and offering loans to help small businesses.[41]

The Post-pandemic Landscape

With the easing of restrictions and the world getting to grips with the 'new normal'—loosely described as an era of economic downturn and related by-products—it is reasonable to expect that criminals would want to make up for their 2020 lost revenues, resume trafficking activities that had been impaired by the pandemic, and capitalize on any new opportunities that might present themselves. In particular, growing levels of unemployment, changes in consumer demand and behaviour, and the possible increase in the number of would-be economic migrants are likely to generate lucrative business avenues for criminal actors.

The shape of the global economy is possibly the greatest determinant of the direction organized crime will take mid and long term. Forecasts are daunting, painting a picture of a global recession worse than in the aftermath of the 2008 financial crisis.

Laundering of Criminal Proceeds

From the experience of post-2008 and other crises, we know criminals will find ways to profit. Yet, unlike the late 2000s when cash transactions were the option of choice for criminals wishing to launder their profits, we are now in an era of growing reliance on cashless payments (especially in advanced economies), which saw a marked increase during the pandemic and is likely to continue. This makes it harder for criminals to rely on cash-intensive businesses such as casinos, restaurants and nail bars for laundering—not to mention that many of those businesses have stopped trading due to the pandemic.[42] Based on that, it is reasonable to expect a doubling of criminal efforts in the real estate sector as well as in using off-shore financial systems. Additionally, we might see growing attempts by criminals to buy troubled legitimate businesses that are unable to continue to operate due to the financial crisis. Prosecutors in Italy are deeply worried that usury will rise with *mafiosi* lending money to struggling businesses unable to secure bank loans. Within a couple of years, deeply indebted restaurant and shop owners will be left with no choice than to hand over their businesses to the mafia to be used in laundering schemes.[43]

Cybercrime and Sales of Counterfeit Medical Supplies

It is fair to expect that cybercrime will represent an even greater share of criminal activities. In the mid-term COVID-19-related scams involving fake vaccines and the sale of substandard medical supplies are likely to continue. More broadly, and in the longer term, the sales of substandard or counterfeit goods are likely to grow at a time when many will feel the pressure of financial hardship and may want or need to opt for cheaper alternatives with less concern regarding their origin.

Criminal Recruitment

This same economic hardship and unemployment will make people vulnerable to recruitment by criminal gangs. Already in the course of the pandemic, it was evident criminals were heavily preying on young adults. The United Kingdom for example, saw the negative implications of youth workers' inability (or reduced ability) to reach vulnerable young adults during the lockdown. Not only did this result in young people not receiving support, it also resulted in their recruitment by criminals (in this regard, girls were particularly targeted by gangs). An additional notable side-effect was the decline in intelligence around criminal activity, such as the sales of drugs, that youth workers would normally be able to gather as part of their interactions.[44]

Smuggling and Trafficking of Persons

Criminal exploitation of vulnerable people across international boundaries is certainly a high risk. Europol forecast the recession linked to COVID-19 to have serious implications for migration,[45] whereas Interpol expects a new wave of illegal migration to hit Europe from Asia and the Middle East post-pandemic.[46] During the lockdown however, illicit migration flows decreased as going undetected became more difficult. Even then, those movements did not completely disappear: smugglers identified new and usually more dangerous routes across the Sahel and migrants were subject to more brutal treatment and were forced to pay higher prices in order to reach Europe from Africa.[47] As fragile economies in Africa, Asia and Latin America are likely to suffer from the economic downturns more severely, prospects for better lives in Europe or North America (notwithstanding the economic problems experienced there) will be strong pull factors. Human smugglers are expected to prey on would-be economic migrants trying, for instance, to reach Europe or the United States. Demand for cheap labour in struggling European economies might also increase the risk of exploitation of vulnerable national and foreign workers. Unions in the UK and Germany, for instance, have highlighted the exploitation of migrant workers in meat processing plants who receive very low wages, often live in crowded or unsanitary conditions and are denied sick leave or any form of financial support if they need to self-isolate as a result of COVID-19. One survey suggested that many would attend work even if unwell because they could not afford to lose their wages, hence increasing the risk of spreading the virus.[48]

Finally, the growing number of vulnerable individuals affected by the economic downturn might result in the rise of trafficking for sexual exploitation and, increasingly, online prostitution sites using trafficked or enslaved women.[49]

Corruption

The economic downturn might also have the side effects of lowering the barriers for engagement in corruption, at all levels.[50] For instance, in countries where public officials might see their salaries cut, the temptation to accept bribes might become higher in the future.[51] These practices not only have immediate effects on resource allocation but also have a long-term impact, as indicated in the earlier discussions regarding mafia's involvement in the Italian health sector, and can diminish the credibility of state institutions as in the Mexican or Brazilian examples.

Unrest

Finally, economic instability might lead to social unrest in some places, especially where there are large informal or criminal economies. A July 2020 study forecasted that 37 countries could be at high risk of instability in the following two to three years. The assessment highlighted how pre-existing grievances coupled with the economic fall-out of the pandemic might create the 'perfect storm' for social unrest. The authors identified Nigeria, Iran, Bangladesh, Algeria and Ethiopia in the highest risk category. Overall, it is Africa and Latin America that were deemed to become the worst affected.[52] To add to the concern, these two regions have some of the most deeply-rooted informal economies in the world and feature criminal and other non-state armed groups that are able to exert territorial control. In order to maintain the peace, local officials and law enforcement might be tempted to strike deals with criminal actors. This approach may reduce the immediate risk of unrest but would further undermine state legitimacy and strengthen illegal groups in the long run.

Going Back to 'Normal'

Some forms of organized crime, trafficking in particular, were impaired by the pandemic but law enforcement agencies expect this to quickly return to pre-COVID-19 levels in the midterm. Narcotics, which represent a very adaptable market—is the prime example of the resilience of trafficking. Whereas the supply chain had been disrupted early on during the pandemic, traffickers identified alternative routes and delivery systems and indeed benefited from shortages of substances to increase prices. As for the latter, however, the picture is varied. Whereas in a number of countries disruptions to the supply chain have resulted in an increase in the price of drugs, e.g. cocaine in Spain, Sweden or Australia, elsewhere they have stayed the same, e.g. Netherlands and France.[53,54]

It is very possible that online individual sales, which have soared during lockdown, will continue owing to their convenience. The same goes for arranging the sales of large consignments, which will also become less reliant on face-to-face interactions and will be conducted instead via secure online channels.[55] Users might struggle to afford drugs as a result of soaring prices and the economic downturn, however. This might result in two risks: users becoming involved in illicit activities themselves to earn an income or opting for cheaper and possibly more damaging substances.

Wildlife trafficking is expected to bounce back as quickly. Travel restrictions in the Mekong region have only temporarily reduced sales. The Wildlife Justice Commission has warned that traffickers in Lao PDR, Cambodia and Vietnam spent lockdown stockpiling pangolin scales and elephant ivory in anticipation of the resumption of international travel.[56] Using the usual distribution channels alongside increased online sales would secure the return to business to pre-COVID-19 levels.

Additionally, the financial crisis and related damage to the tourism industry might undermine community-based anti-poaching efforts where communities in source countries might see poaching as the only viable source of income. This has already been the case in most of South Asia, where poaching for illicit wildlife trade but also for bushmeat has increased as disadvantaged families need ways to sustain themselves.[57] This prospect further endangers species such as rhinos, elephants, and the pangolin.[58]

Overall, the post-pandemic landscape is likely to look reasonably rosy for criminals, with opportunities to make up for any financial losses incurred in the early phases of the pandemic and indeed capitalize on new opportunities. This is especially true for those involved in transnational networks who have the technical know-how and maintain generous reserves.

Conclusion

As evidenced in this chapter, criminals at all levels have not gone unscathed during the COVID-19 pandemic. Like everyone else, they had to rethink their operations, from manufacturing to sales and distribution, and accept some losses. Yet, their ability to face adversity and plan for the post-pandemic has, in some cases, surpassed the reaction time of legitimate businesses and institutions. Their adaptable nature has allowed them to secure revenue streams, even when the most stringent lockdown measures were in place. When walking around empty streets or travelling on empty trains would almost inevitably result in detection, even smaller gangs in the United Kingdom were able to find alternative ways to deliver drugs. As burglary of private homes was no longer an option because residents were always in, burglars would break into business premises. So, if it was relatively easy to stay afloat for the small fish, it is easy to see how the resources and expertise at the disposal of large organized criminal networks made them very resilient in the context of COVID-19-related disruptions.

As cybercrime and cyber-enabled criminality are set to rise, and COVID-19 is likely to have accelerated that process, law enforcement agencies more than ever before need to have the digital tools and the know-how at their disposal to thwart illicit activities, speed up investigations and target suspects. This might require developing even stronger partnerships and synergies with tech companies and other stakeholders such as those in the financial and banking sector. As for the latter, professionals in anti-money laundering and regulators will need to be prepared to deal with higher volumes of cases as criminal enterprises will likely want to exploit volatility in the global economy.[59]

Awareness campaigns and education have a role to play in alerting and sensitizing the general public, as potential victims of cybercrime, to the risk of malware, ever more sophisticated phishing emails and scams that they might encounter online. Whereas some will return to their offices after the pandemic, teleworking is likely to remain the preferred option for many employees and employers. Criminals are likely to exploit and try to gain access to business networks by targeting individual employees working from home.

One area where COVID-19 has produced greater public awareness of the perils of criminal activities is illegal wildlife crime. Specifically, the possible connection between wet markets where trafficked species are sold and the coronavirus outbreak has started to impact consumers' behaviours and highlighted the convergence of the health and security spheres.[60] Sadly, however, demand for wildlife persists and border officers in some of the key hotspots for wildlife trafficking, e.g. the Mekong Sub-Region, arguably lack pandemic preparedness.

Developments in the behaviours and actions of criminals in the course of the pandemic as well as the expected post-COVID-19 trajectory highlight the need for institutions to rapidly adapt. The roles played by gangs, cartels and mafia syndicates as *benefactors* at the time of crisis point to a key underlying issue: state ineffectiveness. These are issues that predate the pandemic and require a long-term approach to strengthen institutions, wean them off corrupt practices and increase their legitimacy in the eyes of their citizens. In the shorter term, however, safety nets that prevent individuals from falling (deeper) into poverty, and therefore becoming more vulnerable to criminal exploitation, ought to be prioritized. Among them are categories that were already marginalized before the pandemic, including sex workers, drug users and labourers in the informal economy. This highlights the fact that, although the issue at hand is organized crime, solutions do not entirely rest in the hands of law enforcement and regulators. An array of actors, including social service providers and civil societies, are needed to implement effective and sustainable responses.

Notes

1. "Serious and Organised Crime Strategy," *UK Home Office*, November 2018, https://assets.publishing.service.gov.uk/government/uploads/system/uploads/attachment_data/file/752850/SOC-2018-web.pdf.
2. Zoe Wood, "Recession Fuels Sharp Rise in Financial Crime," *The Guardian*, May 3, 2009, https://www.theguardian.com/business/2009/may/03/tax-avoidance-financial-crime-recession.
3. Jenny H. Peterson, "The Politics of Crime, Violence and Policy," in *Linking Political Violence and Crime in Latin America*, ed.

Kirsten Howarth and Jenny H. Peterson (Lanham, MD: Lexington Books, 2016), 1–26.
4. Peter Tinti, and Tuesday Reitano, *Migrant, Refugee, Smuggler, Saviour* (London: Hurst, 2016).
5. Ian Ralby, "The Criminal Side of Ebola," *HuffPost*, November 5, 2014, https://www.huffpost.com/entry/the-criminal-side-of-ebol_b_6088206.
6. "Global Trade Update," *United Nations Conference on Trade and Development*, June 2020, https://unctad.org/en/PublicationsLibrary/ditcmisc2020d2_en.pdf.
7. "EU Drug Markets—Impact of COVID-19," *European Monitoring Centre for Drugs and Drug Addiction and Europol*, May 2020, https://www.emcdda.europa.eu/publications/joint-publications/eu-drug-markets-impact-of-COVID-19_en.
8. Darren Guccione, "What Is the Dark Web? How to Access It and What You'll Find," *CSO*, November 18, 2020, https://www.csoonline.com/article/3249765/what-is-the-dark-web-how-to-access-it-and-what-youll-find.html.
9. "Preventing Crime and Protecting Police: INTERPOL's COVID-19 Global Threat Assessment," *Interpol*, April 6, 2020, https://www.interpol.int/en/News-and-Events/News/2020/Preventing-crime-and-protecting-police-INTERPOL-s-COVID-19-global-threat-assessment.
10. "School Closings Due to COVID-19 Present Potential for Increased Risk of Child Exploitation," *FBI National Press Office*, March 23, 2020, https://www.fbi.gov/news/pressrel/press-releases/school-closings-due-to-COVID-19-present-potential-for-increased-risk-of-child-exploitation.
11. "Crime and Contagion: The Impact of a Pandemic on Organized Crime," *Global Initiative Against Transnational Organized Crime*, March 2020, https://globalinitiative.net/wp-content/uploads/2020/03/GI-TOC-Crime-and-Contagion-The-impact-of-a-pandemic-on-organized-crime-1.pdf.
12. "Pandemic Profiteering: How Criminals Exploit the COVID-19 Crisis," *Europol*, March 27, 2020, https://www.europol.europa.eu/publications-documents/pandemic-profiteering-how-criminals-exploit-COVID-19-crisis.
13. Ibid.

14. "Unmasked: International COVID-19 Fraud Exposed," *Interpol*, April 14, 2020, https://www.interpol.int/en/News-and-Events/News/2020/Unmasked-International-COVID-19-fraud-exposed.
15. "Mafia e sanita," *Commissione Parlamentare di Inchiesta sul Fenomeno delle Mafie e sulle altre Associazioni Criminali anche Straniere,* February 7, 2018, http://www.illuminiamolasalute.it/wp-content/uploads/2014/06/commissione-antimafia-2018-mafia-e-sanit%C3%A0.pdf.
16. Alessia Candito, "'Ndrangheta: sciolta l'Asp, l'azienda sanitaria di Reggio Calabria," *La Repubblica*, March 12, 2019, https://www.repubblica.it/cronaca/2019/03/13/news/_ndrangheta_sciolta_azienda_sanitaria_reggio_calabria-221426432/.
17. Jelter Meers, "Italy: Mafia Ran Hospitals with Help of Politicians," *OCCRP*, November 14, 2018, https://www.occrp.org/en/daily/8904-italy-mafia-ran-hospitals-with-help-of-politicians.
18. 'Crime and Contagion: The Impact of a Pandemic on Organized Crime," *Global Initiative Against Transnational Organized Crime*, March 2020, https://globalinitiative.net/wp-content/uploads/2020/03/GI-TOC-Crime-and-Contagion-The-impact-of-a-pandemic-on-organized-crime-1.pdf.
19. Cecilia Anesi, and Matteo Civillini, "Coronavirus Has Only Made the Mafia Stronger," *Vice*, July 15, 2020, https://www.vice.com/en_uk/article/935dgy/mafia-italy-profit-coronavirus.
20. Guido Palazzo, "The Camorra: Europe's Toxic Waste Criminal Entrepreneurs," *RUSI*, September 24, 2018, https://shoc.rusi.org/informer/camorra-europe%E2%80%99s-toxic-waste-criminal-entrepreneurs.
21. "Global Operation Sees a Rise in Fake Medical Products Related to COVID-19," *Interpol*, March 19, 2020, https://www.interpol.int/en/News-and-Events/News/2020/Global-operation-sees-a-rise-in-fake-medical-products-related-to-COVID-19.
22. Lucas Roth, et al., "Global Landscape Assessment of Screening Technologies for Medicine Quality Assurance: Stakeholder Perceptions and Practices from Ten Countries," *Global Health* 14, no. 43 (April 2018): https://doi.org/10.1186/s12992-018-0360-y.
23. "Europol Predictions Correct for Fake COVID-19 Vaccines," *Europol Press Release*, December 4, 2020, https://www.europol.europa.eu/newsroom/news/europol-predictions-correct-for-fake-COVID-19-vaccines.

24. "Pro-kremlin Disinformation: COVID-19 Vaccines," *EEAS*, December 22, 2020, https://eeas.europa.eu/delegations/azerbaijan/90950/pro-kremlin-disinformation-COVID-19-vaccines_en.
25. "EU Drug Markets—Impact of COVID-19," *European Monitoring Centre for Drugs and Drug Addiction and Europol*, May 2020, https://www.emcdda.europa.eu/publications/joint-publications/eu-drug-markets-impact-of-COVID-19_en.
26. Vanda Felbab-Brown, "How COVID-19 Is Changing Law Enforcement Practices by Police and by Criminal Groups," *Brookings*, April 7, 2020, https://www.brookings.edu/blog/order-from-chaos/2020/04/07/how-COVID-19-is-changing-law-enforcement-practices-by-police-and-by-criminal-groups/.
27. Alexander Mallin, and Luke Barr, "Police Implement Sweeping Policy Changes to Prepare for Coronavirus Spread," *ABC News*, March 18, 2020, https://abcnews.go.com/US/police-implement-sweeping-policy-prepare-coronavirus-spread/story?id=69672368.
28. "COVID-19: Afghanistan Freeing Thousands of Inmates; Romania Surpasses 1,000 Cases," *Radio Free Europe/Radio Liberty*, March 26, 2020, https://www.rferl.org/a/COVID-19-russia-bans-flights--iran-halts-intercity-travel/30510223.html.; Vanda Felbab-Brown, "How COVID-19 Is Changing Law Enforcement Practices by Police and by Criminal Groups," *Brookings*, April 7, 2020, https://www.brookings.edu/blog/order-from-chaos/2020/04/07/how-COVID-19-is-changing-law-enforcement-practices-by-police-and-by-criminal-groups/.
29. Labelled Africa's first 'narco-state' owing to the involvement of the highest echelons of government and the armed forces in the cocaine trade.
30. Lorraine Mallinder, "Still a Narco-State? Guinea-Bissau's Illegal Drug Economy," *Global Initiative Against Transnational Organized Crime*, March 27, 2018, https://globalinitiative.net/analysis/guinea-bissau-illegal-drug-economy/.
31. Cecilia Anesi, and Matteo Civillini, "Coronavirus Has Only Made the Mafia Stronger," *Vice*, July 15, 2020, https://www.vice.com/en_uk/article/935dgy/mafia-italy-profit-coronavirus.
32. Falko Ernst, "Mexican Criminal Groups See COVID-19 Crisis as Opportunity to Gain More Power," *The Guardian*, April 20, 2020, https://www.theguardian.com/world/2020/apr/20/mexico-criminal-groups-COVID-19-crisis-opportunity-gain-power.

33. Tim Wyatt, "Coronavirus: Gang Kingpins in South Africa Call Truce to Help Community During Pandemic," *The Independent*, April 20, 2020, https://www.independent.co.uk/news/world/africa/south-africa-coronavirus-lockdown-gangs-cape-town-a9474101.html.
34. Caio Barretto Briso, and Tom Phillips, "Brazil Gangs Impose Strict Curfews to Slow Coronavirus Spread," *The Guardian*, March 25, 2020, https://www.theguardian.com/world/2020/mar/25/brazil-rio-gangs-coronavirus.
35. Caio Barretto Briso, and Tom Phillips, "Brazil Gangs Impose Strict Curfews to Slow Coronavirus Spread," *The Guardian*, March 25, 2020, https://www.theguardian.com/world/2020/mar/25/brazil-rio-gangs-coronavirus.
36. Ryan Berg, and Andrea Varsori, "COVID-19 Is Increasing the Power of Brazil's Criminal Groups," *London School of Economics Blogs*, May 28, 2020, https://blogs.lse.ac.uk/latamcaribbean/2020/05/28/COVID-19-is-increasing-the-power-of-brazils-criminal-groups/.
37. Tom Gillespie, "Coronavirus Couldn't Have Come at a Worse Time for Japan's Yakuza Gangs," *Sky News*, May 14, 2020, https://news.sky.com/story/coronavirus-couldnt-have-come-at-a-worse-time-for-japans-yakuza-gangs-11987535.
38. Camilo Tamayo Gomez, "Coronavirus: Narco Gangs Could See Big Popularity Boost from Helping Residents in Latin America," *The Conversation*, June 22, 2020, https://theconversation.com/coronavirus-narco-gangs-could-see-big-popularity-boost-from-helping-residents-in-latin-america-139613.
39. Matteo Pazzona, "Coronavirus: Crime Cartels Helping Communities Will Extract a High Price in Years to Come," *The Conversation*, May 15, 2020, https://theconversation.com/coronavirus-crime-cartels-helping-communities-will-extract-a-high-price-in-years-to-come-138592.
40. Camilo Tamayo Gomez, "Coronavirus: Narco Gangs Could See Big Popularity Boost From Helping Residents in Latin America," *The Conversation*, June 22, 2020, https://theconversation.com/coronavirus-narco-gangs-could-see-big-popularity-boost-from-helping-residents-in-latin-america-139613.

41. Daniel Verdú, "La mafia es inmune al virus," *El País*, April 18, 2020, https://elpais.com/sociedad/2020-04-18/la-mafia-es-inmune-al-virus.html.
42. "Beyond the Pandemic—How COVID-19 Will Shape the Serious and Organized Crime Landscape in the EU," *Europol*, April 30, 2020, 7; 11–12, https://www.europol.europa.eu/publications-documents/beyond-pandemic-how-COVID-19-will-shape-serious-and-organised-crime-landscape-in-eu.
43. "Gratteri spiega come gli usurai approfitteranno del coronavirus," *AGI Agenzia Italia*, March 31, 2020, https://www.agi.it/cronaca/news/2020-03-31/coronavirus-usura-ndrangheta-gratteri-8033085/.
44. Steve Swann, and Tom Symonds, "Drug Gangs on 'Recruitment Drive" During Lockdown," *BBC News*, June 2, 2020, https://www.bbc.co.uk/news/uk-52892917.
45. "Beyond the Pandemic—How COVID-19 Will Shape the Serious and Organized Crime Landscape in the EU," *Europol*, April 30, 2020, 7; 8.
46. "COVID-19 Impact on Migrant Smuggling and Human Trafficking," INTERPOL, June 11, 2020, https://www.interpol.int/en/News-and-Events/News/2020/COVID-19-impact-on-migrant-smuggling-and-human-trafficking.
47. "Stability in the Time of COVID-19: Implications for the Sahel," *International Institute for Strategic Studies*, June 29, 2020, https://www.iiss.org/blogs/research-paper/2020/06/COVID-19-sahel.
48. "Link Between Migrant Worker Exploitation and COVID-19 Meat Processing Outbreaks 'Must be Addressed'," *United Union*, June 30, 2020, https://unitetheunion.org/news-events/news/2020/june/link-between-migrant-worker-exploitation-and-COVID-19-meat-processing-outbreaks-must-be-addressed/.
49. Vanda Felbab-Brown, "What Coronavirus Means for Online Fraud, Forced Sex, Drug Smuggling and Wildlife Trafficking," *Brookings*, April 3, 2020, https://www.brookings.edu/blog/order-from-chaos/2020/04/03/what-coronavirus-means-for-online-fraud-forced-sex-drug-smuggling-and-wildlife-trafficking/.
50. "EU Drug Markets—Impact of COVID-19," *European Monitoring Centre for Drugs and Drug Addiction and Europol*, May 2020, https://www.emcdda.europa.eu/publications/joint-publications/eu-drug-markets-impact-of-COVID-19_en.

51. To note, this *might* happen but is not a foregone conclusion. The relationship between salary levels and the acceptance of bribes is a complex one and the topic of many studies. See for instance: Samira Lindner, "Salary top-ups and Their Impact on Corruption," *U4 Expert Answer*, 398, December 17, 2013, https://www.transparency.org/files/content/corruptionqas/Salary_top-ups_and_their_impact_on_corruption_2013.pdf; and Caroline Van Rijckeghem, and Beatrice Weder, "Corruption and the Rate of Temptation: Do Low Wages in the Civil Service Cause Corruption?" *IMF Working Paper* WP/ 97/ 73, June 1997, https://www.imf.org/external/pubs/ft/wp/wp9773.pdf.
52. Miha Hribernik, and Tim Campbell, "Emerging Markets Face Acute Instability as Pandemic Fuels Unrest," *Verisk Maplecroft*, July 16, 2020, https://www.maplecroft.com/insights/analysis/emerging-markets-face-unparalleled-civil-unrest-as-economic-impacts-of-pandemic-unfold--study/.
53. "Expert Opinion: Changes in Wholesale Price per kg of Cocaine During the COVID-19 Pandemic," *EMCDDA*, May 2020, https://www.emcdda.europa.eu/media-library/infographic-expert-opinion-changes-wholesale-price-kg-cocaine-during-COVID-19-pandemic_en.
54. Sally Rawsthorne, "Profits 'through the roof' as Drug Dealers Hike Prices Amid Pandemic," *The Sydney Morning Herald*, July 12, 2020, https://www.smh.com.au/national/profits-through-the-roof-as-drug-dealers-hike-prices-amid-pandemic-20200710-p55atw.html.
55. "EU Drug Markets—Impact of COVID-19," *European Monitoring Centre for Drugs and Drug Addiction and Europol*, May 2020, https://www.emcdda.europa.eu/publications/joint-publications/eu-drug-markets-impact-of-COVID-19_en.
56. "Rapid Assessment of the Impact of COVID-19 on Wildlife Trafficking," *Wildlife Justice Commission*, April 2020, https://wildlifejustice.org/wp-content/uploads/2020/04/WJC_Impact-of-COVID19-on-wildlife-trafficking_April2020.pdf.
57. Tanika Godbole, "Coronavirus: South Asia Sees Rise in Poaching During Lockdowns," *DW*, July 8, 2020, https://www.dw.com/en/coronavirus-south-asia-sees-rise-in-poaching-during-lockdowns/a-54090081.

58. "Crime and Contagion: The Impact of a Pandemic on Organized Crime," *Global Initiative Against Transnational Organized Crime*, March 2020, https://globalinitiative.net/wp-content/uploads/2020/03/GI-TOC-Crime-and-Contagion-The-impact-of-a-pandemic-on-organized-crime-1.pdf.
59. "Beyond the Pandemic—How COVID-19 Will Shape the Serious and Organized Crime Landscape in the EU," *Europol*, April 30, 2020, 7, https://www.europol.europa.eu/publications-documents/beyond-pandemic-how-COVID-19-will-shape-serious-and-organised-crime-landscape-in-eu.
60. A. Alonso Aguirre, et al., "Illicit Wildlife Trade, Wet Markets, and COVID-19: Preventing Future Pandemics," *World Medical & Health Policy* 12, no. 3 (June 2020): 256–265, https://doi.org/10.1002/wmh3.348.

Bibliography

"Beyond the Pandemic—How COVID-19 Will Shape the Serious and Organised Crime Landscape in the EU." *Europol*, April 30, 2020. https://www.europol.europa.eu/publications-documents/beyond-pandemic-how-COVID-19-will-shape-serious-and-organised-crime-landscape-in-eu.

"Corruption and the Rate of Temptation: Do Low Wages in the Civil Service Cause Corruption?" *IMF Working Paper* WP/ 97/ 73. June 1997, https://www.imf.org/external/pubs/ft/wp/wp9773.pdf.

"COVID-19: Afghanistan Freeing Thousands of Inmates; Romania Surpasses 1,000 Cases." *Radio Free Europe/Radio Liberty*, March 26, 2020. https://www.rferl.org/a/COVID-19-russia-bans-flights--iran-halts-intercity-travel/30510223.html.

"Crime and Contagion: The Impact of a Pandemic on Organized Crime."*Global Initiative Against Transnational Organized Crime*, March 2020. https://globalinitiative.net/wp-content/uploads/2020/03/GI-TOC-Crime-and-Contagion-The-impact-of-a-pandemic-on-organized-crime-1.pdf.

"EU Drug Markets—Impact of COVID-19." *European Monitoring Centre for Drugs and Drug Addiction and Europol*, May 2020. https://www.emcdda.europa.eu/publications/joint-publications/eu-drug-markets-impact-of-COVID-19_en.

"Europol Predictions Correct for Fake COVID-19 Vaccines." *Europol Press Release*, December 4, 2020. https://www.europol.europa.eu/newsroom/news/europol-predictions-correct-for-fake-COVID-19-vaccines.

"Expert Opinion: Changes in Wholesale Price Per kg of Cocaine During the COVID-19 Pandemic." *EMCDDA*, May 2020. https://www.emcdda.europa.eu/media-library/infographic-expert-opinion-changes-wholesale-price-kg-cocaine-during-COVID-19-pandemic_en.

"Global Operation Sees A Rise in Fake Medical Products Related to COVID-19." *Interpol*, March 19, 2020. https://www.interpol.int/en/News-and-Events/News/2020/Global-operation-sees-a-rise-in-fake-medical-products-related-to-COVID-19.

"Global Trade Update." *United Nations Conference on Trade and Development*, June 2020. https://unctad.org/en/PublicationsLibrary/ditcmisc2020d2_en.pdf.

"Gratteri spiega come gli usurai approfitteranno del coronavirus." *AGI Agenzia Italia*, March 31, 2020. https://www.agi.it/cronaca/news/2020-03-31/coronavirus-usura-ndrangheta-gratteri-8033085/.

"Link Between Migrant Worker Exploitation and COVID-19 Meat Processing Outbreaks 'Must be Addressed.'" *United Union*, June 30, 2020. https://unitetheunion.org/news-events/news/2020/june/link-between-migrant-worker-exploitation-and-COVID-19-meat-processing-outbreaks-must-be-addressed/.

"Mafia e sanita." *Commissione Parlamentare di Inchiesta sul Fenomeno delle Mafie e sulle altre Associazioni Criminali anche Straniere*, February 7, 2018. http://www.illuminiamolasalute.it/wp-content/uploads/2014/06/commissione-antimafia-2018-mafia-e-sanit%C3%A0.pdf.

"Pandemic Profiteering: How Criminals Exploit the COVID-19 Crisis." *Europol*, March 27, 2020. https://www.europol.europa.eu/publications-documents/pandemic-profiteering-how-criminals-exploit-COVID-19-crisis.

"Preventing Crime and Protecting Police: INTERPOL's COVID-19 Global Threat Assessment." *Interpol*, April 6, 2020. https://www.interpol.int/en/News-and-Events/News/2020/Preventing-crime-and-protecting-police-INTERPOL-s-COVID-19-global-threat-assessment.

"Pro-kremlin Disinformation: COVID-19 Vaccines." *EEAS*, December 22, 2020. https://eeas.europa.eu/delegations/azerbaijan/90950/pro-kremlin-disinformation-COVID-19-vaccines_en.

"Rapid Assessment of the Impact of COVID-19 on Wildlife Trafficking." *Wildlife Justice Commission*, April 2020. https://wildlifejustice.org/wp-content/uploads/2020/04/WJC_Impact-of-COVID19-on-wildlife-trafficking_April2020.pdf.

"School Closings Due to COVID-19 Present Potential for Increased Risk of Child Exploitation." *FBI National Press Office*, March 23, 2020. https://www.fbi.gov/news/pressrel/press-releases/school-closings-due-to-COVID-19-present-potential-for-increased-risk-of-child-exploitation.

"Serious and Organised Crime Strategy." *UK Home Office*, November 2018. https://assets.publishing.service.gov.uk/government/uploads/system/uploads/attachment_data/file/752850/SOC-2018-web.pdf.

"Stability in the Time of COVID-19: Implications for the Sahel." *International Institute for Strategic Studies*, June 29, 2020. https://www.iiss.org/blogs/research-paper/2020/06/COVID-19-sahel.

"Unmasked: International COVID-19 Fraud Exposed." *Interpol*, April 14, 2020. https://www.interpol.int/en/News-and-Events/News/2020/Unmasked-International-COVID-19-fraud-exposed.

Aguirre, A. Alonso, Richard Catherina, Hailey Frye, and Louise Shelley. "Illicit Wildlife Trade, Wet Markets, and COVID-19: Preventing Future Pandemics." *World Medical & Health Policy* 12, no. 3 (June 2020): 256–265. https://doi.org/10.1002/wmh3.348.

Anesi, Cecilia, and Matteo Civillini. "Coronavirus Has Only Made the Mafia Stronger." *Vice*, July 15, 2020. https://www.vice.com/en_uk/article/935dgy/mafia-italy-profit-coronavirus.

Berg, Ryan, and Andrea Varsori. "COVID-19 Is Increasing the Power of Brazil's Criminal Groups." *London School of Economics Blogs*, May 28, 2020. https://blogs.lse.ac.uk/latamcaribbean/2020/05/28/COVID-19-is-increasing-the-power-of-brazils-criminal-groups/.

Briso, Caio Barretto, and Tom Phillips. "Brazil Gangs Impose Strict Curfews to Slow Coronavirus Spread." *The Guardian*, March 25, 2020. https://www.theguardian.com/world/2020/mar/25/brazil-rio-gangs-coronavirus.

Candito, Alessia. "'Ndrangheta: sciolta l'Asp, l'azienda sanitaria di Reggio Calabria." *La Repubblica*, March 12, 2019. https://www.repubblica.it/cronaca/2019/03/13/news/_ndrangheta_sciolta_azienda_sanitaria_reggio_calabria-221426432/.

Ernst, Falko. "Mexican Criminal Groups See COVID-19 Crisis as Opportunity to Gain More Power." *The Guardian*, April 20, 2020. https://www.theguardian.com/world/2020/apr/20/mexico-criminal-groups-COVID-19-crisis-opportunity-gain-power.

Felbab-Brown, Vanda. "What Coronavirus Means for Online Fraud, Forced Sex, Drug Smuggling, and Wildlife Trafficking." *Brookings*, April 3, 2020. https://www.brookings.edu/blog/order-from-chaos/2020/04/03/what-coronavirus-means-for-online-fraud-forced-sex-drug-smuggling-and-wildlife-trafficking/.

Felbab-Brown, Vanda. "How COVID-19 Is Changing Law Enforcement Practices by Police and by Criminal Groups." *Brookings*, April 7, 2020. https://www.brookings.edu/blog/order-from-chaos/2020/04/07/how-COVID-19-is-changing-law-enforcement-practices-by-police-and-by-criminal-groups/.

Gillespie, Tom. "Coronavirus Couldn't Have Come at a Worse Time for Japan's Yakuza Gangs." *Sky News*, May 14, 2020. https://news.sky.com/story/

coronavirus-couldnt-have-come-at-a-worse-time-for-japans-yakuza-gangs-119 87535.

Godbole, Tanika. "Coronavirus: South Asia Sees Rise in Poaching During Lockdowns." *DW*, July 8, 2020. https://www.dw.com/en/coronavirus-south-asia-sees-rise-in-poaching-during-lockdowns/a-54090081.

Gomez, Camilo Tamayo. "Coronavirus: Narco Gangs Could See Big Popularity Boost from Helping Residents in Latin America." *The Conversation,* June 22, 2020. https://theconversation.com/coronavirus-narco-gangs-could-see-big-popularity-boost-from-helping-residents-in-latin-america-139613.

Guccione, Darren. "What Is the Dark Web? How to Access It and What You'll Find." *CSO*, November 18, 2020. https://www.csoonline.com/article/324 9765/what-is-the-dark-web-how-to-access-it-and-what-youll-find.html.

Hribernik, Miha, and Tim Campbell. "Emerging Markets Face Acute Instability as Pandemic Fuels Unrest." *Verisk Maplecroft*, July 16, 2020. https://www.maplecroft.com/insights/analysis/emerging-markets-face-unparalleled-civil-unrest-as-economic-impacts-of-pandemic-unfold--study/.

Lindner, Samira. "Salary Top-ups and Their Impact on Corruption." *U4 Expert Answer*, 398, December 17, 2013. https://www.transparency.org/files/con tent/corruptionqas/Salary_top-ups_and_their_impact_on_corruption_2013. pdf

Mallin, Alexander, and Luke Barr. "Police Implement Sweeping Policy Changes to Prepare for Coronavirus Spread." *ABC News*, March 18, 2020. https://abcnews.go.com/US/police-implement-sweeping-policy-prepare-coronavirus-spread/story?id=69672368.

Mallinder, Lorraine. "Still a narco-state? Guinea-Bissau's Illegal Drug Economy." *Global Initiative Against Transnational Organized Crime,* March 27, 2018. https://globalinitiative.net/analysis/guinea-bissau-illegal-drug-economy/.

Meers, Jelter. "Italy: Mafia Ran Hospitals with Help of Politicians." *OCCRP*, November 14, 2018. https://www.occrp.org/en/daily/8904-italy-mafia-ran-hospitals-with-help-of-politicians.

Palazzo, Guido. "The Camorra: Europe's Toxic Waste Criminal Entrepreneurs." *RUSI*, September 24, 2018. https://shoc.rusi.org/informer/camorra-eur ope%E2%80%99s-toxic-waste-criminal-entrepreneurs.

Pazzona, Matteo. "Coronavirus: Crime Cartels Helping Communities Will Extract a High Price in Years to Come." *The Conversation*, May 15, 2020. https://theconversation.com/coronavirus-crime-cartels-helping-communities-will-extract-a-high-price-in-years-to-come-138592.

Peterson, Jenny H. "The Politics of Crime, Violence and Policy." In *Linking Political Violence and Crime in Latin America*, edited by Kirsten Howarth and Jenny H. Peterson. Lanham, MD: Lexington Books, 2016.

Ralby, Ian. "The Criminal Side of Ebola." *HuffPost*, November 5, 2014. https://www.huffpost.com/entry/the-criminal-side-of-ebol_b_6088206.

Rawsthorne, Sally. "Profits 'Through the Roof' as Drug Dealers Hike Prices Amid Pandemic." *The Sydney Morning Herald*, July 12, 2020. https://www.smh.com.au/national/profits-through-the-roof-as-drug-dealers-hike-prices-amid-pandemic-20200710-p55atw.html.

Roth, Lucas, Ameena Nalim, Beth Turesson, and Laura Krech. "Global Landscape Assessment of Screening Technologies For Medicine Quality Assurance: Stakeholder Perceptions and Practices From ten Countries." *Global Health* 14, no. 43 (April 2018): doi: https://doi.org/10.1186/s12992-018-0360-y.

Swann, Steve, and Tom Symonds. "Drug Gangs on 'Recruitment Drive' During Lockdown." *BBC News*, June 2, 2020. https://www.bbc.co.uk/news/uk-52892917.

Tinti, Peter, and Tuesday Reitano. *Migrant, Refugee, Smuggler, Saviour.* London: Hurst, 2016.

Van Rijckeghem, Caroline, and Beatrice Weder. "Corruption and the Rate of Temptation: Do Low Wages in the Civil Service Cause Corruption?" *IMF Working Paper* WP/ 97/ 73, June 1997. https://www.imf.org/external/pubs/ft/wp/wp9773.pdf.

Verdú, Daniel. "La mafia es inmune al virus." *El País*, April 18, 2020. https://elpais.com/sociedad/2020-04-18/la-mafia-es-inmune-al-virus.html.

Wood, Zoe. "Recession Fuels Sharp Rise in Financial Crime." *The Guardian*, May 3, 2009. https://www.theguardian.com/business/2009/may/03/tax-avoidance-financial-crime-recession.

Wyatt, Tim. "Coronavirus: Gang Kingpins in South Africa Call Truce to Help Community During Pandemic." *The Independent*, April 20, 2020. https://www.independent.co.uk/news/world/africa/south-africa-coronavirus-lockdown-gangs-cape-town-a9474101.html.

CHAPTER 12

Health Intelligence Systems and Security

Oliver Geffen Obregon

Introduction

The cholera epidemics of nineteenth-century London brought to the surface the chronic issues that characterized London's routine system of water sanitation and supply: multiple organizations acting on different incentives and responding locally with little or no coordination between them. Although the history of water sanitation in London stretches back to Roman times, the crisis that led to the cholera epidemics began in 1815, the year cesspools and house drains were allowed to flow into the river Thames, from which a number of companies drew water to supply Londoners. Although concerns regarding sanitation and the quality of water provided to households existed, actions in the first half of the nineteenth century tended to be voluntary and ad hoc. For example, in 1829 the Chelsea Water Company, but not the more upstream Grand Junction Water Company at Kew, introduced a filtration protocol for the water it drew from the Thames. It was only in August 1858, the year of the Great Stink of London, that parliament passed a bill allowing Sir Joseph Bazalgette to begin his reform of the London sewage system. In

O. G. Obregon (✉)
Freelance Epidemiologist, London, UK

C. Varin (ed.), *Global Security in Times of Covid-19*, New Security Challenges, https://doi.org/10.1007/978-3-030-82230-9_12

the two months leading to the passing of the bill, the stench rising from the Thames was so noxious, that a number of Members of Parliament officially conveyed their alarm about the negative effects on the health and wellbeing of their colleagues.[1] The system Bazalgette implemented provided a comprehensive infrastructure for the routine collection, transport, treatment and disposal of London sewage, which eventually saw the end of the London cholera outbreaks. This same system serves London to this day.[2]

Victorian London also saw the rise to prominence of John Snow, a physician widely known as the founding father of modern epidemiology. In the summer of 1854, Soho, a neighborhood in London, experienced a particularly bad outbreak of cholera. By talking to local residents, Snow was able to record their behaviors and list the number of cholera deaths by household. The pattern that emerged led him to identify a water pump on Broad Street as the strongest link connecting the deaths he recorded. He subsequently succeeded in disabling the water pump by convincing local authorities to remove the pump handle. At the time, miasma (or 'bad air') was the dominant theory of disease transmission, making Snow's observation of the link between the water pump and cholera deaths an important step towards the establishment of germ theory, which identified the causal link between microorganisms and disease. In fact, the famous removal of the pump handle in Soho did not lead to the end of that particular outbreak—it actually occurred at a point at which the epidemic curve was already on the downturn due to a depletion of 'susceptibles,' a term used by epidemiologists to describe individuals at risk of contracting an infection, probably as a result of the outbreak pushing locals to migrate elsewhere.[3] This is lovingly known as the John Snow Effect, where an epidemiologist successfully intervenes at the point at which the epidemic is already naturally subsiding (and becomes famous for it).

The stories of Dr Snow and Sir Joseph Bazalgette illustrate a number of important points. First, epidemics, although obviously disastrous on the individual level, can expose faults that exist on a systemic level. In the long term, the ability to measure, analyze and map a pattern of an epidemic (or an outbreak) can help identify the faults in the system and contribute to a better understanding of both health and infrastructure design. In the short term, the outcome of a response to an epidemic as it emerges is determined by the extent to which we are able to implement adequate interventions ahead of the epidemic's 'natural' peak.[4] The ability to respond effectively hinges on the availability of strong evidence (technical) and the will to implement policies (political), especially when needed at a scale that involves multiple government agencies acting in coordination and at great expenditure. The will to implement often follows a different rhythm: governments tend to respond to emergencies that are accompanied by growing public pressure, or indeed the rising stench of the Thames, which may well only materialize at a point at which the epidemic is already established and the impact of the response is limited. This dynamic was illustrated in the 2015 Ebola epidemic of West Africa, when international financing grew by approximately 500-fold to 2.3 billion USD over nine months during the time of the crisis, but programmes of emergency preparedness still remained underfunded.[5]

The question of emerging infectious diseases as questions of national security per-se has been long debated, especially with the backdrop of the cold war in the context of bio-weapons. Generations of epidemiologists, including the former head of the WHO's smallpox eradication program Donald A. Henderson, have called for robust epidemic intelligence systems with global coverage that are able to detect emerging infectious diseases and respond to them effectively.[6] The emergence of COVID-19, or perhaps more to the point, the public anxiety around the pandemic, has highlighted a particular impact of global pandemics on civil societies, since it lent governments the legitimacy to extend their powers beyond what is ordinarily considered acceptable. Most saliently, this was manifested in the imposition of restrictions on movement in the form of lockdowns, curfews, individual self-isolation and travel bans. Enforcement measures ranged from the collaborative to the coercive, with a mixture of public messaging, fines, criminal records and tracking of individuals using mobile devices, sometimes without their consent or knowledge.[7] Other measures, such as the postponing of elections[8] and restrictions on the right of assembly, and more specifically on the right to protest,[9] have constrained the ability of citizens in democratic societies to engage in the political process, which has conversely become ever more powerful and present in our day to day lives. Although the epidemiological reasoning at the heart of these decisions is clear,[10] their eventual impact on the spread of the virus remains uncertain given the many different approaches to implementation, and will be the subject of much scholarly writing in years to come.

Future research will inevitably argue that earlier implementation of some policies would have had a positive impact on the (short-term) size of the COVID-19 epidemic nationally. Comparisons of the epidemiological profiles of rich democratic societies with authoritarian states may reflect badly on countries such as the UK and US and positively on countries like China. With confidence in Western governments in decline and political divisions heightened, democracies will have to resist the temptation of maintaining the coercive authorities they are acquiring during the pandemic at the expense of the democratic principles that underpin their systems of government.[11] There is recent precedence to this; Israel, for example, has annually renewed a state of emergency since its war of independence in 1948, allowing its government to routinely pass emergency regulations.[12] Limited by political will and the technical availability of evidence, democracies should instead invest in infrastructure and institutions that would allow them to effectively respond to future health emergencies. As we saw with the story of cholera in nineteenth-century London, the long-term answer to health emergencies is the establishment of comprehensive routine infrastructure. Back then, it was the sewage system, and this time it should be data, or more specifically—a health intelligence system.

From an epidemiological perspective, the most proximate explanation for an outbreak is the presence of a disease agent in circulation in a given group of individuals. If the mode of transmission is understood,[13] then the size and pattern of an outbreak can be predicted based on the frequency of 'risky behavior' in the given group, and based on the current levels of the circulating disease agents. The calculations of these predictions can be complicated, uncertain and their reliability is directly linked to the quality of the evidence (i.e. data) that informs them. This logic, along with its disclaimers, can be reversed; when the mode of transmission is unknown, measuring patterns of disease cases in a population can help infer transmission dynamics. So, when a new infectious disease such as COVID-19 emerges in a population, this iterative cycle of projections and measurements contributes to the understanding of infection dynamics, and is crucial for planning effective responses both in the short and the long term. This planning is typically concerned with questions of capacity, such as the number of hospital beds or Intensive Care Units (ICUs) that may be required when a surge of demand is expected. Data is, if so, essential for designing effective responses, but also plays a role in creating the pressure that generates the political will to act and equally serves to scrutinize the policies of governments. Good data[14] therefore has dual value: epidemiological and democratic.

Mortuaries Management in London: A Case Study

The issue of mortality planning in London during the early stages of the COVID-19 epidemic is a good example of the role that data plays, or rather could have played, in emergency planning during a national crisis. In this case study, based on interviews given on condition of anonymity with a number of senior stakeholders that were involved in the coordination and implementation of mortality planning in London, two themes emerged: a lack of guidance coming from central government alongside an absence of data that could have informed mortuary capacity planning. For context, Under the Civil Contingency Act of 2004, 42 Local Resilience Forums (LRFs) were established as an emergency preparedness instrument to facilitate collaboration between agencies at a local authority level. These LRFs have the authority to establish a Strategic Coordination Group (SCG) to coordinate multi-agency action in the event of a disruptive incident, such as the COVID-19 pandemic. The London SCG was established at the beginning of March 2020, with the added London Local Authority Gold Resolution which '...empowers the nominated "Gold" chief executive to discharge emergency response functions on behalf of the councils which are affected by an incident, when particular triggers are met.'[15] Needless to say, during the COVID-19 epidemic, all 33 London Local Authorities were considered affected.

With an expected surge in COVID-19 related deaths, one of the key missions of the London SCG was to estimate the current capacity of mortuaries in London and establish a plan to create further capacity in order to handle deaths beyond what was already in place. Over the month of March 2020, an early point in the epidemic in the UK, there was still substantial uncertainty in the evidence. This was partly due to the low number of recorded cases in the UK, which was biased by approaches to testing—by 14 March the government decided to test only hospital patients, but not in the community[16]—and partly because it was not clear whether evidence about infection dynamics[17] observed in other countries would be applicable to the UK. With this backdrop and the absence of official guidance, stakeholders involved in mortality planning were naturally concerned with how many excess deaths they should be planning for. Excess deaths can be defined in different ways, but in this context, the term is used to refer to the number of deaths expected to occur beyond what is ordinarily observed in a given setting, typically estimated by looking at the preceding five-year average.

On 29 March 2020, the Cabinet Office circulated a document to its own members of staff titled 'Reasonable Worst-Case Planning Scenario' (RWCPS), which reported epidemiological projections including mortality in the UK from modelling studies reported by the Scientific Advisory Group for Emergencies (SAGE), a committee of leading experts advising the government. The RWCPS document included a figure that would become the core multiplier for all mortuary capacity planning in London: 50,000 expected 'direct' COVID-19 deaths in the UK between 30 March and the end of August.[18] Regional-level projections were not yet available. However, this information was not shared with the SCGs immediately perhaps because the government did not fully trust the SAGE projections, or perhaps because as a Conservative government they did not believe that the London leadership, seen as affiliated to the Labour Party, would remain discreet about the figures. It was only a week after the circulation of the original documents that the London SCG gained informal access to these figures, ahead of them being officially distributed. With an estimated epidemic doubling time of 3.3 days and over 2,300 deaths expected in the first week of April, a week was a long time.

But the London SCG was not completely in the dark for the period before it had access to this report. A publicly available report from Imperial College London published on 16 March set out projections of mortality and other surges in capacity under a multitude of policy scenarios, broadly divided into suppression[19] and mitigation.[20] The report pointed out that even under the most effective *mitigation* strategy, a 'short' pandemic would be expected with up to 250,000 deaths in the UK.[21] At that point the UK Government had already received international criticism for being the only country pursuing a 'herd immunity approach,'[22] which was only emphasized with the following alarm caused by findings of the Imperial College report. The UK government announced it was changing its approach from mitigation to suppression the following day.[23] At any rate, the London SCG already knew, in the middle of March, that when it came to mortality handling it had to plan big.

Given the limited evidence available publicly, the delays in official guidance, the lack of regional-level estimates, and the fact that London was experiencing high transmission ahead of the rest of the country, the London SCG went ahead with its planning for creating extra mortuary capacity required for London. Based on the national 50,000 COVID-19 deaths figure and on the existing London mortuary capacity of 3,500 bodies, the SCG estimated it would need up to 10,000 additional capacity in London, which it could deliver most rapidly by setting up temporary mortuary annexes. These 'flexible pods,' which could be set up and removed within a few days, were in place by early April. As extra mortuary capacity was put in place, the London SCG sought to evaluate the demand for it and its usage to understand whether provision was adequate. However, the data publicly reported at the time included hospital based COVID-19 deaths but not deaths in the community.[24] On 29 April, a month after the initial circulation of the RWCP document and with full excess mortuary capacity in London in place, the UK Government began to officially include COVID-19 deaths in the community in its daily figures, in addition to hospital based COVID-19 deaths.[25]

By then, the London SCG, needing local daily estimates for its mortuary capacity management, had already begun independently collecting data on deaths directly from hospitals trusts and local authorities, where deaths are officially reported to the local deaths registrar. These data indicated that the London SCG's additional mortuary capacity was well in excess of the demand for it.[26] These data allowed the SCG to gradually scale the temporary mortuary annexes back down from early May.

This brief account of how mortuary capacity was handled in the early days of the pandemic in one part of the UK highlights the need of modern governments to have reliable and timely evidence when trying to respond to emergencies. This evidence plays a role both in the ability to plan programmes and also lends legitimacy to government actions when making decisions on how taxpayer funded resources are used. In the case of mortality, the delay in official guidance and evidence from the center led the London SCG to collect its own data from some of the same sources that report their data to central government agencies, like the Office of National Statistics (ONS), Public Health England (PHE), The Department of Health and Social Care (DHSC) and the National Health Service (NHS). This move was understandable under the circumstances since it contributed to the ability to scale down mortuary capacity in London, freeing up resources that could be used for other needs. However, getting hold of the data in a timely manner required the diversion of local resources towards essentially replicating the work of central government agencies, which were collecting the same data concurrently.

Separately, interpretation of the locally generated analyses would have required the kind of specific expertise that was concentrated in central government and would have only been available to local authorities on a voluntary basis, if at all. Finally, the evidence collected by the London SCG is not currently publicly available, preventing scrutiny of its decisions by other parties. Broadly, the ad hoc collection of health data by different agencies, in the absence of timely evidence otherwise provided, may be the best solution to a crisis in the short term but comes at efficiency and transparency costs in the short and long term.

There will have been, without a doubt, multiple government agencies, both local and national, demanding a wide range of data outputs and analyses at any given moment.[27] Initial delays in evidence provision while reporting and analysis mechanisms are being established are understandable, especially as experts need the time to process the data in order to articulate it in a way that is clear for both decision makers and the public. Some of the delays and misunderstandings, though, can be traced back to the way health data is collected routinely in the UK, and indeed elsewhere. The difficulties faced when clear health data is required at a speed and scale never before required from government agencies could led to patterns that characterize the points of weakness in its data infrastructure. The political and policy considerations that affect the timing and quality of evidence clearly play an important role in the contribution of evidence to decision making and deserve their own separate analysis.

Health Data Systems in the UK

The UK's health system has some of the most highly trained health professionals in the world, from medical practitioners through to hospital managers, epidemiologists and modelers. It is privileged for having access to highly granular health data at a scope and scale that represents all parts of society. This coverage is due to its unique design as 'free at the point of use' to all legal residents of the UK.[28] Of course, access to services and health outcomes varies with socio-economic status,[29] a problem of inequality long debated in its own right by health professionals, which also somewhat limits the NHS's coverage and the representativeness of the data it produces. More crucially, though, the way data is routinely collected and processed is such that evidence is often delayed, partial, or difficult to interpret from the user's perspective.

Earlier in this chapter, we saw that the central collection, analysis and reporting of mortality data was not synchronized with the policy needs of the London SCG, leading it to collect and analyze mortality data independently directly from Local Authorities and hospitals. The ONS, NHS and the Demographic Batch Service (which is also part of the NHS), all collect and report death data as well. This presents a type of semi-duplication in datasets in which equivalent records are collected separately but are often not redundant copies of one another, and are sometimes used for cross-referencing or 'enhancing' data.[30] This could be partially up to design, since different agencies may collect data with varying non-overlapping objectives in mind, but it could also be due to a number of other reasons including, for example, different data input interfaces that vary in user friendliness. The issue of user interfaces has broader implications than just the administrative burden it places on analysts centrally piecing data together: it requires health professionals and administrators in health facilities to operate a wide range of different software that change on the basis of hospital trusts, units within hospitals, community care providers, specialists care providers, type of treatment given, surveillance programs etc. This process of scrambling and unscrambling data slows down the ability to produce high quality analysis, partly since it results in associated lengthy and manual processes, which may also cause difficulties in tracing errors in the data, which in turn could make the data difficult to interpret. This is a crucial point—as epidemiologists, we constantly think about how systematic errors are affecting our results and how we might correct for them, but this requires tracing of the regularity of the problem; for example, if COVID-19 deaths are only reported from hospitals, we can reasonably suspect that the number reported is lower relative to the overall number of COVID-19 deaths. Systematic errors that are hard to trace, like those that could potentially be related to the many ways data is processed and entered, make interpreting the data very difficult—we will come back to this point.

Reporting of data to agencies such as the ONS and PHE exists within a statutory landscape that also directly impacts the way in which data is processed. One example of this is the statutory tool of notifiable diseases, that creates the legal duty to all labs in England to report confirmed cases (i.e. positive tests) to PHE via the Second-Generation Surveillance System.[31] (SGSS) The classification of COVID-19 as a notifiable disease on 5 March was a major step in the facilitation of data reporting and analysis of this infection.[32] However, the legal duty of labs was only to report positive test results, but not negative ones. Negative results are essential for measuring the impact of interventions and the size of the epidemic (e.g. in local positivity rates). Negative tests were subsequently reported *separately* from SGSS, on what is technically a voluntary basis. This added step of data processing alone, without the consideration of the absence of a statutory obligation to report negative cases, causes added administrative pressures on analysts and may lead to data loss.

Information loss is an inevitable step of inputting and processing observations due to the need to conform data to a standard format. For example, a classification of severity of an illness may come at the cost of losing some detail about the patient, and similar patients may be classed differently by different individuals. This is a classic issue of epidemiology known to lead to information bias—a type of systematic skewing of the data. The way to deal with biases in data is by understanding their origin, which allows the analyst to correct them in either her analysis or interpretation. For example, if a health provider is known to over-diagnose obesity, the analyst will be able to either quantitatively adjust her analysis of obesity prevalence in that area or say that she believes that the prevalence she is reporting is higher than the 'real' population prevalence. In either case, the key to this is the traceability of the source of information bias. If the points at which data gets potentially skewed are not traceable, the data may be warped in ways that are impossible to interpret or measure, making it less reliable. This is one of the risks of such semi-duplicated processes of data collection where multiple agencies, teams and protocols are involved in data collection, processing and 'enhancing.'

One of the routine approaches to dealing with this type of untraceable data skewing is by using cross validation. In this process, the quality of the evidence is established on the basis of identity between two analyses separately created based on the same protocol; if differences are observed, an investigation into their causes ensues and corrections are applied. When part of a formal process, the same analysis will be conducted by two analysts simultaneously and independently. More informally, analysts will compare their results to, for example, last year's result for consistency but will not have a source of comparison for this year (similar to a game of pinning the tail on the donkey). In any case, this process may prevent the introduction of new biases to an extent, but it ultimately incentivizes analysts to replicate the work of other analysts and does not create the opportunity to trace deeper issues that may be influencing the validity of the data over time. Fundamentally, the best way to minimize the impact of non-traceable biases is the automation of as many manual processing steps as possible, as well as the restriction of redundancies in data collection. These steps are not in themselves immune to skewing data, but have the advantage of relying on rules, or algorithms, which can be interrogated and adjusted on a systematic level, making their origins traceable and interpretable. More broadly, such technical improvements can also translate into gains in time, and may allow official data to be available in a way that better suits dynamic policy needs.

The question of multiple agencies collecting, processing and reporting health related data should also be examined from an institutional perspective. Having multiple agencies, or parts of agencies, involved in the production of similar analyses could prove confusing for the public and could artificially create limitations on the way that data is used. For example, COVID-19 testing data in the UK is reported to PHE via the various testing pillars, which include both privately and publicly provided tests. These data are then processed at PHE and chunks of it are subsequently transferred for analysis to DHSC and separately to the NHS Foundry. Different parts of the same data are reported somewhat separately in three places: the weekly statistics for NHS Test and Trace (England) and Coronavirus Testing (UK), the National COVID-19 Surveillance Report (England) and the COVID-19 Dashboard (UK). With different reporting schedules (daily, weekly), different types of visualizations, different regions included (England as opposed to the UK) at different resolutions (national, regional, local authority level), differences in methodologies over time, and sometimes subtle differences in the way in which similar analyses are defined, even an experienced epidemiologist would struggle to interpret the combined evidence presented coherently. The involvement of a multitude of agencies where different agencies rely on chunks of data provided by other agencies also limits the scope of analysis any one agency can conduct, potentially limiting its ability to interrogate the data usefully, or even disincentivizing it from attempting new analyses. All this reduced the usefulness of the data and its coherence, limiting its contribution to policy planning and research and the ability of the public to scrutinize the government's actions.

Conclusion

An obvious and perhaps ironic limitation of the discussion in this chapter is the difficulty in measuring to what extent the issues raised impact the speed and reliability of evidence provided for policy makers and the public. This is partly due to the technical difficulty in measuring the impact of certain processes (while data is often published, the processes and code underlying rarely are), and partly due to the fact that impact considered was in terms of values such as transparency, accountability, and oversight. In a sense, the analysis presented here is written from the perspective of someone who experienced a number of these large organizations from within as an analyst but is not in itself scientific since it is non-falsifiable. There will doubtless be many other perspectives that could contribute to how data systems in the UK work and how they can be improved.

In the broadest sense, this chapter seeks to draw attention to how structural issues in health data can create the space within which governments can operate without accountability and how this could lead to unsuitable responses to emerging health threats. Although different national health data systems globally will be characterized by different technical issues, the observations raised here about the UK's health data system can be helpful in highlighting why understanding and addressing these should be a major civil society priority, not only to improve the quality of the evidence used for national policy, but to protect the democratic process from lack of transparency and accountability.

In the beginning of the chapter we observed how the cholera outbreaks of Victorian London signaled a deeper issue with the existing sanitation infrastructure in the city. This observation illustrated the importance of how measuring patterns during crises can provide the insight needed for long-term reforms to routine infrastructure. These infrastructures, once established, represent a national security asset not only because they contribute to routine functioning of the state, but also because they directly enhance the wellbeing of citizens. When it comes to the evidence on which political power relies for decision making, its coherent and timely availability is essential both to the policy maker and for members of the public. For the former, in particular, it may constitute as a democratic asset where citizens can scrutinize governments and hold them to their promises while establishing trust through transparency, especially at times of emergency when governments assume powers at the expense of individual rights or proper oversight.

The national infrastructure that should emerge from this crisis should be a singular Health Intelligence Agency with fully automated procedures collecting, processing and reporting evidence to both decision makers and the public, backed by comprehensive statutory mechanisms. This will be critical for improving the way states make health policy in the future, as well as the way they respond to emerging infections with epidemic potential, and would give the public the scope to engage meaningfully with the decision making process. It may well be the case that such an agency would be freer to provide such a service if it were not under the authority of ministerial-lead departments. Instead, it could be bound by its own constitution based on principles such as those laid out in the ONS Code of Practice for Statistics[33] or the Financial Modelers Manifesto,[34] and be regularly scrutinized by an independent regulatory body. This regulatory body should be competent to scrutinize the standard of any health data evidence provided to policy makers, those providing it (including private companies working on behalf of governments), and the appropriateness of the policy decisions based on such evidence. During the days of the London cholera epidemics, the technical know-how and the skilled individuals were already present—the crisis created the political will to act at scale. We are in the very same place today.

Notes

1. A commentator later quipped that 'The Great Stink concentrated minds wonderfully.'
2. Stephen Halliday, *The Great Stink of London* (Stroud: Sutton, 1999).
3. Charles E. Smith, "The Broad Street Pump Revisited," *International Journal of Epidemiology* 11, no. 2 (1982): 99–100, https://doi.org/10.1093/ije/11.2.99.
4. For this reason, well-studied infections with tried and tested responses are better candidates for successful outcomes.
5. "Resources for Results V," *Office of the United Nations Special Envoy on Ebola,* September 1, 2014, https://ebolaresponse.un.org/sites/default/files/resources_for_results_v.pdf.
6. Andrew Lakoff, *Unprepared: Global Health in a Time of Emergency* (Oakland: California, 2017): 81–83.
7. Kelly Servick, "Cellphone Tracking Could Help Stem the Spread of Coronavirus. Is Privacy the Price?" *Science*, March 22, 2020, https://www.sciencemag.org/news/2020/03/cellphone-tracking-could-help-stem-spread-coronavirus-privacy-price.
8. "New Zealand: Jacinda Ardern Delays Election over Coronavirus Fears," *BBC News,* August 17, 2020, https://www.bbc.co.uk/news/world-asia-53796434.

9. Christos Kypraios, and Danilo B. Garrido Alves, "A Human Rights and Rule of Law Assessment of Legislative and Regulatory Responses to the COVID-19 Pandemic across 27 Jurisdictions," *Bonavero Institute of Human*, October 30, 2020, https://www.law.ox.ac.uk/sites/files/oxlaw/bonavero_report_7_2020.pdf; "Derogations by States Parties from Article 21 ICCPR, Article 11 ECHR, and Article 15 ACHR on the Basis of the COVID-19 Pandemic," *The Right of Peaceful Assembly*. November 11, 2020. https://www.rightofassembly.info/assets/downloads/Derogations_from_the_Right_of_Peaceful_Assembly_(at_11_November_2020)_.pdf.
10. I.e. seeking to reduce the average frequency of interactions between individuals, sometimes, but not always, based on an individual's exposure status or risk-group.
11. "2020 Edelman Trust Barometer," *Edelman*, January 19, 2020, https://www.edelman.com/trust/2020-trust-barometer.
12. Aeyal Gross, and Nir Kosti, "The Paradox of Israel's Coronavirus Law," *Verfassungsblog on Matters Constitutional,* January 8, 2021, https://verfassungsblog.de/the-paradox-of-israels-coronavirus-law/.
13. Cholera, for example, follows a faecal-oral path and can be waterborne; J. Glenn Morris Jr, "Cholera--Modern Pandemic Disease of Ancient Lineage," *Emerging Infectious Diseases* 17, no. 11 (November 2011): 2099–2104, https://doi.org/10.3201/eid1711.111109.
14. Reliable, accessible to the public, easily understood, but perhaps above all—timely.
15. "London Resilience Structure," *London Councils,* https://londoncouncils.gov.uk/members-area/civil-resilience-handbook-london-councillors/london-resilience.
16. "Notifiable Diseases and Causative Organisms: How to Report," *Public Health England,* May 1, 2010, https://www.gov.uk/guidance/notifiable-diseases-and-causative-organisms-how-to-report.
17. Infectiousness, severity, mortality, etc.
18. With a mean of approximately 2,100 deaths per week.
19. Aiming to reduce the average number of secondary cases per primary case, or R, with the aim of elimination.

20. Aiming to reduce R to spread out the effects of the pandemic without the object of elimination—this was understood as the 'herd immunity' approach.
21. Neil Ferguson, Daniel Laydon, and Gemma Nedjati-Gilani, "Impact of Non-Pharmaceutical Interventions (NPIs) to Reduce COVID19 Mortality and Healthcare Demand," *Imperial College COVID 19 Response Team* (March 2020): https://doi.org/10.25561/77482.
22. "WHO Director-General's Opening Remarks at the Mission Briefing on COVID-19—12 March 2020," *World Health Organization,* March 12, 2020, https://www.who.int/director-general/speeches/detail/who-director-general-s-opening-remarks-at-the-mission-briefing-on-covid-19---12-march-2020.
23. Owen Matthews, "Britain Drops Its Go-It-Alone Approach to Coronavirus," *Foreign Policy*, March 17, 2020, https://foreignpolicy.com/2020/03/17/britain-uk-coronavirus-response-johnson-drops-go-it-alone/.
24. "The NHS Constitution for England," *NHS England*, January 21, 2009, https://www.gov.uk/government/publications/the-nhs-constitution-for-england/the-nhs-constitution-for-england.
25. "Daily Death Reporting Now Includes All Positive COVID-19 Deaths," *Public Health England*, April 29. 2020, https://www.gov.uk/government/news/daily-death-reporting-now-includes-all-positive-covid-19-deaths.
26. An approximate 800 overall deaths were processed by the excess capacity created, planned to accommodate up to 10,000 deaths.
27. E.g. number of tests provided, number of people tested, number of positive results, ICU bed use, contacts traced, etc.
28. "The NHS Constitution for England," *NHS England*, January 21, 2009, https://www.gov.uk/government/publications/the-nhs-constitution-for-england/the-nhs-constitution-for-england.
29. "Independent Inquiry into Inequalities in Health," *Department of Health and Social Security*, August 1980, https://assets.publishing.service.gov.uk/government/uploads/system/uploads/attachment_data/file/265503/ih.pdf.
30. The process by which some of the details that exist about a record in one system are used to inform the equivalent record existing in another system.

31. "Notifiable Diseases and Causative Organisms: How to Report," *Public Health England,* May 1, 2010, https://www.gov.uk/guidance/notifiable-diseases-and-causative-organisms-how-to-report.
32. "Coronavirus (COVID-19) Listed as a Notifiable Disease," *Department of Health and Social Care,* March 5, 2020, https://www.gov.uk/government/news/coronavirus-covid-19-listed-as-a-notifiable-disease.
33. "Code of Practice for Statistics," *Office for Statistics Regulation,* February 2018, https://code.statisticsauthority.gov.uk/wp-content/uploads/2018/02/Code-of-Practice-for-Statistics.pdf.
34. Emanuel Derman, and Paul Wilmott, "Financial Modelers' Manifesto," *Wilmott*, January 8, 2009, https://wilmott.com/financial-modelers-manifesto/.

Bibliography

"2020 Edelman Trust Barometer." *Edelman*, January 19, 2020. https://www.edelman.com/trust/2020-trust-barometer.

"Code of Practice for Statistics." *Office for Statistics Regulation,* February 2018. https://code.statisticsauthority.gov.uk/wp-content/uploads/2018/02/Code-of-Practice-for-Statistics.pdf.

"Coronavirus (COVID-19) Listed as a Notifiable Disease." *Department of Health and Social Care,* March 5, 2020. https://www.gov.uk/government/news/coronavirus-covid-19-listed-as-a-notifiable-disease.

"Daily Death Reporting Now Includes All Positive COVID-19 Deaths." *Public Health England*, April 29. 2020. https://www.gov.uk/government/news/daily-death-reporting-now-includes-all-positive-covid-19-deaths.

"Derogations by States Parties from Article 21 ICCPR, Article 11 ECHR, and Article 15 ACHR on the Basis of the COVID-19 Pandemic." *The Right of Peaceful Assembly*, November 11, 2020. https://www.rightofassembly.info/assets/downloads/Derogations_from_the_Right_of_Peaceful_Assembly_(at_11_November_2020)_.pdf.

"Independent Inquiry into Inequalities in Health." *Department of Health and Social Security*, August 1980. https://assets.publishing.service.gov.uk/government/uploads/system/uploads/attachment_data/file/265503/ih.pdf.

"London Resilience Structure." *London Councils.* https://londoncouncils.gov.uk/members-area/civil-resilience-handbook-london-councillors/london-resilience.

"New Zealand: Jacinda Ardern Delays Election over Coronavirus Fears." *BBC News,* August 17, 2020. https://www.bbc.co.uk/news/world-asia-53796434.

"Notifiable Diseases and Causative Organisms: How to Report." *Public Health England,* May 1, 2010. https://www.gov.uk/guidance/notifiable-diseases-and-causative-organisms-how-to-report.

"Resources for Results V." *Office of the United Nations Special Envoy on Ebola*, September 1, 2014. https://ebolaresponse.un.org/sites/default/files/resources_for_results_v.pdf.

"The NHS Constitution for England." *NHS England*, January 21, 2009. https://www.gov.uk/government/publications/the-nhs-constitution-for-england/the-nhs-constitution-for-england.

"WHO Director-General's Opening Remarks at the Mission Briefing on COVID-19 - 12 March 2020." *World Health Organization*, March 12, 2020. https://www.who.int/director-general/speeches/detail/who-director-general-s-opening-remarks-at-the-mission-briefing-on-covid-19---12-march-2020.

Andrew Lakoff. *Unprepared: Global Health in a Time of Emergency.* Oakland: California, 2017.

Derman, Emanuel, and Paul Wilmott. "Financial Modelers' Manifesto." *Wilmott*, January 8, 2009. https://wilmott.com/financial-modelers-manifesto/.

Ferguson, Neil, Daniel Laydon, and Gemma Nedjati-Gilani. "Impact of Non-Pharmaceutical Interventions (NPIs) to Reduce COVID19 Mortality and Healthcare Demand." *Imperial College COVID 19 Response Team* (March 2020): https://doi.org/10.25561/77482.

Gross, Aeyal, and Nir Kosti. "The Paradox of Israel's Coronavirus Law." *Verfassungsblog on Matters Constitutional*, January 8, 2021. https://verfassungsblog.de/the-paradox-of-israels-coronavirus-law/.

Halliday, Stephen. *The Great Stink of London.* Stroud: Sutton, 1999.

Kypraios, Christos, and Danilo B. Garrido Alves. "A Human Rights and Rule of Law Assessment of Legislative and Regulatory Responses to the COVID-19 Pandemic across 27 Jurisdictions." *Bonavero Institute of Human*, October 30, 2020. https://www.law.ox.ac.uk/sites/files/oxlaw/bonavero_report_7_2020.pdf.

Matthews, Owen. "Britain Drops Its Go-It-Alone Approach to Coronavirus." *Foreign Policy*, March 17, 2020. https://foreignpolicy.com/2020/03/17/britain-uk-coronavirus-response-johnson-drops-go-it-alone/.

Morris Jr, J. Glenn. "Cholera---Modern Pandemic Disease of Ancient Lineage." *Emerging Infectious Diseases* 17, no. 11 (November 2011): 2099–2104. https://doi.org/10.3201/eid1711.111109.

Servick, Kelly. "Cellphone Tracking Could Help Stem the Spread of Coronavirus. Is Privacy the Price?" *Science*, March 22, 2020. https://www.sciencemag.org/news/2020/03/cellphone-tracking-could-help-stem-spread-coronavirus-privacy-price.

Smith, Charles E. "The Broad Street Pump Revisited." *International Journal of Epidemiology* 11, no. 2 (1982): 99–100. https://doi.org/10.1093/ije/11.2.99.

CHAPTER 13

Brave New World

Caroline Varin

Conclusion

After twelve chapters describing political mistakes, rampant corruption, criminal opportunism and socio-economic devastation that colourfully illustrate the state of global security in the first 18 months of the COVID-19 pandemic, it is easy to view the future as a dystopian universe. In this world, we accept to live with fewer freedoms. Those who can, rely on taking medication, tests and vaccines, they wear protective gear and share their movements and vital stats with the state while restricting social interactions to protect themselves from recurrent diseases. A superficial return to a new 'normal' is lauded by a central government that enforces its control over its citizens. The others, the underprivileged citizens, 'suffer what they must' while toiling on the front lines.[1] Protectionism and nationalism prevail over solidarity, cooperation and institutionalism. The brave new world that was built after World War II, that promoted integration, broke down borders and encouraged a global society that mirrored

C. Varin (✉)
Professors Without Borders, Regent's University London, London, UK
e-mail: varinc@regents.ac.uk

C. Varin (ed.), *Global Security in Times of Covid-19*, New Security Challenges, https://doi.org/10.1007/978-3-030-82230-9_13

Western neoliberal values, failed in 2020. In its wake, disorder, inequality, violence and denial. The future looks grim indeed.

This book was written, nonetheless, with a message of hope. If we can identify what went so horribly wrong and understand the long and short-term consequences of the COVID policies that were adopted in response to the pandemic, then the next step is to rebuild a world better prepared to manage a global crisis. As more will inevitably follow, in the shape of diseases probably but certainly with climate change.

Science for Good and Bad

Science and technology have been at the core of this pandemic. First, the suspicion that the virus was engineered in a laboratory in Wuhan, China. Whether or not this is the case for COVID, scientists have irrevocably created and stored biological agents that can be weaponized by states and non-state actors. The myths that emerged around the origins of COVID are a staunch reminder of the 'demon in the freezer'[2] that can be released onto humanity at any time. Lewis Herrington reminds us in Chapter 10 that terrorists have been inspired by the effects this pandemic has had on modern society. It is more vital than ever that governments continue to invest in protecting such facilities and continue to engage pro-actively with counterterrorism and deradicalization programmes that have largely been demoted over the last 18 months.

Conversely, the speed with which vaccines, tests and treatments were funded, developed and distributed demonstrates the importance of our collective survival instinct and what can be achieved when industry heads, political leaders and especially leaders in the scientific community work together. Improved connectivity has facilitated and accelerated multi-national and multi-disciplinary collaboration. This bodes well for advancing medical progress, and dare one hope scientific solutions to effectively tackle climate change.

Technology has also created new opportunities for governments to oversee their citizens' welfare, gain access to personal medical information, manage their movements and interactions and control their access to information. In Chapter 7, Sipim Sornbanlang reveals that in countries like Thailand and China, technology has empowered politicians who have exploited safeguarding policies to suppress dissent and subdue minority groups. The battle between individual freedoms and public health has been played out in every country, leading to deep distrust between citizens and their governments, as explained by George Richards in Chapter 9 and Oliver Geffen Obregon in Chapter 12. This will have long-term repercussions and can lead to social unrest, rebellions and even civil wars if mismanaged by the powers that be.

Why We Need Strong Institutions

There has been a shocking lack of leadership throughout this crisis, both on the part of established institutions like the United Nations, the European Union and the World Health Organization but equally so from individual nations. This has revealed a significant weakness in the international system: when America doesn't lead, there is no alternative. While this may be due to the exceptional circumstances of Donald Trump's presidency, the world cannot rely on American politics to resolve future crises. It is critical to build institutions that are empowered and funded in order to solve global existential crises, without relying on any one nation or coalition to function.

The G7's 2021 'commitment' to 'prevent any repeat of the human and economic devastation wreaked by coronavirus'[3] excludes the participation of Turkey, Iran, Russia and China. But the world has already moved on (see Chapter 8), with most G7 nations considerably weakened, politically, socially and economically from two years of questionable crisis mismanagement. The balance of powers has shifted and emerging economic and political powerhouses need to be actively integrated into new solutions to avoid a repeat of the political chaos and protectionism we witnessed in 2020 and 2021. Leadership is still necessary, but it can come from many directions.

Security Trends Ahead

As most of the contributors pointed out, COVID-19 did not necessarily create new security problems, but it did accelerate existing trends. Terrorism and transnational crimes were already security threats in December 2019. Violent non-state actors have generally grown in influence throughout the crisis, capitalizing on state failures and growing poverty in Africa and Latin America (Chapters 2 and 5). Civil unrest has been a permanent feature of the twenty-first century, but grew exponentially in 2020 and 2021 (Chapters 3, 7 and 9) as citizens became increasingly frustrated by the inability of their governments to find tangible solutions to this crisis—a consequence of the failure to cooperate regionally and internationally.

Inequality was already on the rise, flagged by the World Economic Forum over the last decade as one of the biggest threats to global security with increasing urgency. COVID-19 has been devastating for human security, exacerbating inequality between the 'haves' and the 'have nots' and demonstrating the colossal differences (and often indifference) between rich and poorer nations. We can expect this to grow in the next decade as nations grapple to stabilize their own economies under the leadership of the same political and economic elite who failed to react competently in 2020.

In a note of optimism, there is clearly much we can improve on. The progress of science and scientific collaborations are encouraging. Weaknesses of the international system have been revealed and can now be addressed. There is a wind of change blowing in the air—less tolerance for corruption, discrimination and inequality, an awareness that freedom and human rights are values worth fighting for, and a very human desire to make our world better, driven in part by a new generation of future economic, political and social leaders who recognize the existential crises facing humanity. After all, what is a good Dystopia for, if not to serve as a warning and a turning point for a better future?

Notes

1. Thucydides, "The Melian Dialogue". *Mtholyoke.Edu*, 2021, https://www.mtholyoke.edu/acad/intrel/melian.htm.
2. Richard Preston. *The Demon in the Freezer* (New York: Ballantine Books, 2003).
3. David Sanger, and Mark Langer, "G7 News: Leaders Turn to Cooperation to Prepare for Next Health Crisis," *Nytimes.Com*, 2021, https://www.nytimes.com/live/2021/06/12/world/g7summit.

Bibliography

Preston, Richard. *The Demon in the Freezer*. New York: Ballantine Books, 2003.

Sanger, David, and Mark Langer. "G7 News: Leaders Turn to Cooperation to Prepare for Next Health Crisis." *Nytimes.Com*, 2021. https://www.nytimes.com/live/2021/06/12/world/g7summit.

Thucydides. "The Melian Dialogue." *Mtholyoke.Edu*, 2021. https://www.mtholyoke.edu/acad/intrel/melian.htm.

Index

C. Varin (ed.), *Global Security in Times of Covid-19*, New Security Challenges, https://doi.org/10.1007/978-3-030-82230-9

M

N

O

P

Q